FOURTH EDITION

Essential Haematology

A.V. Hoffbrand
MA DM FRCP FRCPath FRCP(Edin) DSc FMED Sci
*Emeritus Professor of Haematology, Royal Free
and University College Medical School, London*

J.E. Pettit
MD FRCPA FRCPath
*Haematologist, Medlab South,
Christchurch, New Zealand*

P.A.H. Moss
PhD MRCP MRCPath
*Professor of Haematology,
University of Birmingham*

Blackwell
Science

Editorial Offices:
Osney Mead, Oxford OX2 0EL
25 John Street, London WC1N 2BS
23 Ainslie Place, Edinburgh EH3 6AJ
350 Main Street, Malden
   MA 02148-5018, USA
54 University Street, Carlton
   Victoria 3053, Australia
10, rue Casimir Delavigne
   75006 Paris, France

Other Editorial Offices:
Blackwell Wissenschafts-Verlag GmbH
Kurfürstendamm 57
10707 Berlin, Germany

Blackwell Science KK
MG Kodenmacho Building
7–10 Kodenmacho Nihombashi
Chuo-ku, Tokyo 104, Japan

First published 1980
Reprinted 1981, 1982, 1983 (twice)
Second edition 1984
Reprinted 1985
Reprinted with corrections 1985, 1988 (twice), 1989
German edition 1986 (reprinted 1996)
Japanese edition 1986
Spanish edition 1987 (reprinted twice)
Indonesian edition 1987
Third edition 1993
Four Dragons edition 1993
Hungarian edition 1997
Chinese edition 1998
Reprinted with corrections 1993, 1994, 1995, 1996, 1997,
   1998, 1999, 2000
Fourth edition 2001
Reprinted with corrections 2002

Set by SNP Best-set Typesetter Ltd., Hong Kong
Printed and bound in Italy
by G. Canale & C.S.p.A

DISTRIBUTORS

Marston Book Services Ltd
PO Box 269
Abingdon, Oxon OX14 4YN
(*Orders*: Tel: 01235 465500
         Fax: 01235 465555)

The Americas
Blackwell Publishing
c/o AIDC
PO Box 20
50 Winter Sport Lane
Williston, VT 05495-0020
(*Orders*: Tel: 800 216 2522
         Fax: 802 864 7626)

Australia
Blackwell Science Pty Ltd
54 University Street
Carlton, Victoria 3053
(*Orders*: Tel: 3 9347 0300
         Fax: 3 9347 5001)

A catalogue record for this title
is available from the British Library

ISBN 0-63205-153-1

Library of Congress
Cataloging-in-publication Data

Hoffbrand, A.V.
    Essential haematology / A.V. Hoffbrand,
J.E. Pettit, P. Moss.—4th ed.
      p.; cm.
    Includes bibliographical references and index.
    ISBN 0-63205-153-1
    1. Blood—Diseases. 2. Hematology. I. Pettit,
J.E. II. Moss, P. III. Title. [DNLM: 1. Hemato-
logic Diseases. WH 120 H698e 2000]
RC633 .H627 2000
616.1'5—dc21
                                                    00-023594

For further information on
Blackwell Science, visit our website:
www.blackwell-science.com

Contents

Preface to fourth edition

The vast increase in knowledge of the pathogenesis of blood disorders and the advances in their management since 1995 have necessitated the introduction of new information in every chapter for the fourth edition of *Essential Haematology*. We have reduced or omitted some sections, e.g. those concerning ferrokinetics and red cell survival studies. The new double column format, smaller print and reduction in size of some figures have also helped to keep the fourth edition of the book to a manageable size. New chapters have been added on stem cell transplantation and haematological aspects of pregnancy and childhood. Sections on stem cells, iron metabolism, genetic haemochromatosis, homocysteine, molecular aspects of haematological malignancy, the lymphomas and thrombophilia have been particularly increased to include major advances in these areas.

Like the previous editions, the present book is intended primarily for use by medical students. It includes, however, more information than most medical students can reasonably be expected to know, given the pressures from expansion in knowledge in all areas of medicine and the widening of the undergraduate curriculum. We have, therefore, as in the third edition, indicated those sections which we consider to be core material for medical students taking their final examinations and those intended for honours candidates and for postgraduates specializing in medicine or haematology. We hope the book will also be used by science graduates, medical laboratory technicians and others wishing to gain knowledge in one of the most exciting and rapidly advancing fields of medicine.

For this edition, the two original authors have been joined by Professor Paul Moss, reducing the average age of the authors substantially and bringing additional expertise, particularly in the fields of stem cells, stem cell transplantation, the immune system and the haematological malignancies. We are grateful to all colleagues who have helped in discussions and by provision of illustrative material and particularly to the publishers, Mosby, for their permission to reproduce ten figures from the third edition of the *Clinical Atlas of Haematology* (Hoffbrand A.V. & Pettit J.E., Harcourt Publishers Ltd, 2000). We are grateful to Drs Charles Craddock, Heidi Doughty, Sarah Lawson, David Perry, Peter Rose, Jonathan Wilde and Mr G Hazelhurst for reviewing various sections of the text. The authors also wish to thank Rebecca Huxley and Fiona Goodgame of Blackwell Science for their expert and patient collaboration during the publishing process and Jane Fallow, for the clear, attractive diagrams with which the text is heavily illustrated.

AVH
JEP
PAHM

For the fourth edition we have indicated by a vertical blue line in the margin those sections of text which we consider *less essential* for undergraduate medical students approaching their final examination.

Preface to first edition

The major changes that have occurred in all fields of medicine over the last decade have been accompanied by an increased understanding of the biochemical, physiological and immunological processes involved in normal blood cell formation and function and the disturbances that may occur in different diseases. At the same time, the range of treatment available for patients with diseases of the blood and blood-forming organs has widened and improved substantially as understanding of the disease processes has increased and new drugs and means of support care have been introduced.

We hope the present book will enable the medical student of the 1980s to grasp the essential features of modern clinical and laboratory haematology and to achieve an understanding of how many of the manifestations of blood diseases can be explained with this new knowledge of the disease processes.

We would like to thank many colleagues and assistants who have helped with the preparation of the book. In particular, Dr H.G. Prentice cared for the patients whose haematological responses are illustrated in Figs 5.3 and 7.8 and Dr J. McLaughlin supplied Fig. 8.6. Dr S. Knowles reviewed critically the final manuscript and made many helpful suggestions. Any remaining errors are, however, our own. We also thank Mr J.B. Irwin and R.W. McPhee who drew many excellent diagrams, Mr Cedric Gilson for expert photomicrography, Mrs T. Charalambos, Mrs B. Elliot, Mrs M. Evans and Miss J. Allaway for typing the manuscript, and Mr Tony Russell of Blackwell Scientific Publications for his invaluable help and patience.

AVH, JEP

viii

Bibliography

Bain B., Clark D.M., Lampert I.A. and Wilkins B.S. (2001) *Bone Marrow Pathology*, 2nd edn. Blackwell Science, Oxford.

Beutler E., Kipps T.J., Lichtman M.A., Seligsohn S., Collier B.C., Rosenberg M.N. and Bronfman S. (eds) (2000) *William's Hematology*, 6th edn. McGraw-Hill, New York.

Cox T.M. and Sinclair J. (1997) *Molecular Biology in Medicine*, Blackwell Science, Oxford.

Degos L., Linch D.C. and Lowenberg B. (eds) (2000) *A Textbook of Malignant Hematology*, Martin Dunitz, London.

Hoffbrand A.V. and Pettit J.E. (2000) *Color Atlas of Clinical Hematology*, 3rd edn. Mosby, London.

Hoffbrand A.V., Lewis S.M. and Tuddenham E.G. (eds) (1999) *Postgraduate Hematology*, 4th edn. Butterworth Heinemann, Oxford.

Hoffman R., Benz E.J., Shatill S.J., Furie B., Cohen H.J., Silberstein L.E. and McGlave P. (1999) *Hematology: Basic Principles and Practice*, 3rd edn. Churchill Livingstone, New York.

Jandl J. (1996) *Blood: Textbook of Hematology*, 2nd edn. Little Brown, Boston.

Lee G.R., Foerster J., Kukens J., Paraskewas F., Freer J.P. and Rogers G.M. (eds) (1998) *Wintrobe's Clinical Hematology*, 10th edn. Lippincott, Williams & Wilkins, Philadelphia.

Lichtman M.A., Spivak J.L., Boxer L.A., Shattil S.J. and Henderson E.S. (eds) (2000) *Hematology Landmark Papers of the Twentieth Century*, Academic Press, San Diego.

Provan D. and Gribben J. (eds) (2000) *Molecular Haematology*, Blackwell Science, Oxford.

Stamatoyannopous G., Perlmutter R.M., Majerus P.W. and Varmus H. (eds) (2000) *The Molecular Basis of Blood Diseases*, 3rd edn. W.B. Saunders, Philadelphia.

Blood cell formation (haemopoiesis)

This first chapter mainly concerns general aspects of blood cell formation (haemopoiesis) and the early stages of formation of red cells (erythropoiesis), granulocytes and monocytes (myelopoiesis) and platelets (thrombopoiesis).

SITE OF HAEMOPOIESIS

In the first few weeks of gestation the yolk sac is the main site of haemopoiesis. From 6 weeks until 6–7 months of fetal life the liver and spleen are the main organs involved and they continue to produce blood cells until about 2 weeks after birth (Table 1.1) (see Fig. 6.1b). The bone marrow is the most important site from 6 to 7 months of fetal life and, during normal childhood and adult life, the marrow is the only source of new blood cells. The developing cells are situated outside the bone marrow sinuses and mature cells are released into the sinus spaces, the marrow microcirculation and so into the general circulation.

In infancy all the bone marrow is haemopoietic but during childhood there is progressive fatty replacement of marrow throughout the long bones so that in adult life haemopoietic marrow is confined to the central skeleton and proximal ends of the femurs and humeri (Table 1.1). Even in these haemopoietic areas, approximately 50% of the marrow consists of fat (Fig. 1.1). The remaining fatty marrow is capable of reversion to haemopoiesis and in many diseases there is also expansion of haemopoiesis down the long bones. Moreover, the liver and spleen can resume their fetal haemopoietic role ('extramedullary haemopoiesis').

Table 1.1 Sites of haemopoiesis

Fetus	0–2 months (yolk sac)
	2–7 months (liver, spleen)
	5–9 months (bone marrow)
Infants	Bone marrow (practically all bones)
Adults	Vertebrae, ribs, sternum, skull, sacrum and pelvis, proximal ends of femur

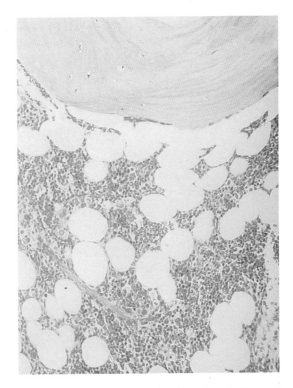

Fig. 1.1 A normal bone marrow trephine biopsy (posterior iliac crest). Haematoxylin and eosin stain; approximately 50% of the intertrabecular tissue is haemopoietic tissue and 50% is fat.

HAEMOPOIETIC STEM AND PROGENITOR CELLS

Haemopoiesis starts with a common, pluripotential stem cell that can give rise to the separate cell lineages. The exact phenotype of the human stem cell is unknown but on immunological testing it is CD34+, CD38– and has the appearance of a small or medium-sized lymphocyte (see Fig. 8.3). Cell differentiation occurs from the stem cell down the erythroid, granulocytic and other lineages via the committed haemopoietic progenitors which are restricted in their developmental potential (Fig. 1.2). The existence of the separate progenitor

cells can be demonstrated by *in vitro* culture techniques. Very early progenitors are assayed by culture on bone marrow stroma as long-term culture initiating cells whereas late progenitors are generally assayed in semi-solid media. An example is the earliest detectable mixed myeloid precursor which gives rise to granulocytes, erythrocytes, monocytes and megakaryocytes and is termed CFU (colony-forming unit in agar culture medium)-GEMM (Fig. 1.2). The bone marrow is also the primary site of origin of lymphocytes (Chapter 10) and there is evidence for a common precursor cell of the myeloid and lymphoid systems.

The stem cell has the capability of self-renewal (Fig. 1.3) so that, although the marrow is a major site of new cell production, its overall cellularity remains constant in a normal healthy steady state. There is considerable amplification in the system: one stem cell is capable of producing about 10^6 mature blood cells after 20 cell divisions (Fig. 1.3). The precursor cells are, however, capable of

Fig. 1.2 Diagrammatic representation of the bone marrow pluripotent stem cell and the cell lines that arise from it. Various progenitor cells can be identified by culture in semi-solid medium by the type of colony they form. baso, basophil; BFU, burst-forming unit; CFU, colony-forming unit; E, erythroid; Eo, eosinophil; GEMM, granulocyte, erythroid, monocyte and megakaryocyte; GM, granulocyte, monocyte; Meg, megakaryocyte; NK, natural killer.

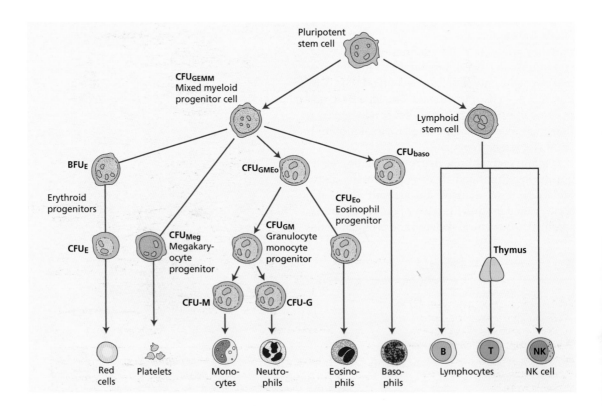

responding to haemopoietic growth factors with increased production of one or other cell line when the need arises.

Haemopoietic stem cells also give rise to osteoclasts which are part of the monocyte–phagocyte system, natural killer (NK) cells and dendritic cells (Chapter 10). The development of the mature cells (red cells, granulocytes, monocytes, megakaryocytes and lymphocytes) is considered further in other sections of this book.

BONE MARROW STROMA

The bone marrow forms a suitable environment for stem cell growth and development. It is composed of stromal cells and a microvascular network (Fig. 1.4). The stromal cells include adipocytes, fibroblasts, reticulum cells, endothelial cells and macrophages and they secrete extracellular molecules such as collagen, glycoproteins (fibronectin and thrombospondin) and

Fig. 1.3 (a) Bone marrow cells are increasingly differentiated and lose the capacity for self-renewal as they mature. (b) A single stem cell gives rise, after multiple cell divisions (shown by vertical lines), to $> 10^6$ mature cells.

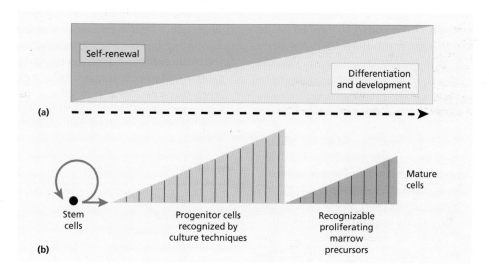

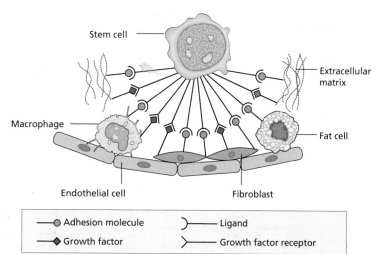

Fig. 1.4 Haemopoiesis occurs in a suitable microenvironment provided by a stromal matrix on which stem cells grow and divide. There are probably specific recognition and adhesion sites (see p. 10); extracellular glycoproteins and other compounds are involved in the binding.

glycosaminoglycans (hyaluronic acid and chondroitin derivatives) to form an extracellular matrix. In addition stromal cells secrete several growth factors necessary for stem cell survival.

HAEMOPOIETIC GROWTH FACTORS

The haemopoietic growth factors are glycoprotein hormones that regulate the proliferation and differentiation of haemopoietic progenitor cells and the function of mature blood cells. The biological effects of the growth factors are mediated through specific receptors on target cells. They may act locally at the site where they are produced by cell–cell contact or circulate in plasma. They may bind to the extracellular matrix to form niches to which stem and progenitor cells adhere. They share a number of common properties (Table 1.2) and act at different stages of haemopoiesis (Table 1.3 and Fig. 1.6). T lymphocytes, monocytes (and macrophages) and stromal cells are the major sources of growth factors except for erythropoietin, 90% of which is synthesized in the kidney, and thrombopoietin, made largely in the liver. Antigens or endotoxins activate T lymphocytes or macrophages to release interleukin-1 (IL-1) and tumour necrosis factor (TNF) which then stimulate other cells including endothelial cells, fibroblasts, other T cells and macrophages to produce granulocyte–macrophage colony-stimulating factor (GM-CSF), G-CSF, M-CSF, IL-6 and other growth factors in an interacting network (Fig. 1.5).

An important feature of growth factor action is that two or more factors may synergize in stimulating a particular cell to proliferate or differentiate. Moreover, the action of one growth factor on a cell may stimulate production of another growth factor or growth factor receptor. IL-1 has a wide variety of biological activities mainly related to inflammation. Stem cell factor and Flt ligand (Flt-L) act locally on the pluripotential stem cells and on early myeloid and lymphoid progenitors (Fig. 1.6). IL-3 and GM-CSF are multipotential growth factors with overlapping activities, IL-3 being more active on the earliest marrow progenitors. G-CSF and thrombopoietin enhance the effects of stem cell factor, Flt-L, IL-3 and GM-CSF on survival and differentiation of the early haemopoietic cells. Together these factors maintain a pool of haemopoietic stem and progenitor cells on which later acting factors erythropoietin, G-CSF, M-CSF, IL-5 (an eosinophilic growth factor) and thrombopoietin act to stimulate increased production of one or other cell lineage in response to the body's needs, e.g. in infection (Fig. 1.5), haemorrhage, hypoxia or thrombocytopenia. The growth factors may cause cell proliferation but

Table 1.3 Haemopoietic growth factors

Act on stromal cells
IL-1
TNF

Act on pluripotential stem cells
Stem cell factor (SCF)
Flt ligand (Flt-L)

Act on multipotential progenitor cells
IL-3
GM-CSF
IL-6
G-CSF
thrombopoietin

Act on committed progenitor cells
G-CSF*
M-CSF
IL-5 (eosinophil-CSF)
erythropoietin
thrombopoietin*

G- and GM-CSF, granulocyte and granulocyte–macrophage colony-stimulating factor; IL, interleukin; M-CSF, macrophage colony-stimulating factor; TNF, tumour necrosis factor.
* These also act synergistically with early acting factors on pluripotential progenitor.

Table 1.2 General characteristics of myeloid and lymphoid growth factors

Glycoproteins that act at very low concentrations
Act hierarchically
Usually produced by many cell types
Usually affect more than one lineage
Usually active on stem/progenitor cells and on functional end cells
Usually show synergistic or additive interactions with other growth factors
Often act on the neoplastic equivalent of a normal cell
Multiple actions: proliferation, differentiation, maturation, functional activation, prevention of apoptosis

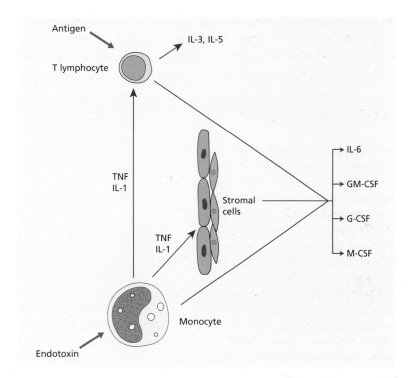

Fig. 1.5 Regulation of haemopoiesis; pathways of stimulation of leucopoiesis by endotoxin, for example from infection. It is likely that endothelial and fibroblast cells release basal quantities of GM-CSF and G-CSF in the normal resting state and that this is enhanced substantially by the monokines tumour necrosis factor (TNF) and interleukin-1 (IL-1).

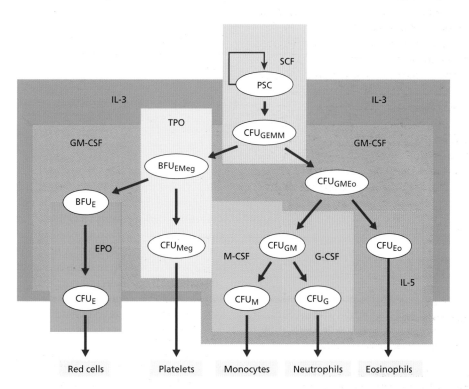

Fig. 1.6 A diagram of the role of growth factors in normal haemopoiesis. Multiple growth factors act on the earlier marrow stem and progenitor cells. EPO, erythropoietin; PSC, pluripotential stem cell; SCF, stem cell factor; TPO, thrombopoietin. For other abbreviations see Fig. 1.2.

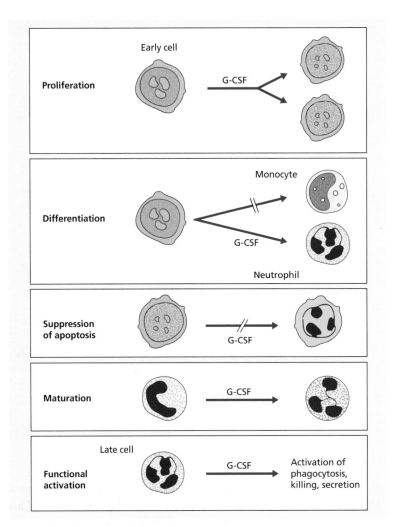

Fig. 1.7 Growth factors may stimulate proliferation of early bone marrow cells, direct differentiation to one or other cell type, stimulate cell maturation, suppress apoptosis or affect the function of mature non-dividing cells, as illustrated here for G-CSF for an early myeloid progenitor and a neutrophil.

also can stimulate differentiation, maturation, prevent apoptosis and affect the function of mature cells (Fig. 1.7).

STEM CELL PLASTICITY

Embryonic stem cells are totipotent since they can generate all the tissues of the body (Fig. 1.8). There is increasing evidence that adult stem cells in different organs are pluripotent and can generate various types of tissue. Bone marrow contains both haemopoietic stem cells (which give rise to the lymphoid and myeloid systems) and mes-

enchymal stem cells. Mesenchymal stem cells can differentiate into muscle, bone (osteoblasts), vascular endothelial tissue, fat cells and fibrous tissue depending on the culture conditions. They may have considerable clinical application for treating diseases of mesenchymal tissue, e.g. osteogenesis imperfecta. Studies in patients and animals who have received haemopoietic stem cell transplants (Chapter 8) have shown that donor cells may contribute to tissues such as neurones, liver and muscle. Although the contribution of adult donor bone marrow cells to non-haemopoietic tissues is small, these findings raise the exciting possibility of using haemopoietic stem cell transplantation to

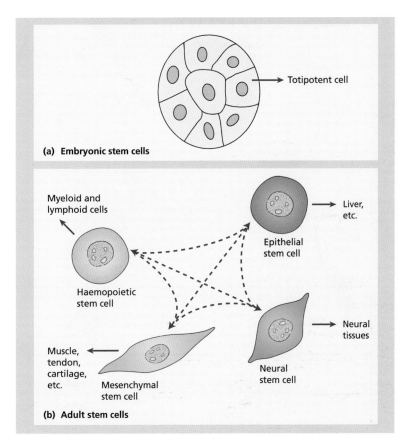

(a) **Embryonic stem cells**

Totipotent cell

Myeloid and
lymphoid cells

Liver,
etc.

Epithelial
stem cell

Haemopoietic
stem cell

Neural
tissues

Muscle,
tendon,
cartilage,
etc.

Neural
stem cell

Mesenchymal
stem cell

(b) **Adult stem cells**

Fig. 1.8 (a) Cells in the early embryo are able to generate all the tissues of the body and are known as totipotent. (b) Specialized adult stem cells of the bone marrow, nervous tissue, epithelial and other tissues give rise to differentiated cells of the same tissue. Under certain circumstances adult stem cells may also contribute to cells of a different lineage. These potential pathways are represented by the dashed lines.

treat a wide range of inherited and acquired disorders such as muscle dystrophy, Parkinson's disease, stroke and diabetes mellitus.

APOPTOSIS

Apoptosis is a regulated process of physiological cell death in which cells are triggered to activate intracellular proteins that lead to the death of the cell. Morphologically it is characterized by cell shrinkage, condensation of the nuclear chromatin, fragmentation of the nucleus and cleavage of DNA at internucleosomal sites. It is an important process for maintaining tissue homeostasis in haemopoiesis and lymphocyte development.

Apoptosis results from the action of intracellular cysteine proteases called caspases which are activated following cleavage and lead to endonuclease digestion of DNA and disintegration of the cell skeleton (Fig. 1.9). There are two major pathways by which caspases can be activated. The first is by signalling through membrane proteins such as Fas or TNF receptor via their intracellular death domain. An example of this mechanism is shown by activated cytotoxic T cells expressing Fas ligand which induce apoptosis in target cells. The second pathway is via the release of cytochrome c from mitochondria. Cytochrome c binds to Apaf-1 which then activates caspases. DNA damage induced by irradiation or chemotherapy may act through this pathway. The protein p53 has an important role in sensing DNA damage. It activates apoptosis by raising the cell level of BAX which then increases cytochrome c release. It also shuts down the cell cycle to stop the damaged cell from dividing (Fig. 1.10). Following death, apoptotic

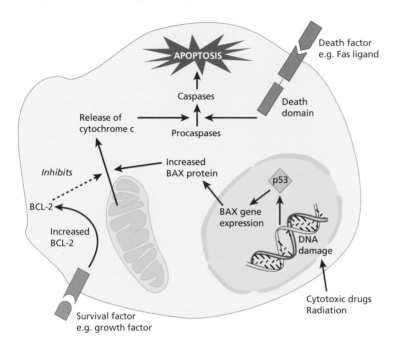

Fig. 1.9 Representation of apoptosis. Apoptosis is initiated via two main stimuli: (i) signalling through cell membrane receptors such as FAS or tumour necrosis factor (TNF) receptor or (ii) release of cytochrome c from mitochondria. Membrane receptors signal apoptosis through an intracellular death domain leading to activation of caspases which digest DNA. Cytochrome c binds to the cytoplasmic protein Apaf-1 leading to activation of caspases. The intracellular ratio of pro- (e.g. BAX) or anti-apoptotic (e.g. BCL-2) members of the BCL-2 family may influence mitochondrial cytochrome c release. Growth factors raise the level of BCL-2 inhibiting cytochrome c release whereas DNA damage, by activating p53, raises the level of BAX which enhances cytochrome c release.

cells display molecules that lead to their ingestion by macrophages.

As well as molecules that mediate apoptosis there are several intracellular proteins that protect cells from apoptosis. The best characterized example is BCL-2. BCL-2 is the prototype of a family of related proteins, some of which are anti-apoptotic and some, like BAX, pro-apoptotic. The intracellular ratio of BAX and BCL-2 determines the relative susceptibility of cells to apoptosis and may act through regulation of cytochrome c release from mitochondria.

Many of the genetic changes associated with malignant disease lead to a reduced rate of apoptosis and hence prolonged cell survival. The clearest example is the translocation of the *BCL-2* gene to the immunoglobulin heavy chain locus in the t(14; 18) translocation in follicle centre lymphoma. Overexpression of the BCL-2 protein makes the malignant B cells less susceptible to apoptosis.

Apoptosis is the normal fate for most B cells undergoing selection in the lymphoid germinal centres. Several translocations leading to the generation of fusion proteins such as t(9; 22), t(1; 14)

and t(15; 17) also result in inhibition of apoptosis (Chapter 11). In addition, genes encoding proteins that are involved in mediating apoptosis following DNA damage, such as p53 and ATM are also frequently mutated and therefore inactivated in haemopoietic malignancies.

GROWTH FACTOR RECEPTORS AND SIGNAL TRANSDUCTION

Growth factors bind with high affinity to their corresponding receptors on target cells (Table 1.3). The majority of the receptors belong to a set of structurally related transmembrane glycoproteins. The intracellular domains of the receptors associate with members of a family of tyrosine-specific protein kinases, the Janus associated kinase (JAK) family (Fig. 1.10). A growth factor molecule binds simultaneously to the extracellular domains of two or three receptor molecules, resulting in their aggregation. Receptor aggregation induces activation of the JAKs which now phosphorylate members of the signal transducer and activator of transcription (STAT) family of tran-

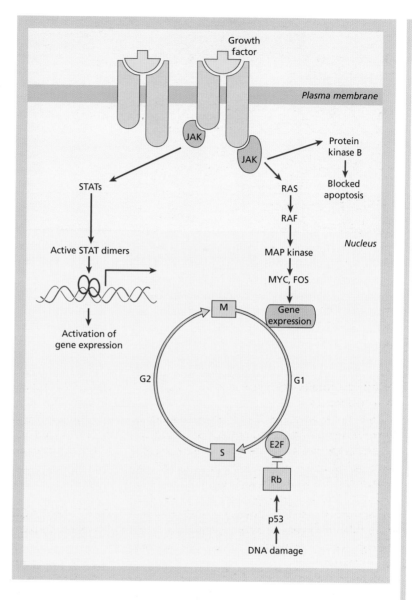

Fig. 1.10 Control of haemopoiesis by growth factors. The factors act on cells expressing the corresponding receptors. Binding of a growth factor to its receptor activates by phosphorylation Janus associated kinases (JAKs) which then phosphorylate signal transducer and activators of transcription (STATs) which translocate to the nucleus and activate transcription of specific genes (see text). JAKs may also activate other pathways, e.g. RAS/RAF/MAP kinase, concerned with cell proliferation by activating nuclear transcription factors which stimulate the cell to enter the cell cycle. E2F is a transcription factor needed for cell transition from G1 to S phase. E2F is inhibited by the tumour suppressor gene *Rb* (retinoblastoma) which can be indirectly activated by p53. The synthesis and degradation of different cyclins (not shown) stimulates the cell to pass through the different phases of the cell cycle. The growth factors may also suppress apoptosis by activating protein kinase B.

scription factors. This results in their dimerization and translocation from the cell cytoplasm across the nuclear membrane to the cell nucleus. Within the nucleus STAT dimers activate transcription of specific genes. A model for control of gene expression by a transcription factor is shown in Fig. 1.11. Growth factors thus regulate the function of myeloid and lymphoid cells via the JAK/STAT pathways which in turn control expression of specific genes.

JAK activation may also initiate pathways which result in cell proliferation. The RAS G protein (guanine nucleotide-binding protein), the protein kinases RAF and mitogen-activated protein kinase (MAPK) and increased expression of a set of transcription factors, including MYC and FOS, have crucial roles in proliferation signalling (Fig. 1.10). The cyclin protein family also plays an important part in the transition of cells through cell cycle control points located at the G0/G1,

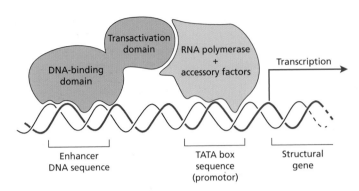

Fig. 1.11 Model for control of gene expression by a transcription factor. The DNA-binding domain of a transcription factor binds a specific enhancer sequence adjacent to a structural gene. The transactivation domain then binds a molecule of RNA polymerase, thus augmenting its binding to the TATA box. The RNA polymerase now initiates transcription of the structural gene to form messenger RNA. Translation of the mRNA by the ribosomes generates the protein encoded by the gene.

G1/S, S/G2 and G2/M boundaries (Fig. 1.10). Growth factors also promote cell survival by blocking apoptotic cell death (Fig. 1.9). JAK-mediated activation of protein kinase B and the consequent phosphorylation and functional inactivation of the pro-apoptotic BAD protein may mediate this anti-apoptotic signalling. Different domains of the intracellular receptor protein may signal for the different processes, e.g. proliferation or suppression of apoptosis mediated by growth factors.

A second smaller group of growth factors, including stem cell factors (SCF) and M-CSF (Table 1.3), bind to receptors which have an extracellular immunoglobulin-like domain linked via a transmembrane bridge to a cytoplasmic tyrosine kinase domain. Growth factor binding results in dimerization of these receptors and consequent activation of the tyrosine kinase domain. Phosphorylation of tyrosine residues in the receptor itself generates binding sites for a set of signalling proteins which initiate complex cascades of biochemical events resulting in changes in gene expression, cell proliferation and prevention of apoptosis.

ADHESION MOLECULES

A large family of glycoprotein molecules termed adhesion molecules mediate the attachment of marrow precursors, leucocytes and platelets to various components of the extracellular matrix, to endothelium, to other surfaces and to each other. The adhesion molecules on the surface

of leucocytes are termed receptors and these interact with molecules (termed ligands) on the surface of potential target cells. Three main families exist:

1 Immunoglobulin superfamily. This includes receptors which react with antigens (the T-cell receptors and the immunoglobulins) and antigen-independent surface adhesion molecules.

2 Selectins. These are mainly involved in leucocyte and platelet adhesion to endothelium during inflammation and coagulation.

3 Integrins. These are involved in cell adhesion to extracellular matrix, e.g. to collagen in wound healing and in leucocyte and platelet adhesion.

The adhesion molecules are thus important in the development and maintenance of inflammatory and immune responses, and in platelet–vessel wall and leucocyte–vessel wall interactions. Expression of adhesion molecules can be modifed by extracellular and intracellular factors and this alteration of expression may be quantitative or functional. IL-1, TNF, γ-interferon, T-cell activation, adhesion to extracellular proteins and viral infection may all up-regulate expression of these molecules.

The pattern of expression of adhesion molecules on tumour cells may determine their mode of spread and tissue localization, e.g. the pattern of metastasis of carcinoma cells or non-Hodgkin's lymphoma cells into a follicular or diffuse pattern. The adhesion molecules may also determine whether or not cells circulate in the bloodstream or remain fixed in tissues. They may also partly determine whether or not tumour cells are susceptible to the body's immune defences.

BIBLIOGRAPHY

Armitage J.O. (1998) Emerging applications for recombinant human granulocyte–macrophage colony-stimulating factor. *Blood* **92**, 4491–508.

Metcalf D. (2000) Summon up the Blood—In dogged persuit of the blood cell regulators. *Alpha Med Press*, Dayton, OH, USA.

Metcalf D. and Nicola N.A. (1995) *The Haemopoietic Colony Stimulating Factors.* Cambridge University Press, Cambridge.

Miller L.J. and Marx J. (1998) Apoptosis reviews. *Science* **281**, 1301–26.

Moore M.A.S. (1999) 'Turning brain into blood.' Clinical applications of stem-cell research in neurobiology and hematology. *Clin. Implicat. Basic Res.* **341**, 605–7.

Potten C.S. (ed.) (1997) *Stem Cells.* Academic Press, San Diego.

Welte K. (1996) Filgastrin (r-metHuG-CSF): the first 10 years. *Blood* **88**, 1907–29.

Whetton A.D. (ed.) (1997) Molecular haemopoiesis. *Clin. Haematol.* **10**, 429–619.

Wickremasinghe R.G. and Hoffbrand A.V. (1999) Biochemical and genetic control of apoptosis: relevance to normal hematopoiesis and hematological malignancies. *Blood* **93**, 3587–600.

CHAPTER 2

Erythropoiesis and general aspects of anaemia

We each make around 10^{12} new erythrocytes (red cells) each day by the complex and finely regulated process of erythropoiesis. Erythropoiesis passes from the stem cell through the progenitor cells CFU_{GEMM} (colony-forming unit granulocyte, erythroid, monocyte and megakaryocyte), BFU_E (burst-forming unit erythroid) and erythroid CFU (CFU_E) (see Figs 1.2 and 2.2) to the first recognizable erythrocyte precursor in the bone marrow, the pronormoblast. This is a large cell with dark blue cytoplasm, a central nucleus with nucleoli and slightly clumped chromatin (Fig. 2.1). The pronormoblast gives rise to a series of progressively smaller normoblasts by a number of cell divisions. They also contain progressively more haemoglobin (which stains pink) in the cytoplasm; the cytoplasm stains paler blue as it loses its RNA and protein synthetic apparatus while nuclear chromatin becomes more condensed (Figs 2.1 and 2.2). The nucleus is finally extruded from the late normoblast within the marrow and a reticulocyte stage results which still contains some ribosomal RNA and is still able to synthesize haemoglobin (Fig. 2.3). This cell is slightly larger than a mature red cell, spends 1–2 days in the marrow and also circulates in the peripheral blood for 1–2 days before maturing, mainly in the spleen, when RNA is completely lost. A completely pink-staining, mature erythrocyte results which is a non-nucleated biconcave disc. A single pronormoblast usually gives rise to 16 mature red cells (Fig. 2.2). Nucleated red cells (normoblasts) appear in the blood if erythropoiesis is occurring outside the marrow (extramedullary erythro-poiesis) and also with some marrow diseases. Normoblasts are not present in normal human peripheral blood.

ERYTHROPOIETIN

Erythropoiesis is regulated by the hormone erythropoietin. It is a heavily glycosylated polypeptide of 165 amino acids with a molecular weight of 30 400. Normally 90% of the hormone is produced in the peritubular interstitial cells of the kidney and 10% in the liver and elsewhere. There are no preformed stores and the stimulus to erythropoietin production is the oxygen (O_2) tension in the tissues of the kidney (Fig. 2.4). Erythropoietin production therefore increases in anaemia, when haemoglobin for some metabolic or structural reason is unable to give up O_2 normally, when atmospheric O_2 is low or when defective cardiac or pulmonary function or damage to the renal circulation affects O_2 delivery to the kidney. It stimulates erythropoiesis by increasing the number of progenitor cells committed to erythropoiesis. Late BFU_E and CFU_E which have erythropoietin receptors are stimulated to proliferate, differentiate and produce haemoglobin. The proportion of erythroid cells in the marrow increases and, in the chronic state, there is anatomical expansion of erythropoiesis into fatty marrow and sometimes into extramedullary sites. In infants, the marrow cavity may expand into cortical bone resulting in bone deformities with frontal bossing and protrusion of the maxilla (p. 77).

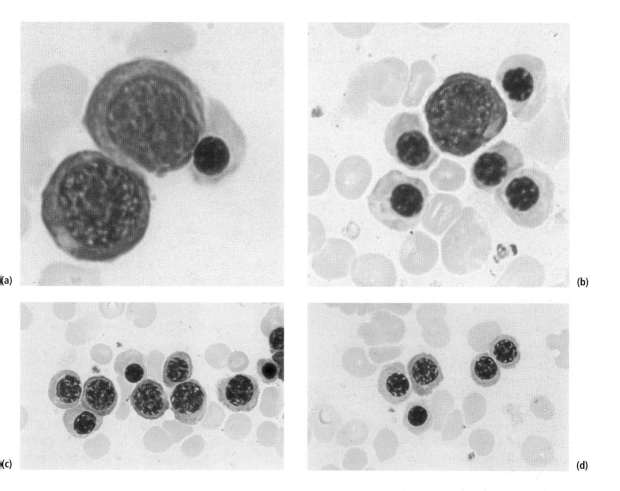

(a)

(b)

(c)

(d)

Fig. 2.1 Erythroblasts (normoblasts) at varying stages of development. The earlier cells are larger, with more basophilic cytoplasm and a more open nuclear chromatin pattern. The cytoplasm of the later cells is more eosinophilic as a result of haemoglobin formation.

Conversely, increased O_2 supply to the tissues (due to an increased red cell mass or because haemoglobin is able to release its O_2 more readily than normal) reduces the erythropoietin drive.

Plasma erythropoietin levels can be valuable in clinical diagnosis. They are high if a tumour-secreting erythropoietin is causing poly-cythaemia but low in severe renal disease or polycythaemia rubra vera (Fig. 2.5).

Indications for erythropoietin therapy

Recombinant erythropoietin is proving of great value in treating anaemia due to renal disease or various other causes. It may be given intravenous-ly or, more effectively, subcutaneously. The main indication is end-stage renal disease (with or with-out dialysis) and in this situation intravenous iron supplementation is often also needed to get the best response. Other uses are pre-autologous blood transfusions; the anaemia of chronic disor-ders, e.g. in rheumatoid arthritis or cancer; some cases of myelodysplasia or myeloma; and ac-quired immune deficiency syndrome (AIDS) (see also p. 289). A low serum erythropoietin level

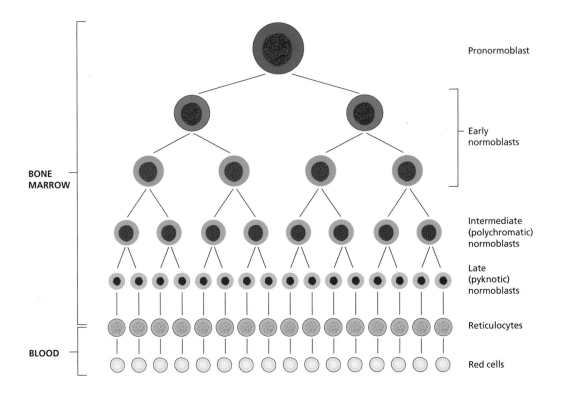

Fig. 2.2 The amplification and maturation sequence in the development of mature red cells from the pronormoblast.

	Normoblast	Reticulocyte	Mature RBC
Nuclear DNA	Yes	No	No
RNA in cytoplasm	Yes	Yes	No
In marrow	Yes	Yes	Yes
In blood	No	Yes	Yes

Fig. 2.3 Comparison of the DNA and RNA content, and marrow and peripheral blood distribution of the erythroblast (normoblast), reticulocyte and mature red blood cell (RBC).

prior to treatment is valuable in predicting an effective response.

The marrow requires many other precursors for effective erythropoiesis. These include metals such as iron or cobalt, vitamins (especially vitamin B_{12}, folate, vitamin C, vitamin E, vitamin B_6, thiamine and riboflavin) and hormones such as androgens and thyroxine. Deficiency in any of these may be associated with anaemia.

HAEMOGLOBIN

Haemoglobin synthesis

The main function of red cells is to carry O_2 to the tissues and to return carbon dioxide (CO_2) from the tissues to the lungs. In order to achieve this gaseous exchange they contain the specialized protein haemoglobin. Each red cell contains approximately 640 million haemoglobin molecules.

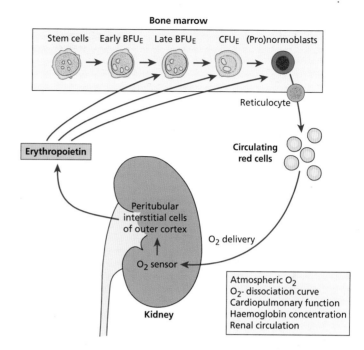

Fig. 2.4 The production of erythropoietin by the kidney in response to its oxygen (O_2) supply. Erythropoietin stimulates erythropoiesis and so increases O_2 delivery. (From A.J. Erslev and F. Gabuzda 1985.)

Each molecule of normal adult haemoglobin (Hb) A (the dominant haemoglobin in blood after the age of 3–6 months) consists of four polypeptide chains $\alpha_2\beta_2$, each with its own haem group. The molecular weight of Hb A is 68 000. Normal adult blood also contains small quantities of two other haemoglobins, Hb F and Hb A_2. These also contain α chains, but with γ and δ chains, respectively, instead of β (Table 2.1). The synthesis of the various globin chains in the fetus and adult is discussed in more detail in Chapter 6. The major switch from fetal to adult haemoglobin occurs 3–6 months after birth (see Fig. 6.1a).

Haem synthesis occurs largely in the mitochondria by a series of biochemical reactions commencing with the condensation of glycine and succinyl coenzyme A under the action of the key rate-limiting enzyme δ-aminolaevulinic acid (ALA) synthase (Fig. 2.6). Pyridoxal phosphate (vitamin B_6) is a coenzyme for this reaction which is stimulated by erythropoietin. Ultimately, protoporphyrin combines with iron in the ferrous (Fe^{2+}) state to form haem (Fig. 2.7), each molecule of which combines with a globin chain made on the

Table 2.1 Normal haemoglobins in adult blood

	Hb A	Hb F	Hb A_2
Structure	$\alpha_2\beta_2$	$\alpha_2\gamma_2$	$\alpha_2\delta_2$
Normal (%)	96–98	0.5–0.8	1.5–3.2

polyribosomes (Fig. 2.6). A tetramer of four globin chains each with its own haem group in a 'pocket' is then formed to make up a haemoglobin molecule (Fig. 2.8).

Haemoglobin function

The red cells in systemic arterial blood carry O_2 from the lungs to the tissues and return in venous blood with CO_2 to the lungs. As the haemoglobin molecule loads and unloads O_2, the individual globin chains in the haemoglobin molecule move on each other (Fig. 2.8). The $\alpha_1\beta_1$ and $\alpha_2\beta_2$ contacts stabilize the molecule. The β chains slide on the $\alpha_1\beta_2$ and $\alpha_2\beta_1$ contacts during oxygenation and

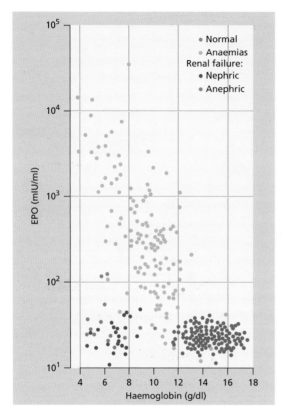

Fig. 2.5 The relation between radioimmunoassay estimates of erythropoietin (EPO) in plasma and haemoglobin concentration. Anaemias exclude conditions shown to be associated with impaired production of EPO. (From M. Pippard *et al.* 1992.)

deoxygenation. When O_2 is unloaded the β chains are pulled apart, permitting entry of the metabolite 2,3-diphosphoglycerate (2,3-DPG) resulting in a lower affinity of the molecule for O_2. This movement is responsible for the sigmoid form of the haemoglobin O_2 dissociation curve (Fig. 2.9). The P_{50} (i.e. the partial pressure of O_2 at which haemoglobin is half saturated with O_2) of normal blood is 26.6 mmHg. With increased affinity for O_2, the curve shifts to the left (i.e. the P_{50} falls) while, with decreased affinity for O_2, the curve shifts to the right (i.e. the P_{50} rises).

Normally *in vivo*, O_2 exchange operates between 95% saturation (arterial blood) with a mean arterial O_2 tension of 95 mmHg and 70% saturation (venous blood) with a mean venous O_2 tension of 40 mmHg.

The normal position of the curve depends on the concentration of 2,3-DPG, H^+ ions and CO_2 in the red cell and on the structure of the haemoglobin molecule. High concentrations of 2,3-DPG, H^+ or CO_2, and the presence of certain haemoglobins, e.g. sickle haemoglobin (Hb S), shift the curve to the right (oxygen is given up more easily) whereas fetal haemoglobin (Hb F)—which is unable to bind 2,3-DPG—and certain rare abnormal haemoglobins associated with polycythaemia shift the curve to the left because they give up O_2 less readily than normal.

Methaemoglobinaemia

This is a clinical state in which circulating haemoglobin is present with iron in the oxidized (Fe^{3+}) instead of the usual Fe^{2+} state. It may arise because of a hereditary deficiency of reduced nicotinamide adenine dinucleotide (NADH), diaphorase or inheritance of a structurally abnormal haemoglobin (Hb M). These contain an amino acid substitution affecting the haem pocket of the globin chain. Toxic methaemoglobinaemia (and/or sulphaemoglobinaemia) occurs when a drug or other toxic substance oxidizes haemoglobin. In all these states, the patient is likely to show cyanosis.

THE RED CELL

In order to carry haemoglobin into close contact with the tissues and for successful gaseous exchange, the red cell, 8 μm in diameter, must be able to pass repeatedly through the microcirculation whose minimum diameter is 3.5 μm, to maintain haemoglobin in a reduced (ferrous) state and to maintain osmotic equilibrium despite the high concentration of protein (haemoglobin) in the cell. Its total journey throughout its 120-day lifespan has been estimated to be 480 km (300 miles). To fulfil these functions, the cell is a flexible, biconcave disc with an ability to generate energy as adenosine triphosphate (ATP) by the anaerobic, glycolytic (Embden–Meyerhof) pathway (Fig. 2.10) and to generate reducing power as NADH

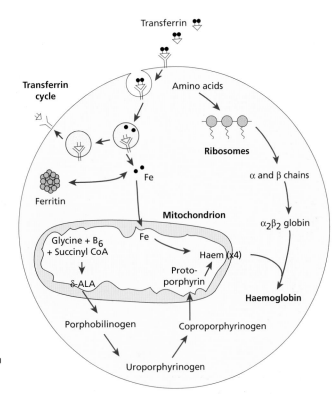

Fig. 2.6 Haemoglobin synthesis in the developing red cell. The mitochondria are the main sites of protoporphyrin synthesis, iron (Fe) is supplied from circulating transferrin; globin chains are synthesized on ribosomes. δ-ALA, δ-aminolaevulinic acid; CoA, coenzyme A.

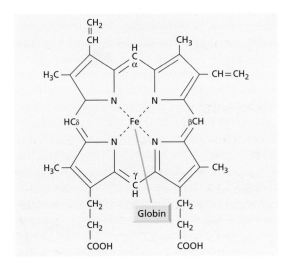

Fig. 2.7 The structure of haem.

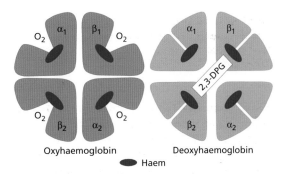

Fig. 2.8 The oxygenated and deoxygenated haemoglobin molecule. α, β, globin chains of normal adult haemoglobin (Hb A); 2,3-DPG, 2,3-diphosphoglycerate.

Red cell metabolism

Embden–Meyerhof pathway

In this series of biochemical reactions glucose is metabolized to lactate (Fig. 2.10). For each molecule of glucose used, two molecules of ATP and thus two high-energy phosphate bonds are gener-

by this pathway and as reduced nicotinamide adenine dinucleotide phosphate (NADPH), by the hexose monophosphate shunt (Fig. 2.11).

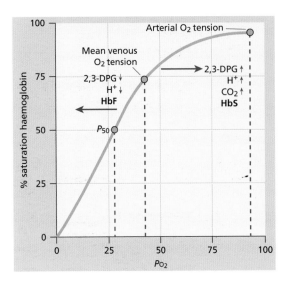

Fig. 2.9 The haemoglobin oxygen (O_2) dissociation curve.

ated. This ATP provides energy for maintenance of red cell volume, shape and flexibility. The red cell has an osmotic pressure five times that of plasma and an inherent weakness of the membrane results in continual Na^+ and K^+ movement. A membrane ATPase sodium pump is needed, and this uses one molecule of ATP to move three sodium ions out and two potassium ions into the cell.

The Embden–Meyerhof pathway also generates NADH which is needed by the enzyme methaemoglobin reductase to reduce functionally dead methaemoglobin (oxidized haemoglobin) containing ferric iron (produced by oxidation of about 3% of haemoglobin each day) to functionally active, reduced haemoglobin. 2,3-DPG which is generated in the Luebering–Rapoport shunt, or side arm, of this pathway (Fig. 2.10b) forms a 1:1 complex with haemoglobin and, as mentioned above, is important in the regulation of haemoglobin's oxygen affinity.

Hexose monophosphate (pentose phosphate) pathway

About 5% of glycolysis occurs by this oxidative pathway in which glucose-6-phosphate is converted to 6-phosphogluconate and so to ribulose-5-phosphate (Fig. 2.11). NADPH is generated and is linked with glutathione which maintains sulphydril (SH) groups intact in the cell including

those in haemoglobin and the red cell membrane. NADPH is also used by another methaemoglobin reductase to maintain haemoglobin iron in the functionally active Fe^{2+} state. In one of the most common inherited abnormalities of red cells, glucose-6-phosphate dehydrogenase (G6PD) deficiency, the red cells are extremely susceptible to oxidant stress (see p. 63).

Red cell membrane

The red cell membrane comprises a lipid bilayer, integral membrane proteins and a membrane skeleton (Fig. 2.12). About 50% of the membrane is protein, 40% is fat and up to 10% is carbohydrate. Carbohydrates occur only on the external surface while proteins are either peripheral or integral, penetrating the lipid bilayer. Several red cell proteins have been numbered accordingly to their mobility on polyacrylamide gel electrophoresis (PAGE).

The membrane skeleton is formed by structural proteins that include α and β spectrin, ankyrin, protein 4.1 and actin. These proteins form an horizontal lattice on the internal side of the red cell membrane and are important in maintaining the biconcave shape. Spectrin is the most abundant and consists of two chains, α and β, wound around each other to form heterodimers which then self-associate head-to-head to form tetramers. These tetramers are linked at the tail end to actin and are attached to protein band 4.1. At the head end, the β-spectrin chains attach to ankyrin which connects to band 3, the transmembrane protein that acts as an anion channel ('vertical connections') (Fig. 2.12). Protein 4.2 enhances this interaction.

Defects of the proteins may explain some of the abnormalities of shape of the red cell membrane, e.g. hereditary spherocytosis and elliptocytosis (Chapter 5), while alterations in lipid composition because of congenital or acquired abnormalities in plasma cholesterol or phospholipid may be associated with other membrane abnormalities. For instance, an increase in cholesterol and phospholipid has been suggested as one cause of target cells whereas a large selective increase in cholesterol may cause acanthocyte formation (see Fig. 2.15).

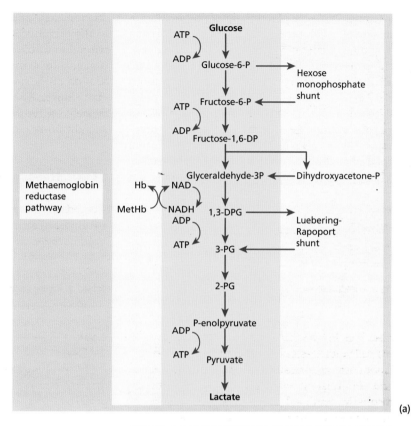

(a)

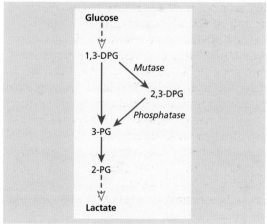

(b)

Fig. 2.10 (a) The Embden–Meyerhof glycolytic pathway. (b) The Luebering–Rapoport shunt which regulates the concentration of 2,3-DPG (2,3-diphosphoglycerate) in the red cell. ADP, adenosine diphosphate; ATP, adenosine triphosphate; Hb, haemoglobin; NAD, NADH, nicotinamide adenine dinucleotide; PG, phosphoglycerate.

ANAEMIA

This is defined as a reduction in the haemoglobin concentration of the blood. Although normal values can vary between laboratories typical values would be less than 13.5 g/dl in adult males and less than 11.5 g/dl in adult females. From the age of 3 months to puberty, less than 11.0 g/dl indicates anaemia. As newborn infants have a high haemoglobin level, 15.0 g/dl is taken as the lower limit at birth (Table 2.2). Reduction of haemoglobin is usually accompanied by a fall in red cell count and packed cell volume (PCV) but these may be normal in some patients with subnormal haemoglobin levels (and therefore by definition anaemic). Alterations in total circulating plasma volume as well as of total circulating haemoglobin mass determine the haemoglobin concentration. Reduction in plasma volume (as in dehydration) may mask anaemia or even cause (pseudo) polycythaemia (see p. 232); conversely, an increase in plasma volume (as with splenomegaly or pregnancy) may cause anaemia even with a normal total circulating red cell and haemoglobin mass.

After acute major blood loss, anaemia is not immediately apparent because the total blood volume is reduced. It takes up to a day for the plasma volume to be replaced and so for the degree of anaemia to become apparent (see p. 318). Regeneration of the haemoglobin mass takes substantially longer. The initial clinical features of major blood loss are therefore a result of reduction in blood volume rather than anaemia.

Clinical features of anaemia

The major adaptations to anaemia are in the cardiovascular system (with increased stroke volume and tachycardia) and in the haemoglobin

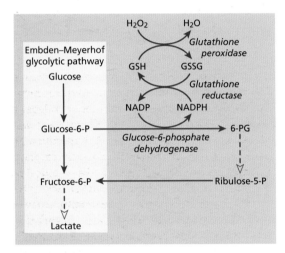

Fig. 2.11 The hexose monophosphate shunt pathway. GSH, GSSG, glutathione; NADP, NADPH, nicotinamide adenine dinucleotide phosphate; P, phosphate; PG, phosphoglycerate.

Table 2.2 Normal adult red cell values

	Male	Female
Haemoglobin* (g/dl)	13.5–17.5	11.5–15.5
Haematocrit (PCV) (%)	40–52	36–48
Red cell count ($\times 10^{12}$/l)	4.5–6.5	3.9–5.6
Mean cell haemoglobin (pg)	27–34	
Mean cell volume (fl)	80–95	
Mean cell haemoglobin concentration (g/dl)	30–35	
Reticulocyte count ($\times 10^9$/l)	25–125	

*In children normal haemoglobin values are: newborn, 15.0–21.0 g/dl; 3 months, 9.5–12.5 g/dl; 1 year to puberty, 11.0–13.5 g/dl. PCV, packed cell volume.

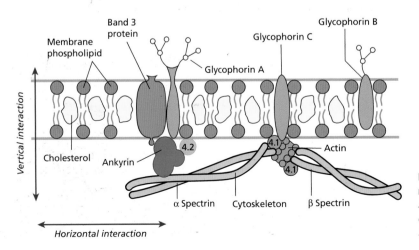

Fig. 2.12 The structure of the red cell membrane. Some of the penetrating and integral proteins carry carbohydrate antigens; other antigens are attached directly to the lipid layer.

O_2 dissociation curve. In some patients with quite severe anaemia there may be no symptoms or signs, whereas others with mild anaemia may be severely incapacitated. The presence or absence of clinical features can be considered under four major headings.

1 Speed of onset. Rapidly progressive anaemia causes more symptoms than anaemia of slow onset because there is less time for adaptation in the cardiovascular system and in the O_2 dissociation curve of haemoglobin.

2 Severity. Mild anaemia often produces no symptoms or signs but these are usually present when the haemoglobin is less than 9–10 g/dl. Even severe anaemia (haemoglobin concentration as low as 6.0 g/dl) may produce remarkably few symptoms, however, when there is very gradual onset in a young subject who is otherwise healthy.

3 Age. The elderly tolerate anaemia less well than the young because of the effect of lack of oxygen on organs when normal cardiovascular compensation (increased cardiac output caused by increased stroke volume and tachycardia) is impaired.

4 Haemoglobin O_2 dissociation curve. Anaemia, in general, is associated with a rise in 2,3-DPG in the red cells and a shift in the O_2 dissociation curve to the right so that oxygen is given up more readily to tissues. This adaptation is particularly marked in some anaemias which either affect red cell metabolism directly, e.g. in the anaemia of pyruvate kinase deficiency (which causes a rise in 2,3-DPG concentration in the red cells), or which are associated with a low affinity haemoglobin (e.g. Hb S) (Fig. 2.9).

Symptoms

If the patient does have symptoms, these are usually shortness of breath particularly on exercise, weakness, lethargy, palpitation and headaches. In older subjects symptoms of cardiac failure, angina pectoris or intermittent claudication or confusion may be present. Visual disturbances because of retinal haemorrhages may complicate very severe anaemia, particularly of rapid onset.

Signs

These may be divided into general and specific. General signs include pallor of mucous membranes which occurs if the haemoglobin level is less than 9–10 g/dl (Fig. 2.13). Conversely, skin colour is not a reliable sign. A hyperdynamic circulation may be present with tachycardia, a bounding pulse, cardiomegaly and a systolic flow murmur especially at the apex. Particularly in the elderly, features of congestive heart failure may be present. Retinal haemorrhages are unusual (Fig. 2.14). Specific signs are associated with particular types of anaemia, e.g. koilonychia (spoon nails) with iron deficiency, jaundice with haemolytic or megaloblastic anaemias, leg ulcers with sickle cell and other haemolytic anaemias, bone deformities with thalassaemia major and other severe congenital haemolytic anaemias.

Fig. 2.13 Pallor of the conjunctival mucosa (a) and of the nail bed (b) in two patients with severe anaemia (haemoglobin 6.0 g/dl).

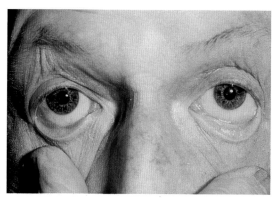

(a)

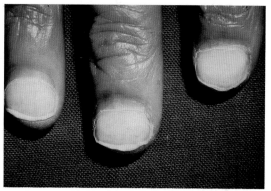

(b)

Table 2.3 Classification of anaemia

Microcytic, hypochromic	Normocytic, normochromic	Macrocytic
MCV < 80 fl	MCV 80–95 fl	MCV > 95 fl
MCH < 27 pg	MCH > 26 pg	Megaloblastic: vitamin B$_{12}$ or folate deficiency
Iron deficiency	Many haemolytic anaemias	Non-megaloblastic: alcohol, liver disease, myelodysplasia, aplastic anaemia, etc. (see p. 55)
Thalassaemia	Anaemia of chronic disease (some cases)	
Anaemia of chronic disease (some cases)	After acute blood loss	
	Renal disease	
Lead poisoning	Mixed deficiencies	
Sideroblastic anaemia (some cases)	Bone marrow failure, e.g. post-chemotherapy, infiltration by carcinoma, etc.	

MCH, mean corpuscular haemoglobin; MCV, mean corpuscular volume.

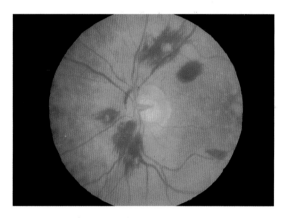

Fig. 2.14 Retinal haemorrhages in a patient with severe anaemia (haemoglobin 2.5 g/dl) caused by severe chronic haemorrhage.

The association of features of anaemia with excess infections or spontaneous bruising suggest that neutropenia or thrombocytopenia may be present possibly due to bone marrow failure.

Classification and laboratory findings in anaemia

Red cell indices

The most useful classification is that based on red cell indices (Table 2.3) and divides the anaemia into microcytic, normocytic and macrocytic. As well as suggesting the nature of the primary defect this approach may also indicate an underlying abnormality before overt anaemia has developed.

In two common physiological situations, the mean corpuscular volume (MCV) may be outside the normal adult range. In the newborn for a few weeks the MCV is high but, in infancy, it is low (e.g. 70 fl at 1 year of age) and rises slowly throughout childhood to the normal adult range. In normal pregnancy there is a slight rise in MCV, even in the absence of other causes of macrocytosis, e.g. folate deficiency.

Other laboratory findings

Although the red cell indices will indicate the type of anaemia, further useful information can be obtained from the initial blood sample.

Leucocyte and platelet counts

Measurement of these helps to distinguish 'pure' anaemia from 'pancytopenia' (a drop in red cells, granulocytes and platelets) which suggests a more general marrow defect, e.g. caused by marrow hypoplasia, infiltration or general destruction of cells (e.g. hypersplenism). In anaemias caused by haemolysis or haemorrhage the neutrophil and platelet counts are often raised; in infections and leukaemias the leucocyte count is also often raised and there may be abnormal leucocytes or neutrophil precursors present.

Reticulocyte count

The normal count is 0.5–2.5%, and the absolute count $25–125 \times 10^9/l$. This should rise in anaemia because of erythropoietin increase and be higher the more severe the anaemia. This is particularly so when there has been time for erythroid hyperplasia to develop in the marrow as in chronic haemolysis. After an acute major haemorrhage, there is an erythropoietin response in 6 h, the reticulocyte count rises within 2–3 days, reaches a maximum in 6–10 days and remains raised until the haemoglobin returns to the normal level. If the reticulocyte count is not raised in an anaemic pa-

tient this suggests impaired marrow function or lack of erythropoietin stimulus (Table 2.4).

Blood film

It is essential to examine the blood film in all cases of anaemia. Abnormal red cell morphology (Fig.

Table 2.4 Factors impairing the normal reticulocyte response to anaemia

Marrow diseases, e.g. hypoplasia, infiltration by carcinoma, lymphoma, myeloma, acute leukaemia, tuberculosis
Deficiency of iron, vitamin B_{12} or folate
Lack of erythropoietin, e.g. renal disease
Reduced tissue O_2 consumption, e.g. myxoedema, protein deficiency
Ineffective erythropoiesis, e.g. thalassaemia major, megaloblastic anaemia, myelodysplasia, myelofibrosis, congenital dyserythropoietic anaemia
Chronic inflammatory or malignant disease

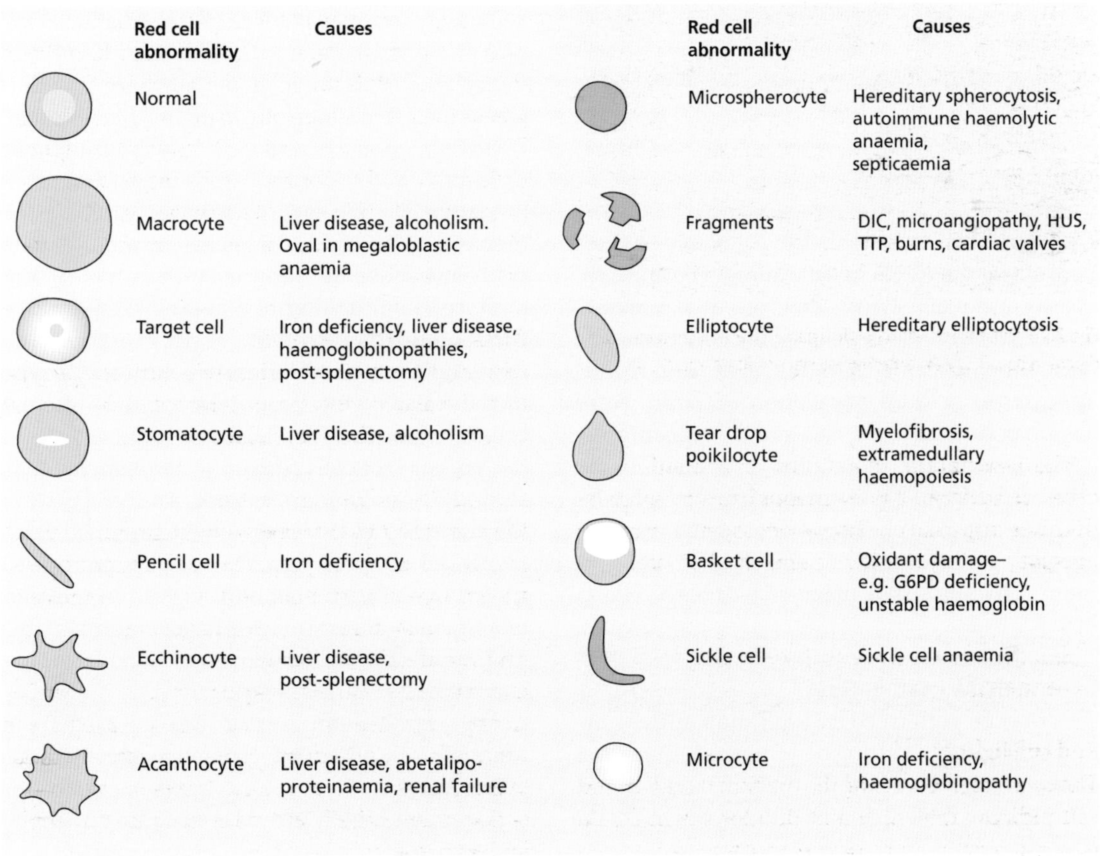

Fig. 2.15 Some of the more frequent variations in size (anisocytosis) and shape (poikilocytosis) that may be found in different anaemias. DIC, disseminated intravascular coagulopathy; G6PD, glucose-6-phosphate dehydrogenase; HUS, haemolytic uraemic syndrome; TTP, thrombotic thrombocytopenic purpura.

Red cell abnormality	Causes		Red cell abnormality	Causes
Normal			Microspherocyte	Hereditary spherocytosis, autoimmune haemolytic anaemia, septicaemia
Macrocyte	Liver disease, alcoholism. Oval in megaloblastic anaemia		Fragments	DIC, microangiopathy, HUS, TTP, burns, cardiac valves
Target cell	Iron deficiency, liver disease, haemoglobinopathies, post-splenectomy		Elliptocyte	Hereditary elliptocytosis
Stomatocyte	Liver disease, alcoholism		Tear drop poikilocyte	Myelofibrosis, extramedullary haemopoiesis
Pencil cell	Iron deficiency		Basket cell	Oxidant damage– e.g. G6PD deficiency, unstable haemoglobin
Ecchinocyte	Liver disease, post-splenectomy		Sickle cell	Sickle cell anaemia
Acanthocyte	Liver disease, abetalipo-proteinaemia, renal failure		Microcyte	Iron deficiency, haemoglobinopathy

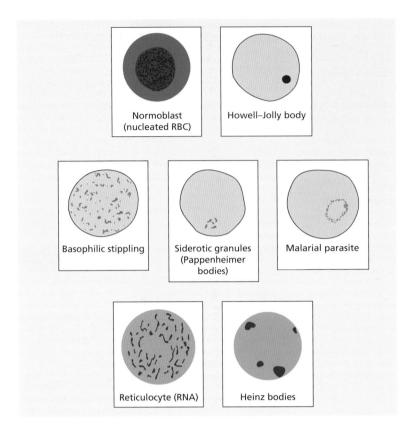

Fig. 2.16 Red blood cell (RBC) inclusions which may be seen in the peripheral blood film in various conditions. The reticulocyte RNA and Heinz bodies are only demonstrated by supravital staining, e.g. with new methylene blue. Heinz bodies are oxidized denatured haemoglobin. Siderotic granules (Pappenheimer bodies) contain iron. They are purple on conventional staining but blue with Perls' stain. The Howell–Jolly body is a DNA remnant. Basophilic stippling is denatured RNA.

2.15) or red cell inclusions (Fig. 2.16) may suggest a particular diagnosis. When causes of both microcytosis and macrocytosis are present, e.g. mixed iron and folate or B_{12} deficiency, the indices may be normal but the blood film reveals a 'dimorphic' appearance (a dual population of large, well-haemoglobinized cells and small, hypochromic cells). During the blood film examination the white cell differential count is performed, platelet number and morphology are assessed and the presence or absence of abnormal cells, e.g. normoblasts, granulocyte precursors or blast cells, is noted.

Bone marrow examination

This may be performed by aspiration or trephine biopsy (Fig. 2.17). During bone marrow aspiration a needle is inserted into the marrow and a liquid sample of marrow is sucked into a syringe. This is then spread on a slide for microscopy and stained by the usual Romanowsky technique. A great deal of morphological information can be obtained by examining aspirate slides. The detail of the developing cells can be examined (e.g. normoblastic or megaloblastic), the proportion of the different cell lines assessed (myeloid : erythroid ratio) and the presence of cells foreign to the marrow (e.g. secondary carcinoma) observed. The cellularity of the marrow can also be viewed provided fragments are obtained. An iron stain is performed routinely so that the amount of iron in reticuloendothelial stores (macrophages) and as fine granules ('siderotic' granules) in the developing erythroblasts can be assessed.

An aspirate sample may also be used for a number of other specialized investigations (Table 2.5).

A trephine biopsy provides a solid core of bone

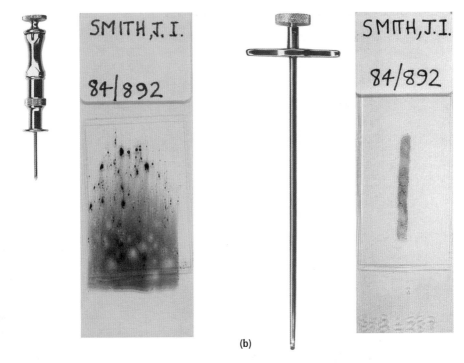

Fig. 2.17 (a) The Salah bone marrow aspiration needle and a smear made from a bone marrow aspirate. (b) The Jamshidi bone marrow trephine needle and normal trephine section.

Table 2.5 Comparison of bone marrow aspiration and trephine biopsy

	Aspiration	Trephine
Site	Posterior iliac crest or sternum (tibia in infants)	Posterior iliac crest
Stains	Romanowsky; Perls' reaction (for iron)	Haematoxylin and eosin; reticulin (silver stain)
Result available	1–2 h	1–7 days (according to decalcification method)
Main indications	Investigation of anaemia, pancytopenia, suspected leukaemia or myeloma, neutropenia, thrombocytopenia, etc.	Indications for additional trephine: suspicion of polycythaemia vera, myelofibrosis and other myeloproliferative disorders, aplastic anaemia, malignant lymphoma, secondary carcinoma, cases of splenomegaly or pyrexia of undetermined cause. Any case where aspiration gives a 'dry' tap
Special tests	Cytogenetics, microbiological culture, biochemical analysis, immunological and cytochemical markers, immunoglobulin or T-cell receptor gene analysis, DNA or RNA analysis for gene abnormalities, progenitor cell culture	Immunophenotyping

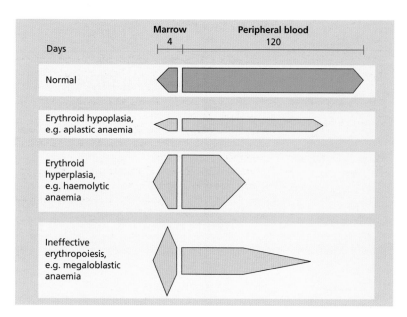

Fig. 2.18 The relative proportions of marrow erythroblastic activity, circulating red cell mass and red cell lifespan in normal subjects and three types of anaemia.

including marrow and is examined as a histological specimen after fixation in formalin, decalcification and sectioning. It is less valuable than aspiration when individual cell detail is to be examined but provides a panoramic view of the marrow from which overall marrow architecture, cellularity and presence of fibrosis or abnormal infiltrates can be reliably determined.

Ineffective erythropoiesis

Erythropoiesis is not entirely efficient because about 10–15% of developing erythroblasts die within the marrow without producing mature cells. This is termed ineffective erythropoiesis and it is substantially increased in a number of chronic anaemias (Table 2.4). The serum unconjugated bilirubin (derived from breaking down haemoglobin) and lactate dehydrogenase (LDH, derived from breaking down cells) are usually raised when ineffective erythropoiesis is marked. The reticulocyte count is low in relation to the degree of anaemia and to the proportion of erythroblasts in the marrow.

Assessment of erythropoiesis

Total erythropoiesis and the amount of erythropoiesis that is effective in producing circulating red cells can be assessed by examining the bone marrow, haemoglobin level and reticulocyte count.

Total erythropoiesis is assessed from the marrow cellularity and the myeloid : erythroid ratio (i.e. the proportion of granulocyte precursors to red cell precursors in the bone marrow, normally 2.5 : 1 to 12 : 1). This ratio falls and may be reversed when total erythropoiesis is selectively increased.

Effective erythropoiesis is assessed by the reticulocyte count. This is raised in proportion to the degree of anaemia when erythropoiesis is effective, but is low when there is ineffective erythropoiesis or an abnormality preventing normal marrow response (Table 2.4).

RED CELL LIFESPAN

This is measured by ^{51}Cr-labelled red cell survival. A sample of the subject's blood is incubated with ^{51}Cr which binds firmly to haemoglobin and the labelled cells are reinjected into the circulation. The disappearance of ^{51}Cr from the blood is measured sequentially over the next 3 weeks. The sites of red cell destruction are determined by surface counting over the spleen, liver and heart (as an index of blood activity). Typical results in haemolytic anaemias are shown in Fig. 5.2. Figure 2.18 shows typical changes in marrow erythropoiesis and circulating red cell mass in some of the different types of anaemia.

BIBLIOGRAPHY

Adamson J.W. (1994) The relationship of erythropoietin and iron metabolism to red blood cell production in humans. *Semin. Oncol.* **21**, 9–15.

Bain B.J. (1995) *Blood Cellls: A Practical Guide,* 2nd edn. Blackwell Science, Oxford.

Lewis S.M., Bain B.J. and Bates I. (eds) (2001) Dacie and Lewis *Practical Haematology.* 9th edn. Churchill Livingston, Edinburgh.

Cazzola M. (1998) How and when to use erythropoietin. *Curr. Opin. Haematol.* **5**, 103–8.

Hsia C.C.W. (1998) Respiratory function of haemoglobin. *N. Engl. J. Med.* **338**, 239–47.

Hypochromic anaemias and iron overload

Iron deficiency is the most common cause of anaemia in every country of the world. It is the most important cause of a microcytic hypochromic anaemia, in which all three red cell indices (the MCV, MCH and MCHC—mean corpuscular volume, haemoglobin and haemoglobin concentration, respectively) are reduced and the blood film shows small (microcytic) and pale (hypochromic) red cells. This appearance is caused by a defect in haemoglobin synthesis (Fig. 3.1). The major differential diagnosis in microcytic hypochromic anaemia is thalassaemia which is considered in Chapter 6 and anaemia of chronic disease which is dealt with in this chapter.

NUTRITIONAL AND METABOLIC ASPECTS OF IRON

Iron is one of the most common elements in the earth's crust, yet iron deficiency is the most common cause of anaemia affecting about 500 million people worldwide. This is because the body has a limited ability to absorb iron and excess loss of iron as a result of haemorrhage is frequent.

Body iron distribution and transport

The transport and storage of iron is largely mediated by three proteins—transferrin, the transferrin receptor and ferritin. Transferrin may contain up to two atoms of iron. It delivers iron to tissues which have transferrin receptors, especially erythroblasts in the bone marrow which incorporate the iron into haemoglobin (Fig. 3.2). The transferrin is then reutilized. At the end of their life, red cells are broken down in the macrophages of the reticuloendothelial system and the iron is released from haemoglobin, enters the plasma and provides most of the iron on transferrin. Only a small proportion of plasma transferrin iron comes from dietary iron, absorbed through the duodenum and jejunum.

Some iron is stored in the reticuloendothelial cells as ferritin and haemosiderin, the amount varying widely according to overall body iron status. Ferritin is a water-soluble protein–iron complex of molecular weight 465 000. It is made up of an outer protein shell, apoferritin, consisting of 22 subunits and an iron–phosphate–hydroxide core. It contains up to 20% of its weight as iron and is not visible by light microscopy. Each molecule of apoferritin may bind up to 4000–5000 atoms of iron. Haemosiderin is an insoluble protein–iron complex of varying composition containing about 37% of iron by weight. It is derived from partial lysosomal digestion of aggregates of ferritin molecules and is visible in macrophages and other cells by light microscopy after staining by Perls' (Prussian blue) reaction. Iron in ferritin and haemosiderin is in the ferric form. It is mobilized after reduction to the ferrous form, vitamin C being involved. A copper-containing enzyme, caeruloplasmin, catalyses oxidation of the iron to the ferric form for binding to plasma transferrin.

Iron is also present in muscle as myoglobin and in most cells of the body in iron-containing enzymes, e.g. cytochromes, succinic dehydrogenase, catalase, etc. (Table 3.1). This tissue iron is

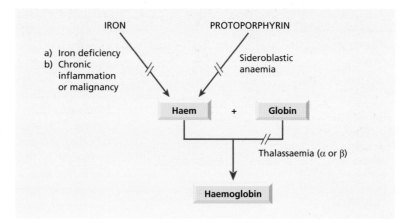

Fig. 3.1 The causes of a hypochromic microcytic anaemia. These include lack of iron (iron deficiency) or of iron release from macrophages to serum (anaemia of chronic inflammation or malignancy), failure of protoporphyrin synthesis (sideroblastic anaemia) or of globin synthesis (α- or β-thalassaemia). Lead also inhibits haem and globin synthesis.

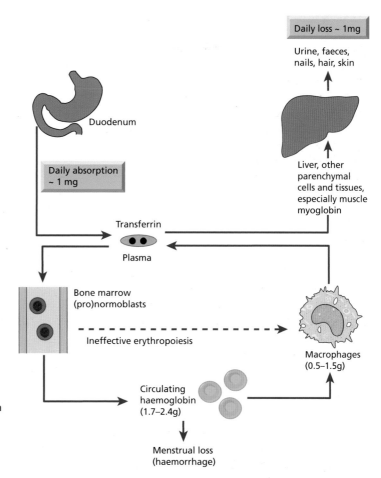

Fig. 3.2 Daily iron cycle. Most of the iron in the body is contained in circulating haemoglobin (Table 3.1) and is reutilized for haemoglobin synthesis after the red cells die. Iron is transferred from macrophages to plasma transferrin and so to bone marrow erythroblasts. Iron absorption is normally just sufficient to make up for iron loss. The dashed line indicates ineffective erythropoiesis.

Table 3.1 The distribution of body iron

Amount of iron in average adult	Male (g)	Female (g)	Percentage of total
Haemoglobin	2.4	1.7	65
Ferritin and haemosiderin	1.0 (0.3–1.5)	0.3 (0–1.0)	30
Myoglobin	0.15	0.12	3.5
Haem enzymes (e.g. cytochromes, catalase, peroxidases, flavoproteins)	0.02	0.015	0.5
Transferrin-bound iron	0.004	0.003	0.1

less likely to become depleted than haemosiderin, ferritin and haemoglobin in states of iron deficiency, but some reduction of haem-containing enzymes may occur.

The levels of ferritin and transferrin receptor (TfR) are linked to iron status so that iron overload causes a rise in tissue ferritin and a fall in TfR, whereas in iron deficiency ferritin is low and TfR increased. This linkage arises through the binding of an iron regulatory protein (IRP) to iron response elements (IREs) on the ferritin and TfR messenger (m)RNA molecules. Iron deficiency increases the ability of IRP to bind to the IREs whereas iron overload reduces the binding. The site of IRP binding to IREs, whether upstream (5′) or downstream (3′) from the coding gene, determines whether the amount of mRNA and so protein produced is increased or decreased (Fig. 3.3). Upstream binding reduces translation whereas downstream binding stabilizes the mRNA, increasing protein translation.

When plasma iron is raised and transferrin is saturated the amount of iron transferred to parenchymal cells, e.g. those of the liver, endocrine organs, pancreas and heart, is increased and this is the basis of the pathological changes associated with iron loading conditions.

Dietary iron

Iron is present in food as ferric hydroxides,

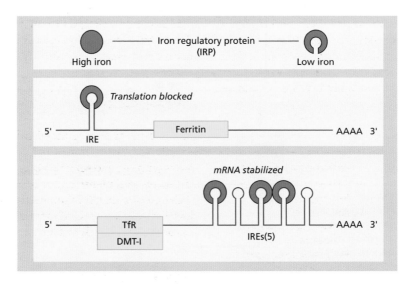

Fig. 3.3 Regulation of transferrin receptor (TfR), DMT-1 (divalent metal transporter), ferroportin and ferritin expression by iron regulatory protein (IRP) sensing of intracellular iron levels. IRPs (⬤) are able to bind to stem-loop structures called iron response elements (IREs) (⎧) in transferrin receptor or ferritin messenger RNAs (mRNAs). IRP binding to the IRE within the 3′ untranslated region of the former leads to stabilization of mRNA levels and increased protein synthesis whereas IRP binding to the IRE within the 5′ untranslated region of ferritin mRNA reduces translation. IRPs can exist in two states—at times of high iron levels the IRP binds iron and exhibits a reduced affinity for the IREs whereas when iron levels are low the binding of IRPs to IREs is increased. In this way synthesis of TfR, DMT-1 and ferritin is coordinated to physiological requirements.

ferric–protein complexes and haem–protein complexes. Both the iron content and the proportion of iron absorbed differ from food to food; in general, meat and, in particular, liver is a better source than vegetables, eggs or dairy foods. The average Western diet contains 10–15 mg of iron from which only 5–10% is normally absorbed. The proportion can be increased to 20–30% in iron deficiency or pregnancy (Table 3.2) but, even in these situations, most dietary iron remains unabsorbed.

Iron absorption

Organic dietary iron is partly absorbed as haem and partly broken down in the gut to inorganic iron. Absorbtion occurs through the duodenum and is favoured by factors such as acid and reducing agents that keep iron in the gut lumen in the Fe^{2+} rather than the Fe^{3+} state (Table 3.2). The protein DMT-1 (divalent metal transporter) is involved in transfer of iron from the lumen of the gut across the enterocyte microvilli (Fig. 3.4). Ferroportin at the basolateral surface controls exit of iron from the cell into portal plasma. The amount of iron absorbed is regulated according to the body's needs by changing the levels of DMT-1 and probably of ferroportin according to the iron status of the duodenal villous crypt enterocyte. Iron is incorporated into the crypt enterocyte from plasma transferrin which binds to transferrin re-

ceptor in association with the protein HFE at the basal surface of the cell. In iron deficiency less iron is delivered to the crypt cell from transferrin which is largely unsaturated with iron. The consequent iron deficiency in the crypt cell results in increased expresssion of DMT-1. This occurs by the same mechanism (IRP/IRE binding) by which transferrin receptor is increased in iron deficiency (Fig. 3.3). The increased expression of DMT-1 results, when the enterocyte reaches the apical absorptive surface of the duodenal villous 24–48 h later, in increased transfer of iron from the gut lumen into the enterocyte. Increased ferroportin in iron deficiency has not yet been shown but as the mRNA has an IRE, like that of DMT-1,3' from the coding portion, it is likely that ferroportin levels also rise in iron deficiency. This would result in increased transfer of iron from the enterocyte to portal blood.

An enzyme is present at the apical surface which converts iron from the Fe^{3+} to Fe^{2+} state and another enzyme, hephaestin (which contains copper), converts Fe^{2+} to Fe^{3+} at the basal surface prior to binding to transferrin. The mechanism by which increased ineffective erythropoiesis, e.g. in thalassaemia intermedia (see p. 81) results in increased iron absorption remains unclear. The defect of iron absorption in primary haemochromatosis is discussed on p. 41.

Iron requirements

The amount of iron required each day to compensate for losses from the body and growth varies with age and sex; it is highest in pregnancy, adolescent and menstruating females (Table 3.3). These groups therefore are particularly likely to develop iron deficiency if there is additional iron loss or prolonged reduced intake.

IRON DEFICIENCY

Clinical features

When iron deficiency is developing the reticuloendothelial stores (haemosiderin and ferritin) be-

Table 3.2 Iron absorption

Factors favouring absorption	Factors reducing absorption
Haem iron	Inorganic iron
Ferrous form (Fe^{2+})	Ferric form (Fe^{3+})
Acids (HCl, vitamin C)	Alkalis — antacids, pancreatic secretions
Solubilizing agents (e.g. sugars, amino acids)	Precipitating agents — phytates, phosphates
Iron deficiency	Iron excess
Increased erythropoiesis	Decreased erythropoiesis
Pregnancy	Infection
Hereditary haemochromatosis	Tea
Increased expression of DMT-1 and ferroportin in duodenal enterocytes	Decreased expression of DMT-1 and ferroportin in duodenal enterocytes

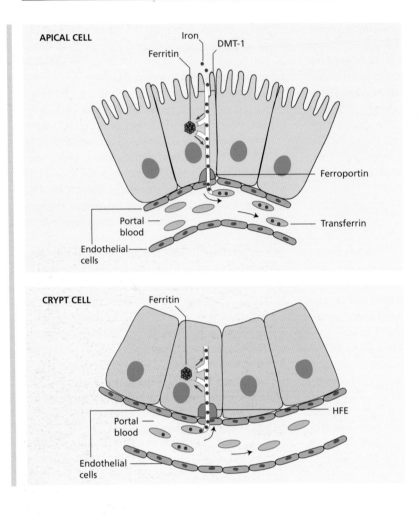

Fig. 3.4 The regulation of iron absorption. The protein DMT-1 transports iron across the duodenal microvillus brush border at the apex of the villus. Exit of iron from the cell is controlled by ferroportin. The haemochromatosis protein HFE is expressed at the basolateral surface of crypt cells and binds to the transferrin receptor where it seems to control uptake of iron into the cell from portal blood. In the normal situation iron is incorporated into crypt enterocytes from transferrin and the adequate supply of iron leads to physiological levels of DMT-1 and ferroportin expression. In iron deficiency there is reduced delivery of iron to the enterocytes leading to greater expression of DMT-1 and probably of ferroportin (Fig. 3.3) and consequently increased iron absorption and transfer of iron to portal plasma. In hereditary haemochromatosis HFE is mutated, preventing iron incorporation into the crypt enterocytes so iron levels within enterocytes are low in relation to body iron stores. DMT-1 expression is consequently high and iron absorption increased.

Table 3.3 Estimated daily iron requirements. Units are mg/day

	Urine, sweat, faeces	Menses	Pregnancy	Growth	Total
Adult male	0.5–1				0.5–1
Postmenopausal female	0.5–1				0.5–1
Menstruating female*	0.5–1	0.5–1			1–2
Pregnant female*	0.5–1		1–2		1.5–3
Children (average)	0.5			0.6	1.1
Female (age 12–15)*	0.5–1	0.5–1		0.6	1.6–2.6

*These groups more likely to develop iron deficiency.

come completely depleted before anaemia occurs (Fig. 3.5). As the condition develops the patient may develop the general symptoms and signs of anaemia and also show a painless glossitis, angular stomatitis, brittle, ridged or spoon nails (koilonychia), dysphagia as a result of pharyngeal webs (Paterson–Kelly or Plummer–Vinson syndrome) (Fig. 3.6) and unusual dietary cravings

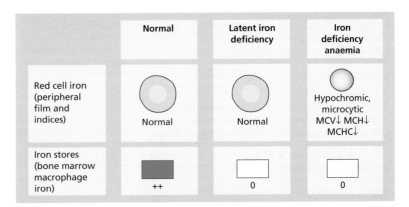

		Normal	Latent iron deficiency	Iron deficiency anaemia
	Red cell iron (peripheral film and indices)	Normal	Normal	Hypochromic, microcytic MCV↓ MCH↓ MCHC↓
	Iron stores (bone marrow macrophage iron)	++	0	0

Fig. 3.5 The development of iron deficiency anaemia. Reticuloendothelial (macrophage) stores are lost completely before anaemia develops. MCH, mean corpuscular haemoglobin; MCHC, mean corpuscular haemoglobin concentration; MCV, mean corpuscular volume.

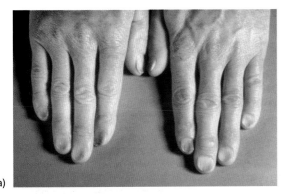

(a)

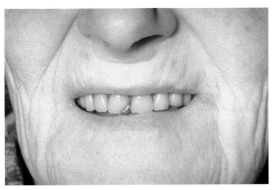

(b)

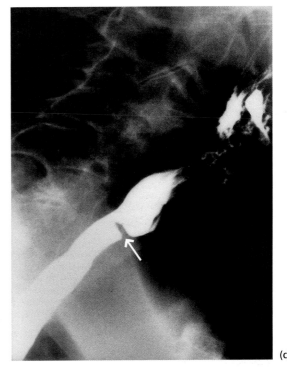

(c)

Fig. 3.6 Iron deficiency anaemia. (a) Koilonychia: typical 'spoon' nails. (b) Angular cheilosis: fissuring and ulceration of the corner of the mouth. (c) Paterson–Kelly (Plummer–Vinson) syndrome: barium swallow X-ray showing a filling defect (arrow) caused by a postcricoid web.

(pica). The cause of the epithelial cell changes is not clear but may be related to reduction of iron in iron-containing enzymes. In children iron deficiency is particularly significant as it can cause irritability, poor cognitive function and a decline in psychomotor development.

Causes of iron deficiency

Chronic blood loss, especially uterine or from the gastrointestinal tract, is the dominant cause (Table 3.4). In contrast, in developed countries dietary

Table 3.4 Causes of iron deficiency

Chronic blood loss
Uterine
Gastrointestinal, e.g. peptic ulcer, oesophageal varices, aspirin (or
   other non-steroidal anti-inflammatory drugs) ingestion, partial
   gastrectomy, carcinoma of the stomach, caecum, colon or rectum,
   hookworm, angiodysplasia, colitis, piles, diverticulosis, etc.
Rarely haematuria, haemoglobinuria, pulmonary haemosiderosis,
   self-inflicted blood loss

Increased demands (see also Table 3.3)
Prematurity
Growth
Pregnancy
Erythropoietin therapy

Malabsorption
For example gluten-induced enteropathy, gastrectomy

Poor diet
A contributory factor in many developing countries but rarely the
   sole cause except in infants and children

deficiency is rarely a cause on its own. Half a litre of whole blood contains approximately 250 mg of iron and, despite the increased absorption of food iron at an early stage of iron deficiency, negative iron balance is usual in chronic blood loss.

Increased demands during infancy, adolescence, pregnancy, lactation and in menstruating women account for the high risk of anaemia in these particular clinical groups. Newborn infants have a store of iron derived from the breakdown of excess red cells. From 3 to 6 months there is a tendency for negative iron balance due to growth. From 6 months supplemented formula milk and mixed feeding, particularly with iron-fortified foods, prevents iron deficiency.

In pregnancy, increased iron is needed for an increased maternal red cell mass of about 35%, transfer of 300 mg of iron to the fetus, and because of blood loss at delivery. Although iron absorption is also increased, iron therapy is often needed if the haemoglobin (Hb) falls below 10 g/dl or the MCV is below 82 fl in the third trimester.

Menorrhagia (a loss of 80 ml or more of blood at each cycle) is difficult to assess clinically, although the loss of clots, the use of large numbers of pads or tampons, or prolonged periods all suggest excessive loss.

It has been estimated to take 8 years for a normal adult male to develop iron deficiency anaemia solely as a result of a poor diet or malabsorption resulting in no iron intake at all. In clinical practice, inadequate intake or malabsorption are only rarely the sole cause of iron deficiency anaemia, although in developing countries iron deficiency may occur as a result of a life-long poor diet, consisting mainly of cereals and vegetables. Gluten-induced enteropathy, partial or total gastrectomy and atrophic gastritis may, however, predispose to iron deficiency.

Laboratory findings

These are summarized and contrasted with those in other hypochromic anaemias in Table 3.7.

Red cell indices and blood film
Even before anaemia occurs, the red cell indices fall and they fall progressively as the anaemia becomes more severe. The blood film shows hypochromic, microcytic cells with occasional target cells and pencil-shaped poikilocytes (Fig. 3.7). The reticulocyte count is low in relation to the degree of anaemia. When iron deficiency is associated with severe folate or vitamin B_{12} deficiency a 'dimorphic' film occurs with a dual population of red cells of which one is macrocytic and the other microcytic and hypochromic; the indices may be normal. A dimorphic blood film is also seen in patients with iron deficiency anaemia who have received recent iron therapy and produced a population of new well-filled normal-sized red cells (Fig. 3.8) and when the patient has been transfused. The platelet count is often moderately raised in iron deficiency, particularly when haemorrhage is continuing.

Bone marrow iron
Bone marrow examination is not essential to assess iron stores except in complicated cases. In iron deficiency anaemia there is a complete absence of iron from stores (macrophages) and from developing erythroblasts (Fig. 3.9). The erythroblasts are small and have a ragged cytoplasm.

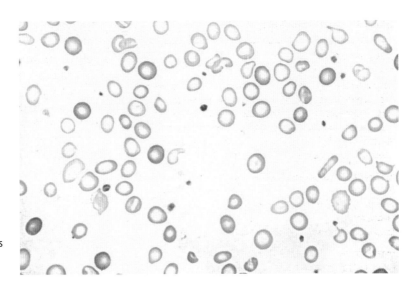

Fig. 3.7 The peripheral blood film in severe iron deficiency anaemia. The cells are microcytic and hypochromic with occasional target cells.

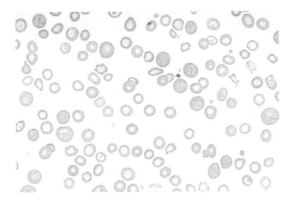

Fig. 3.8 Dimorphic blood film in iron deficiency anaemia responding to iron therapy. Two populations of red cells are present, one microcytic and hypochromic, the other normocytic and well haemoglobinized.

Serum iron and total iron-binding capacity

The serum iron falls and total iron-binding capacity (TIBC) rises so that the TIBC is less than 10% saturated (Fig. 3.10). This contrasts both with the anaemia of chronic disorders (see below) when the serum iron and the TIBC are both reduced and with other hypochromic anaemias where the serum iron is normal or even raised.

Serum transferrin receptor (sTfR)

Transferrin receptor is shed from cells into plasma. The level of sTfR is increased in iron deficiency anaemia but not in the anaemia of chronic disease or thalassaemia trait. The level is also raised if the overall level of erythropoiesis is increased.

Serum ferritin

A small fraction of body ferritin circulates in the serum, the concentration being related to tissue, particularly reticuloendothelial, iron stores. The normal range in men is higher than in women (Fig. 3.10). In iron deficiency anaemia the serum ferritin is very low while a raised serum ferritin indicates iron overload or excess release of ferritin from damaged tissues or an acute phase response, e.g. in inflammation. The serum ferritin is normal or raised in the anaemia of chronic disorders.

Investigation of the cause of iron deficiency
(Table 3.4)

In premenopausal women, menorrhagia and/or repeated pregnancies are the usual causes of the deficiency although other causes must be sought if these are not present. In some patients with menorrhagia a clotting or platelet abnormality, e.g. von Willebrand's disease, is present. In men and postmenopausal women, gastrointestinal blood loss is the main cause of iron deficiency and the exact site is sought from the clinical history,

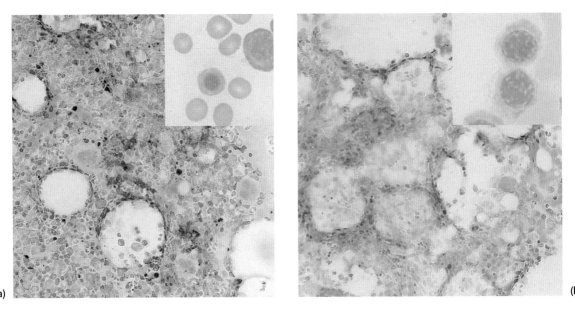

(a)   (b)

Fig. 3.9 Bone marrow iron assessed by Perls' stain. (a) Normal iron stores indicated by blue staining in the macrophages. Inset: normal siderotic granule in erythroblast. (b) Absence of blue staining (absence of haemosiderin) in iron deficiency. Inset: absence of siderotic granules in erythroblasts.

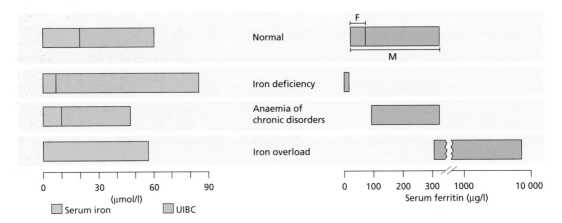

Fig. 3.10 The serum iron, unsaturated serum iron-binding capacity (UIBC) and serum ferritin in normal subjects and in those with iron deficiency, anaemia of chronic disorders and iron overload. The total iron-binding capacity (TIBC) is made up of the serum iron and the UIBC. In some laboratories, the transferrin content of serum is measured directly by immunodiffusion, rather than by its ability to bind iron, and is expressed as g/l. Normal serum contains 2–4 g/l of transferrin (1 g/l transferrin ≃20 μmol/l binding capacity). Normal ranges for serum iron are 10–30 μmol/l; for TIBC, 40–75 μmol/l; for serum ferritin, male, 40–340 μg/l; female, 14–150 μg/l.

physical and rectal examination, by occult blood tests, and by appropriate use of upper and lower gastrointestinal endoscopy and/or radiology (Figs 3.11 and 3.12). Tests for endomysial and gluten antibodies and duodenal biopsy to look for gluten-induced enteropathy can be valuable.

Hookworm ova are sought in stools of subjects from areas where this infestation occurs. Rarely, a coeliac axis angiogram is needed to demonstrate angiodysplasia.

If gastrointestinal blood loss is excluded, loss of iron in the urine as haematuria or haemosiderin-

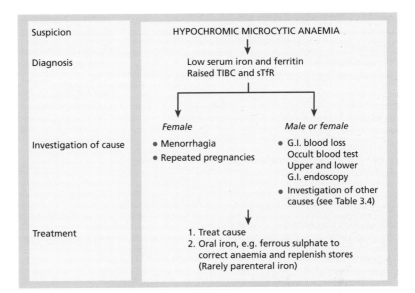

Suspicion	HYPOCHROMIC MICROCYTIC ANAEMIA
Diagnosis	Low serum iron and ferritin Raised TIBC and sTfR

	Female	*Male or female*

Investigation of cause	• Menorrhagia
	• Repeated pregnancies
		• G.I. blood loss
		  Occult blood test
		  Upper and lower
		  G.I. endoscopy
		• Investigation of other
		  causes (see Table 3.4)

Treatment		1. Treat cause
		2. Oral iron, e.g. ferrous sulphate to
		   correct anaemia and replenish stores
		   (Rarely parenteral iron)

Fig. 3.11 Investigation and management of iron deficiency anaemia. GI, gastrointestinal; sTfR, serum transferrin receptor; TIBC, total iron-binding capacity.

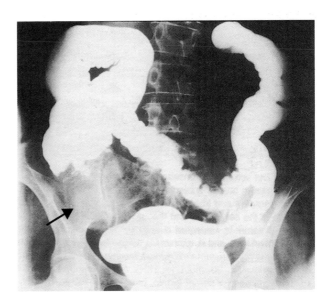

Fig. 3.12 Barium enema of a male patient aged 63 years who presented with iron deficiency anaemia. There is a filling defect of the caecum and barium does not enter the terminal ileum. Carcinoma of the caecum was found at laparotomy.

uria (due to chronic intravascular haemolysis) is considered. A normal chest X-ray excludes the rare condition of pulmonary haemosiderosis. Rarely, patients bleed themselves producing iron deficiency.

Treatment

The underlying cause is treated as far as possible.

In addition, iron is given to correct the anaemia and replenish iron stores.

Oral iron

The best preparation is ferrous sulphate which is cheap, contains 67 mg of iron in each 200 mg (anhydrous) tablet and is best given on an empty stomach in doses spaced by at least 6 h. If side-effects occur (e.g. nausea, abdominal pain, constipation or diarrhoea), these can be reduced by giv-

Table 3.5 Failure of response to oral iron

Continuing haemorrhage
Failure to take tablets
Wrong diagnosis — especially thalassaemia trait, sideroblastic
   anaemia
Mixed deficiency — associated folate or vitamin B_{12} deficiency
Another cause for anaemia, e.g. malignancy, inflammation
Malabsorption — this is a rare cause
Use of slow-release preparation

Table 3.6 Causes of the anaemia of chronic disorders

Chronic inflammatory diseases
Infections, e.g. pulmonary abscess, tuberculosis, osteomyelitis,
   pneumonia, bacterial endocarditis
Non-infectious, e.g. rheumatoid arthritis, systemic lupus
   erythematosus and other connective tissue diseases, sarcoidosis,
   Crohn's disease

Malignant diseases
For example carcinoma, lymphoma, sarcoma

ing iron with food or by using a preparation of lower iron content, e.g. ferrous gluconate which contains less iron (37 mg) per 300 mg tablet. An elixir is available for children. Slow-release preparations should not be used.

Oral iron therapy should be given for long enough both to correct the anaemia and to replenish body iron stores, which usually means for at least 6 months. The haemoglobin should rise at the rate of about 2 g/dl every 3 weeks. There is a reticulocyte response, the height of which is related to the degree of anaemia. Failure of response to oral iron has several possible causes (Table 3.5) which should all be considered before parenteral iron is used.

Parenteral iron

Iron–sorbitol–citrate (Jectofer) is given as repeated deep intramuscular injections whereas ferric hydroxide–sucrose (Venofer) is administered by slow intravenous injection or infusion. There may be hypersensitivity or anaphylactoid reactions and parenteral iron is therefore only given when it is considered necessary to replenish body iron rapidly, for example in late pregnancy or patients on haemodialysis and erythropoietin therapy or when oral iron is ineffective (e.g. severe malabsorption) or impractical (e.g. active Crohn's disease). The haematological response to parenteral iron is no faster than to adequate dosage of oral iron but the stores are replenished much faster.

ANAEMIA OF CHRONIC DISORDERS

One of the most common anaemias occurs in patients with a variety of chronic inflammatory and malignant diseases (Table 3.6). The characteristic features are:

1 normochromic, normocytic or mildly hypochromic (MCV rarely <75 fl) indices and red cell morphology;
2 mild and non-progressive anaemia (haemoglobin rarely less than 9.0 g/dl) — the severity being related to the severity of the disease;
3 both the serum iron and TIBC are reduced; sTfR levels are normal;
4 the serum ferritin is normal or raised; and
5 bone marrow storage (reticuloendothelial) iron is normal but erythroblast iron is reduced (Table 3.7).

The pathogenesis of this anaemia appears to be related to decreased release of iron from macrophages to plasma, reduced red cell lifespan and an inadequate erythropoietin response to anaemia caused by the effects of cytokines such as IL-1 and TNF on erythropoiesis. The anaemia is only corrected by successful treatment of the underlying disease and does not respond to iron therapy despite the low serum iron. Recombinant erythropoietin improves the anaemia in some cases. In many conditions this anaemia is complicated by anaemia resulting from other causes, e.g. iron, vitamin B_{12} or folate deficiency, renal failure, bone marrow failure, hypersplenism, endocrine abnormality, leucoerythroblastic anaemia, etc. and these are discussed in Chapter 20.

Table 3.7 Laboratory diagnosis of a hypochromic anaemia

	Iron deficiency	Chronic inflammation or malignancy	Thalassaemia trait (α or β)	Sideroblastic anaemia
MCV MCH	Reduced in relation to severity of anaemia	Normal or mild reduction	Reduced; very low for degree of anaemia	Usually low in congenital type but MCV often raised in acquired type
Serum iron	Reduced	Reduced	Normal	Raised
TIBC	Raised	Reduced	Normal	Normal
Serum transferrin receptor	Raised	Normal/low	Variable	Normal
Serum ferritin	Reduced	Normal or raised	Normal	Raised
Bone marrow iron stores	Absent	Present	Present	Present
Erythroblast iron	Absent	Absent	Present	Ring forms
Haemoglobin electrophoresis	Normal	Normal	Hb A$_2$ raised in β form	Normal

MCH, mean corpuscular haemoglobin; MCV, mean corpuscular volume; TIBC, total iron-binding capacity.

SIDEROBLASTIC ANAEMIA

This is a refractory anaemia with hypochromic cells in the peripheral blood and increased marrow iron; it is defined by the presence of many pathological ring sideroblasts in the bone marrow (Fig. 3.13). These are abnormal erythroblasts containing numerous iron granules arranged in a ring or collar around the nucleus instead of the few randomly distributed iron granules seen when normal erythroblasts are stained for iron. Sideroblastic anaemia is diagnosed when 15% or more of marrow erythroblasts are ring sideroblasts but they can be found at lower numbers in a variety of haematological conditions.

Sideroblastic anaemia is classified into different types (Table 3.8) and the common link is a defect in haem synthesis. In the hereditary forms, the anaemia is characterized by a markedly hypochromic and microcytic blood picture. The most common mutations are in the δ-aminolaevulinic acid synthase (ALA-S) gene which is on the X chromosome. Pyridoxal-6-phosphate is a co-enzyme for ALA-S. Other rare types include mitochondrial defects, thiamine-responsive and other autosomal defects. The much more common primary acquired form is one subtype of

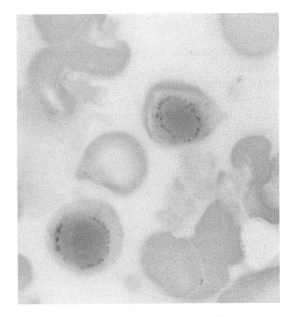

Fig. 3.13 Ring sideroblasts with a perinuclear ring of iron granules in sideroblastic anaemia.

myelodysplasia. It is also termed 'refractory anaemia with ring sideroblasts'. This condition is discussed together with the other types of myelodysplasia in Chapter 13.

Table 3.8 Classification of sideroblastic anaemia

Hereditary

Usually occurs in males, transmitted by females; also occurs rarely in females (see text)

Acquired

Primary
Myelodysplasia (refractory anaemia with ring sideroblasts) (see p. 186)

Secondary
Ring sideroblast formation may also occur in the bone marrow in:
other malignant diseases of the marrow, e.g. other types of
  myelodysplasia, myelofibrosis, myeloid leukaemia, myeloma
drugs, e.g. antituberculous (isoniazid, cycloserine), alcohol, lead
other benign conditions, e.g. haemolytic anaemia, megaloblastic
  anaemia, malabsorption, rheumatoid arthritis

In some patients, particularly with the hereditary type, there is a response to pyridoxine therapy. Folate deficiency may occur and folic acid therapy may also be tried. In many severe cases, however, repeated blood transfusions are the only method of maintaining a satisfactory haemoglobin concentration and transfusional iron overload becomes a major problem. Other treatments which have been tried in myelodysplasia, e.g. erythropoietin, may be tried in the primary acquired form (Chapter 13).

Lead poisoning

Lead inhibits both haem and globin synthesis at a number of points. In addition it interferes with the breakdown of RNA by inhibiting the enzyme pyrimidine 5′ nucleotidase, causing accumulation of denatured RNA in red cells, the RNA giving an appearance called basophilic stippling on the ordinary (Romanowsky) stain (see Fig. 2.16). The anaemia may be hypochromic or predominantly haemolytic, and the bone marrow may show ring sideroblasts. Free erythrocyte protoporphyrin is raised.

Differential diagnosis of hypochromic anaemia

Table 3.7 lists the laboratory investigations that may be necessary. The clinical history is particularly important as the source of the haemorrhage leading to iron deficiency or the presence of a chronic disease may be revealed. The country of origin and the family history may suggest a possible diagnosis of thalassaemia or other haemoglobinopathy. Physical examination may also be helpful in determining a site of haemorrhage, features of a chronic inflammatory or malignant disease, koilonychia or, in some haemoglobinopathies, an enlarged spleen or bony deformities.

In thalassaemia trait, the red cells tend to be small, often with an MCV of 70 fl or less, even when anaemia is mild or absent; the red cell count usually being over $5.5 \times 10^{12}/l$. Conversely, in iron deficiency anaemia the indices fall progressively with the degree of anaemia and when anaemia is mild the indices are often only just reduced below normal (e.g. MCV 75–80 fl). In the anaemia of chronic disorders, the indices are also not markedly low, an MCV in the range 75–82 fl being usual.

It is usual to perform a serum iron and TIBC measurement or, alternatively, serum ferritin estimation to confirm a diagnosis of iron deficiency. sTfR assay is also useful in distinguishing iron deficiency anaemia from anaemia of chronic disease. Haemoglobin electrophoresis with an estimation of Hb A_2 and Hb F is carried out in all patients suspected of thalassaemia or other haemoglobinopathy because of the family history, country of origin, red cell indices and blood film. Iron deficiency or the anaemia of chronic disorders may also occur in these subjects. β-thalassaemia trait is characterized by a raised Hb A_2 above 3.5%, but in α-thalassaemia trait there is no abnormality on simple haemoglobin studies so the diagnosis is usually made by exclusion of all other causes of hypochromic red cells and by the presence of a red cell count $>5.5 \times 10^{12}/l$. DNA studies can be used to confirm the diagnosis. In some α-thalassaemia patients, however, occasional red cells show

Table 3.9 The causes of iron overload

Increased iron absorption	Hereditary (primary) haemochromatosis
	Ineffective erythropoiesis, e.g. thalassaemia intermedia, sideroblastic anaemia
	Chronic liver disease
Increased iron intake	African siderosis (dietary and genetic)
Repeated red cell transfusions	Transfusion siderosis

deposits of Hb H (β^4) in reticulocyte preparations (Chapter 6).

Bone marrow examination is essential if a diagnosis of sideroblastic anaemia is suspected, but is not usually needed in diagnosis of the other hypochromic anaemias.

IRON OVERLOAD

There is no physiological mechanism for eliminating excess iron from the body and so iron absorption is normally carefully regulated to avoid accumulation. Accumulation can occur in disorders associated with excessive absorption or chronic blood transfusion. Excessive iron deposition in tissues can cause serious damage to organs, particularly the heart, liver and endocrine organs. The causes of iron overload are listed in Table 3.9. Iron chelation therapy is discussed on p. 80.

Hereditary (genetic, primary) haemochromatosis

In this autosomally recessive condition there is excessive absorption of iron from the gastrointestinal tract. The gene involved is *HFE* and most patients are homozygous for a missense mutation (845G to A) in the *HFE* gene which leads to insertion of a tyrosine residue rather than a cysteine in the mature protein (C282Y). This allele has a prevalence of around one in 300 within the white population. The *HFE* gene is situated close to the major histocompatibility complex (MHC) locus on chromosome 6 and associated with human leucocyte antigen (HLA)-A3 and -B8. A second mutation resulting in an histidine to aspartic acid substitution H63D is found with the C282Y mutation in about 5% of patients but homozygotes for H63D do not have the disease. Mutations in other genes (e.g. HFE_2) account for other types of genetic haemochromatosis, e.g. a juvenile form which presents before the age of 30.

The C282Y mutation leads to failure of *HFE* to be expressed on the basolateral surface of the crypt cell. The consequence of this appears to be that duodenal crypt cells are unable to incorporate iron from plasma transferrin and are therefore rendered iron deficient. Iron deficiency in the crypt enterocyte increases expression of DMT-1 protein which, when the cell reaches the villous tip, leads to increased intestinal iron absorption in relation to body iron stores (Fig. 3.4).

The consequent iron overload damages parenchymal cells and patients present with hepatic disease, endocrine disturbances such as diabetes or impotence, cardiac disease, skin pigmentation (see also Chapter 6) and arthropathy (due to pyrophosphate deposition). Presentation is usually in adults over the age of 40 years. Diagnosis is shown by increased serum transferrin saturation and ferritin accompanied by testing for *HFE* mutation. Liver biopsy is performed to quantify the degree of iron overload and assess liver damage.

Treatment is with regular venesection, each unit of blood lost removing 200–250 mg iron, and is monitored by serum iron, TIBC and serum ferritin assays as well as tests of organ function.

BIBLIOGRAPHY

Anderson G.J. and Powell L.W. (1999) Haemochromatosis and control of intestinal iron absorption. *Lancet* **353**, 2089–90.

Andrews N.C. (1999) Disorders of iron metabolism. *N. Engl. J. Med.* **341**, 1986–95.

Andrews N.C. (2000) Iron metabolism and absorption. *Rev. Clin. Exp. Hematol.* **4**, 283–301.

Barton J.C. and Edwards C.Q. (eds) (2000) *Hemochromatosis.* Cambridge University Press, Cambridge.

Brittenham G.M. (1991) Disorders of iron metabolism: iron deficiency and overload. In: *Hematology: Basic Principles and Practice* (eds R. Hoffman, E.J. Benz, S.J. Shattil, B. Furie and H.J. Cohen). Churchill Livingstone, New York, pp. 329–49.

Camaschella C., De Gobbi M. and Roetto A. (2000) Hereditary hemochromatosis: progress and perspectives. *Rev. Clin. Exp. Hematol.* **4**, 302–21.

Feder J.N. *et al.* (1996) A novel MHC class I-like gene is mutated in patients with hereditary haemochromatosis. *Nat. Genet.* **13**, 399–408.

Kuhn L.C. (1991) mRNA–protein interactions regulate critical pathways in cellular iron metabolism. *Br. J. Haematol.* **79**, 1–6.

Zoller M., Pietroangelo A., Vogel W. *et al.* (1999) Duodenal metal transporter (DMT-1, NRAMP-2) expression in patients with hereditary haemochromatosis. *Lancet* **353**, 2120–3.

Megaloblastic anaemias and other macrocytic anaemias

INTRODUCTION TO MACROCYTIC ANAEMIA

In macrocytic anaemia the red cells are abnormally large (mean corpuscular volume, MCV >95 fl). There are several causes (see Table 2.3) but they can be broadly subdivided into megaloblastic and non-megaloblastic, based on the appearance of developing erythroblasts in the bone marrow.

MEGALOBLASTIC ANAEMIAS

This is a group of anaemias in which the erythroblasts in the bone marrow show a characteristic abnormality—maturation of the nucleus being delayed relative to that of the cytoplasm. The nuclear chromatin maintains an open, stippled, lacy appearance despite normal haemoglobin formation in the cytoplasm of the erythroblasts as they mature. The underlying defect accounting for the asynchronous maturation of the nucleus is defective DNA synthesis and, in clinical practice, this is usually caused by deficiency of vitamin B_{12} or folate. Less commonly, abnormalities of metabolism of these vitamins or other lesions in DNA synthesis may cause an identical haematological appearance (Table 4.1). Dietary and metabolic aspects of the two vitamins are reviewed before considering the anaemia.

VITAMIN B_{12} (B_{12}, COBALAMIN)

This vitamin is synthesized in nature by microorganisms; animals acquire it by eating other animal foods, by internal production from intestinal bacteria (not in humans) or by eating bacterially contaminated foods. The vitamin consists of a small group of compounds, the cobalamins, which have the same basic structure, with a cobalt atom at the centre of a corrin ring which is attached to a nucleotide portion (Fig. 4.1). The vitamin is found in foods of animal origin such as liver, meat, fish and dairy produce but does not occur in fruit, cereals or vegetables. Table 4.2 compares nutritional aspects of B_{12} and folate.

Absorption

A normal diet contains a large excess of B_{12} compared with daily needs (Table 4.2). B_{12} is combined with the glycoprotein intrinsic factor (IF) (molecular weight, MW 45 000) which is synthesized by the gastric parietal cells. The IF–B_{12} complex can then bind to a specific surface receptor, cubilin, for IF in the distal ileum where B_{12} is absorbed (Fig. 4.2).

Transport: the transcobalamins

Vitamin B_{12} is absorbed into portal blood where it becomes attached to the plasma-binding protein transcobalamin II (TC II) which delivers B_{12} to bone marrow and other tissues. Although TC II is the essential plasma protein for transferring B_{12} into the cells of the body, the amount of B_{12} on TC II is normally very low (<50 ng/l). TC II deficiency causes megaloblastic anaemia because of failure of B_{12} to enter marrow (and other cells) from plasma but the serum B_{12} level in TC II deficiency is normal. This is because most B_{12} in plasma is bound to another transport protein, TC I. This is a glycoprotein largely synthesized by granulocytes and macrophages. In myeloproliferative diseases where granulocyte production is greatly in-

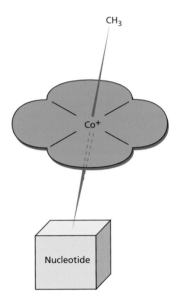

Fig. 4.1 The structure of methylcobalamin (methyl B_{12}), the main form of vitamin B_{12} in human plasma. Other forms include deoxyadenosylcobalamin (ado B_{12}), the main form in human tissues; hydroxocobalamin (hydroxo B_{12}), the main form in treatment; and cyanocobalamin (cyano B_{12}), the radioactively labelled ([57]Co or [58]Co) form used to study vitamin B_{12} absorption or metabolism.

Table 4.1 Causes of megaloblastic anaemia

Vitamin B_{12} deficiency
Folate deficiency
Abnormalities of vitamin B_{12} or folate metabolism, e.g.
    transcobalamin II deficiency, nitrous oxide, antifolate drugs
Other defects of DNA synthesis
   congenital enzyme deficiencies, e.g. orotic aciduria
   acquired enzyme deficiencies, e.g. alcohol, therapy with
     hydroxyurea, cytosine arabinoside

Table 4.2 Vitamin B_{12} and folate: nutritional aspects

	Vitamin B_{12}	Folate
Normal daily dietary intake	7–30 µg	200–250 µg
Main foods	Animal produce only	Most, especially liver, greens and yeast
Cooking	Little effect	Easily destroyed
Minimal adult daily requirement	1–2 µg	100–150 µg
Body stores	2–3 mg (sufficient for 2–4 years)	10–12 mg (sufficient for 4 months)
Absorption		
Site	Ileum	Duodenum and jejunum
Mechanism	Intrinsic factor	Conversion to methyltetrahydrofolate
Limit	2–3 µg daily	50–80% of dietary content
Enterohepatic circulation	5–10 µg/day	90 µg/day
Transport in plasma	Most bound to TC I; TC II essential for cell uptake	Weakly bound to albumin
Major intracellular physiological forms	Methyl- and deoxyadenosylcobalamin	Reduced polyglutamate derivatives
Usual therapeutic form	Hydroxocobalamin	Folic (pteroylglutamic) acid

TC, transcobalamin.

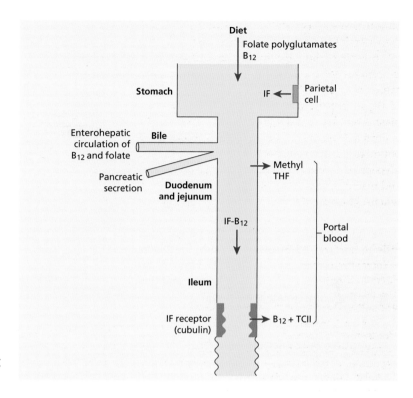

Fig. 4.2 The absorption of dietary vitamin B_{12} after combination with intrinsic factor (IF), through the ileum. Folate absorption occurs through the duodenum and jejunum after conversion of all dietary forms to methyltetrahydrofolate (methyl THF). TC II, transcobalamin II.

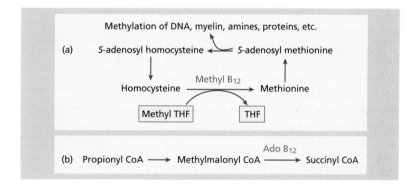

Fig. 4.3 The biochemical reactions of vitamin B_{12} in humans. Ado B_{12}, deoxyadenosylcobalamin; CoA, coenzyme A; THF, tetrahydrofolate.

creased, the TC I and B_{12} levels in serum both rise considerably. B_{12} bound to TC I does not transfer readily to marrow; it appears to be functionally 'dead'. Related glycoproteins are present in gastric juice, milk and other body fluids.

Biochemical function

Vitamin B_{12} is a coenzyme for two biochemical reactions in the body: first, as methyl B_{12} it is a cofactor for methionine synthase, the enzyme responsible for methylation of homocysteine to methionine using methyl tetrahydrofolate (THF) as methyl donor (Fig. 4.3a); and second, as deoxyadenosyl B_{12} (ado B_{12}) it assists in conversion of methylmalonyl coenzyme A (CoA) to succinyl CoA (Fig. 4.3b). Assay of homocysteine in plasma and of methylmalonic acid in urine or plasma may be used as tests for B_{12} deficiency.

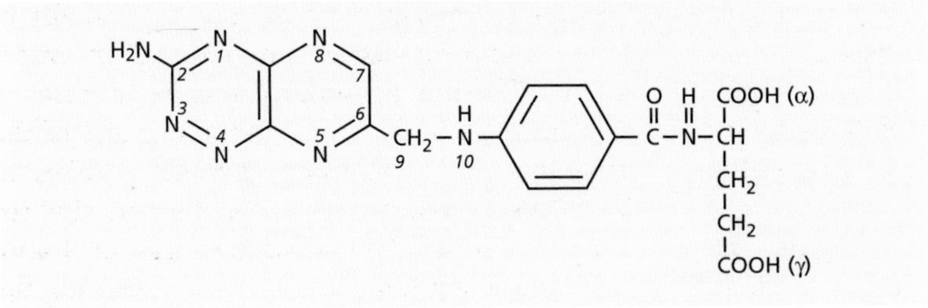

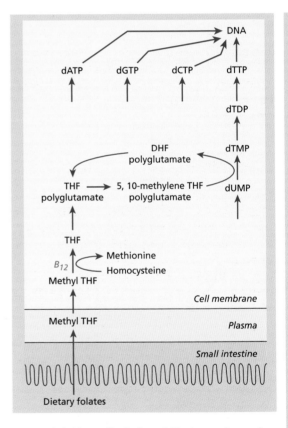

Fig. 4.4 The structure of folic (pteroyl-glutamic) acid. Dietary folates may contain: (a) additional hydrogen atoms at positions 7 and 8 (dihydrofolate) or 5, 6, 7 and 8 (tetrahydrofolate); (b) a formyl group at N_5 or N_{10}, a methyl group at N_5 or other 1-carbon groups; and (c) additional glutamate moiety attached to the γ-carboxyl group of the glutamate moiety.

FOLATE

Folic (pteroylglutamic) acid is the parent compound of a large group of compounds, the folates, which are derived from it (Fig. 4.4). Humans are unable to synthesize the folate structure and thus require preformed folate as a vitamin.

Absorption, transport and function

Dietary folates are converted to methyl THF (which, like folic acid, contains only one glutamate moiety) during absorption through the upper small intestine. Once inside the cell they are converted to folate polyglutamates (Fig. 4.5).

Folates are needed in a variety of biochemical reactions in the body involving single carbon unit transfer (Fig. 4.5) in amino acid interconversions, e.g. homocysteine conversion to methionine and serine to glycine or in synthesis of purine or pyrimidine precursors of DNA.

Biochemical basis for megaloblastic anaemia

DNA is formed by polymerization of the four deoxyribonucleoside triphosphates (Fig. 4.5). Folate deficiency is thought to cause megaloblastic anaemia by inhibiting thymidylate synthesis, a rate-limiting step in DNA synthesis in which thymidine monophosphate is synthesized. This reaction needs 5,10-methylene THF polyglutamate as coenzyme.

All body cells including those of the bone marrow receive folate from plasma as methyl THF.

Fig. 4.5 The biochemical basis of megaloblastic anaemia caused by vitamin B_{12} or folate deficiency. Folate is required in one of its coenzyme forms, 5,10-methylene tetrahydrofolate (THF) polyglutamate, in the synthesis of thymidine monophosphate from its precursor deoxyuridine monophosphate. Vitamin B_{12} is needed to convert methyl THF, which enters the cells from plasma, to THF, from which polyglutamate forms of folate are synthesized. Dietary folates are all converted to methyl THF (a monoglutamate) by the small intestine. A, adenine; C, cytosine; d, deoxyribose; DHF, dihydrofolate; DP, diphosphate; G, guanine; MP, monophosphate; T, thymine; TP, triphosphate; U, uracil.

B_{12}, by its involvement in the methylation of homocysteine to methionine, is needed in the conversion of this methyl THF to THF. THF (but not methyl THF) is a substrate for folate polyglutamate synthesis inside cells. The folate polyglutamates act as intracellular folate coenzymes, including 5,10-methylene THF polyglutamate, the coenzyme form of folate involved in the thymidylate synthase reaction (Fig. 4.5). Lack of B_{12}, therefore, prevents the demethylation of methyl THF thus depriving cells of THF and so of folate polyglutamate coenzymes.

Other congenital or acquired causes of megaloblastic anaemia (e.g. antimetabolite drug therapy) inhibit purine or pyrimidine synthesis at one or other step. The result is a reduced supply of one or other of the four precursors needed for DNA synthesis.

Folate reduction

During thymidylate synthesis, the folate polyglutamate coenzyme becomes oxidized from the THF state to dihydrofolate (DHF) (Fig. 4.5). Regeneration of active THF requires the enzyme DHF reductase. Inhibitors of this enzyme (e.g. methotrexate) therefore inhibit all folate coenzyme reactions, and so DNA synthesis. Methotrexate is a useful drug mainly in the treatment of malignant or inflammatory disease, e.g. of the skin, with excessive cell turnover. The weaker antagonist, pyrimethamine, is used primarily against malaria. Trimethoprim, active against bacterial DHF reductase but only very weakly against the human enzyme, is used in antibacterial combination with a sulphonamide, as co-trimoxazole. Toxicity caused by methotrexate or pyrimethamine is reversed by giving the patient the stable fully reduced folate, folinic acid (5-formyl THF).

VITAMIN B_{12} DEFICIENCY

In Western countries, the deficiency is usually caused by (Addisonian) pernicious anaemia (Table 4.3). Less commonly it may be caused by veganism in which the diet lacks B_{12} (usually in Hindu Indians), gastrectomy or small intestinal lesions. There is no syndrome of B_{12} deficiency as a result of increased utilization or loss of the vitamin, so the deficiency inevitably takes at least 2 years to develop, i.e. the time needed for body stores to deplete at the rate of $1–2\mu g$ each day when there is no new B_{12} entering the body from the diet. Nitrous oxide, however, may rapidly inactivate body B_{12} (p. 55).

Pernicious anaemia

This is caused by autoimmune attack on the gastric mucosa leading to atrophy of the stomach. The wall of the stomach becomes thin, with a plasma cell and lymphoid infiltrate of the lamina propria. Intestinal metaplasia may occur. There is achlorhydria and secretion of IF is absent or almost absent.

More females than males are affected (1.6:1) with a peak occurrence at 60 years, and there may be associated autoimmune disease (Table 4.4). The disease is found in all races but is most common

Table 4.3 Causes of vitamin B_{12} deficiency

Nutritional
Especially vegans

Malabsorption
Gastric causes
    Pernicious anaemia
    Congenital lack or abnormality of intrinsic factor
    Total or partial gastrectomy

Intestinal causes
    Intestinal stagnant loop syndrome—jejunal diverticulosis, blind-loop, stricture, etc.
    Chronic tropical sprue
    Ileal resection and Crohn's disease
    Congenital selective malabsorption with proteinuria (autosomal recessive megaloblastic anaemia)
    Fish tapeworm

NB. Other causes of malabsorption of vitamin B_{12}, e.g. severe pancreatitis, gluten-induced enteropathy, HIV infection, or therapy with metformin, do not usually lead to clinically important vitamin B_{12} deficiency.

Table 4.4 Pernicious anaemia: associations

Female	Vitiligo
Blue eyes	Myxoedema
Early greying	Hashimoto's disease
Northern European	Thyrotoxicosis
Familial	Addison's disease
Blood group A	Hypoparathyroidism
	Hypogammaglobulinaemia
	Carcinoma of the stomach

Table 4.5 Causes of folate deficiency

Nutritional
Especially old age, institutions, poverty, famine, special diets, goat's milk anaemia, etc.

Malabsorption
Tropical sprue, gluten-induced enteropathy (adult or child). Possible contributory factor to folate deficiency in some patients with partial gastrectomy, extensive jejunal resection or Crohn's disease

Excess utilization
Physiological
Pregnancy and lactation, prematurity
Pathological
Haematological diseases: haemolytic anaemias, myelofibrosis
Malignant disease: carcinoma, lymphoma, myeloma
Inflammatory diseases: Crohn's disease, tuberculosis, rheumatoid arthritis, psoriasis, exfoliative dermatitis, malaria

Excess urinary folate loss
Active liver disease, congestive heart failure

Drugs
Anticonvulsants, sulfasalazine

Mixed
Liver disease, alcoholism, intensive care

in northern Europeans and tends to occur in families. There is also an increased incidence of carcinoma of the stomach (about 2–3% of all cases of pernicious anaemia).

Antibodies

Ninety per cent of patients show parietal cell antibody directed against gastric H^+/K^+-ATPase in the serum, and 50% type I or blocking antibody to IF which inhibits IF binding to B_{12}. Thirty-five per cent show a second (type II or precipitating) antibody to IF which inhibits its ileal binding site. IF antibodies are virtually specific for pernicious anaemia but occur in the serum of only half the patients, whereas the more common parietal cell antibody is less specific and occurs quite commonly in older subjects (e.g. 16% of normal women over 60 years).

Congenital lack of IF usually presents at about 2 years of age when stores of B_{12} which were derived from the mother *in utero* have been used up. There is also a form of autoimmune pernicious anaemia which presents in childhood. Congenital lack of ileal receptors for IF may also present in infancy or childhood. Specific malabsorbtion of B_{12} is due to mutation of the IF-B_{12} receptor, cubilin, and usually presents at the same age.

FOLATE DEFICIENCY

This is most often a result of a poor dietary intake of folate alone or in combination with a condition of increased folate utilization or malabsorption (Table 4.5). Excess cell turnover of any sort, including pregnancy, is the main cause of an increased need for folate, since the folate molecule becomes degraded when DNA synthesis is increased. The mechanism by which anticonvulsants and barbiturates cause the deficiency is still controversial. Alcohol, sulfasalazine and other drugs may have multiple effects on folate metabolism.

CLINICAL FEATURES OF MEGALOBLASTIC ANAEMIA

The onset is usually insidious with gradually progressive symptoms and signs of anaemia (Chapter 2). The patient may be mildly jaundiced (lemon yellow tint) (Fig. 4.6) due to the excess breakdown of haemoglobin resulting from increased ineffective erythropoiesis in the bone marrow. Glossitis (a beefy-red, sore tongue) (Fig. 4.7), angular stomatitis (Fig. 4.8) and mild symptoms of malabsorption with loss of weight may be present caused by the epithelial abnormality. Purpura as a result of thrombocytopenia and widespread melanin pigmentation (the cause for which is unclear) are

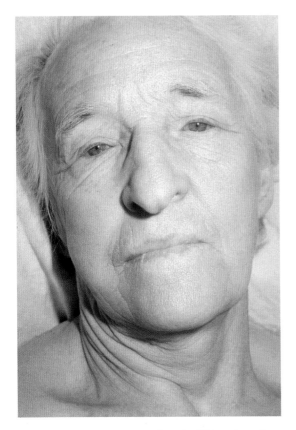

Fig. 4.6 Megaloblastic anaemia: pallor and mild icterus in a patient with a haemoglobin count of 7.0 g/dl and a mean corpuscular volume of 132 fl.

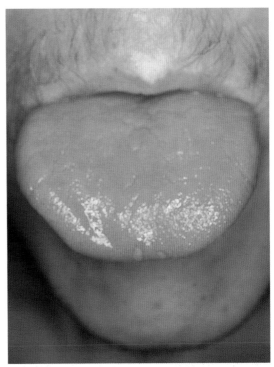

Fig. 4.7 Megaloblastic anaemia: glossitis — the tongue is beefy-red and painful.

less frequent presenting features (Table 4.6). Many asymptomatic patients are diagnosed when a blood count that has been performed for another reason reveals macrocytosis.

Vitamin B$_{12}$ neuropathy (subacute combined degeneration of the cord)

Severe B$_{12}$ deficiency may cause a progressive neuropathy affecting the peripheral sensory nerves, and posterior and lateral columns (Fig. 4.9). The neuropathy is symmetrical and affects the lower limbs more than the upper limbs. The patient notices tingling in the feet, difficulty in walking and may fall over in the dark. Rarely, optic atrophy or severe psychiatric symptoms are

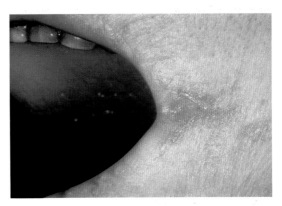

Fig. 4.8 Megaloblastic anaemia: angular cheilosis (stomatitis).

present. Anaemia may be severe, mild or even absent, but the blood film and bone marrow appearances are always abnormal. The cause of the neuropathy is likely to be related to the accumulation of S-adenosyl homocysteine and reduced levels of S-adenosyl methionine in nervous tissue

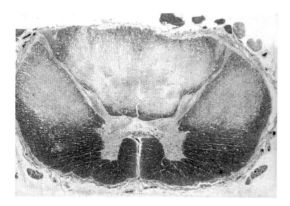

Fig. 4.9 Cross-section of the spinal cord in a patient who died with subacute combined degeneration of the cord (Weigert–Pal stain). There is demyelination of the dorsal and dorsolateral columns.

Table 4.6 Effects of vitamin B_{12} or folate deficiency

Megaloblastic anaemia
Macrocytosis of epithelial cell surfaces
Neuropathy (for vitamin B_{12} only)
Sterility
Rarely, reversible melanin skin pigmentation
Decreased osteoblast activity
Neural tube defects in the fetus are related to folate or B_{12} deficiency
Cardiovascular disease (see text and Chapter 21)

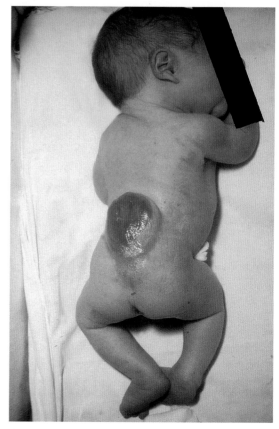

Fig. 4.10 A baby with neural tube defect (spina bifida) (courtesy of Professor C.J. Schorah).

resulting in defective methylation of myelin and other substrates. The evidence that folate deficiency in the adult can cause a neuropathy is conflicting although there are more substantial data suggesting it causes psychiatric changes.

Neural tube defect

Folate or B_{12} deficiency in the mother predisposes to neural tube defect (NTD) (anencephaly, spina bifida or encephalocoele) in the fetus (Fig. 4.10). The lower the maternal serum or red cell folate or serum B_{12} levels (even when these are in the normal range) the higher the incidence of NTDs. Moreover, supplementation of the diet with folic acid at the time of conception and in early pregnancy reduces the incidence of NTD by 75%. The exact mechanism is uncertain but is thought to be related to build-up of homocysteine and *S*-adenosyl homocysteine in the fetus which may impair methylation of various proteins and lipids. A common polymorphism in the enzyme 5,10-methylene tetrahydrofolate reductase (5,10-MTHFR) (677C → T) (see p. 278) results in higher serum homocysteine and lower serum and red cell folate levels compared to controls. The incidence of the mutation is higher in the parents and fetus with NTD than in controls.

Cardiovascular disease

Raised serum homocysteine levels are associated with an increased incidence of myocardial infarct, peripheral and cerebral vascular disease and venous thrombosis (Chapter 21). Raised serum homocysteine levels are associated with low serum and red cell folate and low serum B_{12} or vitamin B_6 levels. In addition homocysteine levels tend to be higher in men than in premenopausal women, in old age, in heavy smokers and those with excess alcohol consumption, with impaired renal function and with some drugs. Although folate deficiency (and in some studies, the presence of the polymorphism in the 5,10-MTHFR gene) has been associated with an increased incidence of cardiovascular disease, results of studies showing a reduction in the rate of myocardial infarction or stroke by the use of prophylactic folic acid have yet to be reported (see p. 279).

Other tissue abnormalities

Sterility is frequent in either sex with severe B_{12} or folate deficiency. Macrocytosis, excess apoptosis and other morphological abnormalities of cervical, buccal, bladder and other epithelia occurs. Widespread reversible melanin pigmentation may also occur. B_{12} deficiency is associated with reduced osteoblastic activity. Uncontrolled trials suggest folate deficiency may predispose to colon cancer.

Laboratory findings

The anaemia is macrocytic (MCV >95 fl and often as high as 120–140 fl in severe cases) and the macrocytes are typically oval in shape (Fig. 4.11). The reticulocyte count is low and the total white cell and platelet counts may be moderately re-duced, especially in severely anaemic patients. A proportion of the neutrophils show hyperseg-mented nuclei (with six or more lobes). The bone marrow is usually hypercellular and the erythro-blasts are large and show failure of nuclear maturation maintaining an open, fine, primitive chromatin pattern but normal haemoglobiniza-tion (Fig. 4.12). Giant and abnormally shaped metamyelocytes are characteristic.

The serum unconjugated bilirubin, hydroxybu-tyrate and lactate dehydrogenase (LDH) are all raised as a result of marrow cell breakdown.

DIAGNOSIS OF VITAMIN B_{12} OR FOLATE DEFICIENCY

It is usual to assay serum B_{12}, serum and red cell folate (Table 4.7). The serum B_{12} is low in megalo-blastic anaemia or neuropathy caused by B_{12}

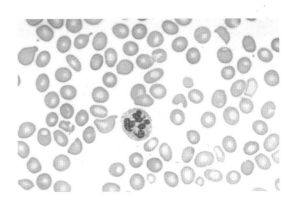

Fig. 4.11 Megaloblastic anaemia: peripheral blood film showing oval macrocytes and hypersegmented neutrophil.

Table 4.7 Laboratory tests for vitamin B_{12} and folate deficiency

Test	Normal value*		Result in	
			Vitamin B_{12} deficiency	Folate deficiency
Serum vitamin B_{12}	160–925 ng/l	120–680 pmol/l	Low	Normal or borderline
Serum folate	3.0–15.0 µg/l	4–30 nmol/l	Normal or raised	Low
Red cell folate	160–640 µg/l	360–1460 nmol/l	Normal or low	Low

* Normal values differ slightly with different commercial kits.

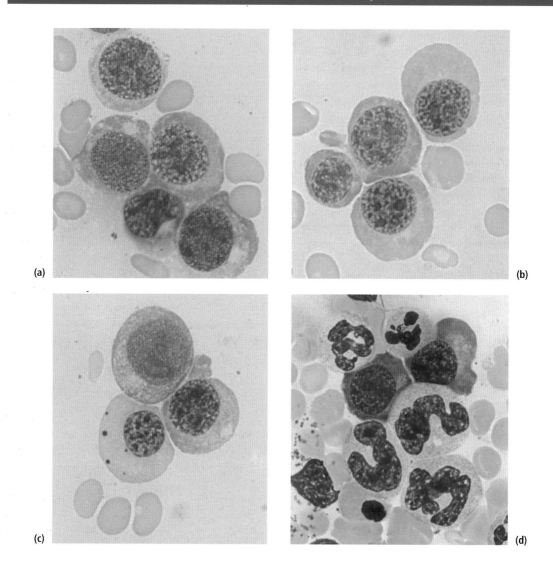

Fig. 4.12 Megaloblastic changes in the bone marrow in a patient with severe megaloblastic anaemia. (a–c) Erythroblasts showing fine, open stippled (primitive) appearance of the nuclear chromatin even in late cells (pale cytoplasm with some haemoglobin formation). (d) Abnormal giant metamyelocytes and band forms.

deficiency. The serum and red cell folate are both low in megaloblastic anaemia caused by folate deficiency. In B_{12} deficiency the serum folate tends to rise but the red cell folate falls. In the absence of B_{12} deficiency, however, the red cell folate is a more accurate guide than the serum folate of tissue folate status.

The deoxyuridine (dU) suppression test may be used to diagnose megaloblastic anaemia. It assesses the integrity of the thymidylate synthase reaction. It measures the degree to which unlabelled dU suppresses uptake of radioactive thymidine into the DNA of bone marrow cells *in vitro*. The test is abnormal (less suppression of thymidine uptake by dU) in megaloblastic anaemia caused by B_{12} or folate deficiency. It can be corrected in B_{12} deficiency by B_{12} but not by methyl THF; in folate deficiency by methyl THF but not by B_{12}.

Tests for cause of vitamin B$_{12}$ or folate deficiency

For B$_{12}$ deficiency, absorption tests (Table 4.8) using an oral dose of radioactive cobalt (^{57}Co)-labelled cyanocobalamin are valuable in distinguishing malabsorption from an inadequate diet. When the test is repeated with an active IF preparation gastric lesions such as those associated with pernicious anaemia can be distinguished from intestinal lesions (Table 4.9). Absorption is most frequently measured indirectly by the urinary excretion (Schilling) technique in which absorbed radio-labelled B$_{12}$ is 'flushed' into a 24-h urine sample by a large (1 mg) dose of non-radioactive B$_{12}$ given simultaneously with the labelled oral dose. The 'DICOPAC' test uses two isotopes of B$_{12}$, Co^{57} and Co^{58}, simultaneously; one attached to IF.

Other useful tests are listed in Table 4.8. These are mainly concerned with assessing gastric function and testing for antibodies to gastric antigens. In all cases of pernicious anaemia, endoscopy studies should be performed to confirm the presence of gastric atrophy and exclude carcinoma of the stomach.

For folate deficiency, the dietary history is most important, although it is difficult to estimate folate intake accurately. Unsuspected gluten-induced enteropathy or other underlying conditions should also be considered (Table 4.5).

Treatment

Most cases only need therapy with the appropriate vitamin (Table 4.10). If large doses of folic acid (e.g. 5 mg daily) are given in B$_{12}$ deficiency they cause a haematological response but may aggravate the neuropathy. They should therefore not be given alone unless B$_{12}$ deficiency has been excluded. In severely anaemic patients who need treatment urgently it may be safer to initiate treatment with both vitamins after blood has been taken for B$_{12}$ and folate examinations and a bone marrow test has been performed. In the elderly, the presence of heart failure should be corrected with diuretics and oral potassium supplements given for 10 days (because hypokalaemia has been found to occur during the response in some cases). Blood transfusion should be avoided if possible as it may cause circulatory overload.

Response to therapy

The patient feels better after 24–48 h of correct vitamin therapy with increased appetite and well-being. A reticulocyte response begins on the second or third day with a peak at 6–7 days — its height is inversely proportional to the initial red cell count (Fig. 4.13). The haemoglobin should rise by 2–3 g/dl each fortnight. The white cell and platelet counts become normal in 7–10 days

Table 4.8 Tests for cause of vitamin B$_{12}$ or folate deficiency

Vitamin B$_{12}$	Folate
Diet history	Diet history
B$_{12}$ absorption ±IF	Tests for intestinal malabsorption
IF, parietal cell antibodies	Anti-gliadin and endomysial
Endoscopy or barium meal	antibodies
and follow through	Duodenal biopsy
Gastric function (acid, IF)	Underlying disease

IF, intrinsic factor.

Table 4.9 Results of absorption tests of radioactive vitamin B$_{12}$

	Dose of labelled B$_{12}$ given alone	Dose of labelled B$_{12}$ given with IF
Vegan	Normal	Normal
Pernicious anaemia or gastrectomy	Low	Normal
Ileal lesion	Low	Low
Intestinal blind-loop syndrome	Low*	Low*

* Corrected by antibiotic therapy.
IF, intrinsic factor.

Table 4.10 Treatment of megaloblastic anaemia

	Vitamin B$_{12}$ deficiency	Folate deficiency
Compound	Hydroxocobalamin	Folic acid
Route	Intramuscular*	Oral
Dose	1000 µg	5 mg
Initial dose	6 × 1000 µg over 2–3 weeks	Daily for 4 months
Maintenance	1000 µg every 3 months	Depends on underlying disease; life-long therapy may be needed in chronic inherited haemolytic anaemias, myelofibrosis, renal dialysis
Prophylactic	Total gastrectomy Ileal resection	Pregnancy, severe haemolytic anaemias, dialysis, prematurity

* Some authors have recommended daily oral or sublingual therapy of vitamin B$_{12}$ deficiency.

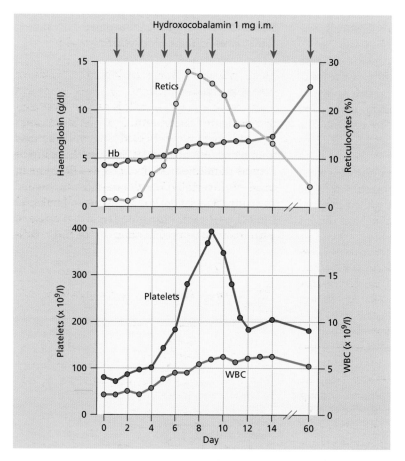

Fig. 4.13 Typical haematological response to vitamin B$_{12}$ (hydroxocobalamin) therapy in pernicious anaemia. Hb, haemoglobin; Retics, reticulocytes; WBC, white blood cells.

and the marrow is normoblastic in about 48 h, although giant metamyelocytes persist for up to 12 days.

The peripheral neuropathy may partly improve but spinal cord damage is irreversible.

Prophylactic therapy

Vitamin B_{12} is given to patients who have total gastrectomy or ileal resection. Folic acid is given in pregnancy at a recommended dose of 400 μg daily and all women of child-bearing age are recommended to have an intake of at least 400 μg daily (by increased intake of folate-rich or folate-supplemented foods or as folic acid) to prevent a first occurrence of an NTD in the fetus. Folic acid is also given to patients undergoing chronic dialysis and with severe haemolytic anaemias and chronic myelofibrosis, and to premature babies. Food fortification with folic acid, e.g. in flour, is currently being considered in Britain to reduce the incidence of NTDs and potentially of cardiovascular disease and is already practised in the USA.

OTHER MEGALOBLASTIC ANAEMIAS

See Table 4.1.

Abnormalities of vitamin B_{12} or folate metabolism

These include congenital deficiencies of enzymes concerned in B_{12} or folate metabolism or of the serum transport protein for B_{12}, TC II. Nitrous oxide (N_2O) anaesthesia causes rapid inactivation of body B_{12} by oxidizing the reduced cobalt atom of methyl B_{12}. Megaloblastic marrow changes occur with several days of N_2O administration and can cause pancytopenia. Chronic exposure (as in dentists and anaesthetists) has been associated with neurological damage resembling B_{12}-deficiency neuropathy. Antifolate drugs, particularly those which inhibit DHF reductase (e.g. methotrexate and pyrimethamine) may also cause megaloblastic change. Trimethoprim, which inhibits bacterial DHF reductase, has only a slight action against the human enzyme and causes

megaloblastic change only in patients already B_{12} or folate deficient.

Defects of DNA synthesis not related to vitamin B_{12} or folate

Congenital deficiency of one or other enzyme concerned in purine or pyrimidine synthesis may cause megaloblastic anaemia identical in appearance to that caused by a deficiency of B_{12} or folate. The best known is orotic aciduria. Therapy with drugs which inhibit purine or pyrimidine synthesis (such as hydroxyurea, cytosine arabinoside, 6-mercaptopurine and zidovudine (AZT)) and some forms of acute myeloid leukaemia or myelodysplasia also cause megaloblastic anaemia.

OTHER MACROCYTIC ANAEMIAS

There are many non-megaloblastic causes of macrocytic anaemia (Table 4.11). The exact mechanisms creating large red cells in each of these conditions is not clear although increased lipid deposition on the red cell membrane or alterations of erythroblast maturation time in the marrow may be implicated. Alcohol is the most frequent cause of a raised MCV in the absence of anaemia. Reticulocytes are bigger than mature red cells and so haemolytic anaemia is an important cause of macrocytic anaemia. The other underlying condi-

Table 4.11 Causes of macrocytosis other than megaloblastic anaemia

Alcohol
Liver disease
Myxoedema
Myelodysplastic syndromes
Cytotoxic drugs
Aplastic anaemia
Pregnancy
Smoking
Reticulocytosis
Myeloma
Neonatal

tions listed in Table 4.11 are usually easily diagnosed provided that they are considered and the appropriate investigations to exclude B_{12} or folate deficiency are carried out.

Differential diagnosis of macrocytic anaemias

The clinical history and physical examination may suggest B_{12} or folate deficiency as the cause. Diet, drugs, alcohol intake, family history, history suggestive of malabsorption, presence of autoimmune diseases or other associations with pernicious anaemia (Table 4.4), previous gastrointestinal disease or operations, are all important. The presence of jaundice, glossitis or a neuropathy are also valuable indications of megaloblastic anaemia.

The laboratory features of particular importance are the shape of macrocytes (oval in megaloblastic anaemia), the presence of hypersegmented neutrophils and of leucopenia and thrombocytopenia in megaloblastic anaemia and the bone marrow appearance. Assay of B_{12} and folate is straightforward. Exclusion of alcoholism (particularly if the patient is not anaemic), liver and thyroid function tests and bone marrow examination for myelodysplasia, aplasia or myeloma are important in the investigation of macrocytosis not caused by B_{12} or folate deficiency.

BIBLIOGRAPHY

Bailey L.B. (ed.) (1995) *Folate in Health and Disease*. Marcel Dekker, New York.

Chanarin I. (1969, 1979, 1990) *The Megaloblastic Anaemias*, 1st, 2nd, 3rd edns. Blackwell Scientific Publications, Oxford.

Green R. and Miller J.W. (1999) Folate deficiency beyond megaloblastic anemia: hyperhomocysteinemia and other manifestations of dysfunctional folate status. *Semin. Hematol.* **36**, 47–64.

Rosenblatt D.S. and Hoffbrand A.V. (1999) Megaloblastic anaemia and disorders of cobalamin and folate metabolism. In: *Pediatric Hematology* (eds J. Lilleyman, I. Hann, V. Blanchette). Churchill Livingstone, London, pp. 167–84.

Rothenberg S.P. (1999) Increasing the dietary intake of folate: pros and cons. *Semin. Hematol.* **36**, 65–74.

Toh B.-H., van Driel I.R. and Gleeson P.A. (1997) Pernicious anemia. *N. Engl. J. Med.* **337**, 1441–8.

Wickramasinghe S.N. (ed.) (1995) Megaloblastic anaemia. *Clin. Haematol.* **8**, 441–703.

Wickramasinghe S.N. (1999) The wide spectrum and unresolved issues of megaloblastic anemia. *Semin. Hematol.* **36**, 3–18.

Zittoun J. and Zittoun R. (1999) Modern clinical testing strategies in cobalamin and folate deficiency. *Semin. Hematol.* **36**, 35–46.

Haemolytic anaemias

NORMAL RED CELL DESTRUCTION

Red cell destruction usually occurs after a mean lifespan of 120 days when the cells are removed extravascularly by the macrophages of the reticuloendothelial (RE) system, especially in the marrow but also in the liver and spleen. As the cells have no nucleus, red cell metabolism gradually deteriorates as enzymes are degraded and not replaced and the cells become non-viable. The breakdown of haem from red cells liberates iron for recirculation via plasma transferrin to marrow erythroblasts, and protoporphyrin which is broken down to bilirubin. This circulates to the liver where it is conjugated to glucuronides which are excreted into the gut via bile and converted to stercobilinogen and stercobilin (excreted in faeces) (Fig. 5.1). Stercobilinogen and stercobilin are partly reabsorbed and excreted in urine as urobilinogen and urobilin. Globin chains are broken down to amino acids which are reutilized for general protein synthesis in the body. Haptoglobins are proteins present in normal plasma capable of binding haemoglobin. The haemoglobin–haptoglobin complex is removed from plasma by the RE system. Intravascular haemolysis (breakdown of red cells within blood vessels) plays little or no part in normal red cell destruction.

INTRODUCTION TO HAEMOLYTIC ANAEMIAS

Haemolytic anaemias are defined as those anaemias which result from an increase in the rate of red cell destruction. Because of erythropoietic hyperplasia and anatomical extension of bone marrow, red cell destruction may be increased several-fold before the patient becomes anaemic—compensated haemolytic disease. The normal adult marrow, after full expansion, is able to produce red cells at six to eight times the normal rate providing this is 'effective'. It leads to a marked reticulocytosis, particularly in the more anaemic cases. Therefore haemolytic anaemia may not be seen until the red cell lifespan is less than 30 days. Sometimes ^{51}Cr-labelled red cell survival studies are useful to confirm haemolysis and to determine sites of destruction by surface counting over different organs (Fig. 5.2).

Classification

Table 5.1 is a simplified classification of the haemolytic anaemias. Hereditary haemolytic anaemias are the result of 'intrinsic' red cell defects whereas acquired haemolytic anaemias are usually the result of an 'extracorpuscular' or 'environmental' change. Paroxysmal nocturnal haemoglobinuria (PNH) is the exception because although it is an acquired disorder the PNH red cells have an intrinsic defect.

Clinical features

The patient may show pallor of the mucous membranes, mild fluctuating jaundice and splenomegaly. There is no bilirubin in urine but this may turn dark on standing because of excess urobilinogen. Pigment (bilirubin) gallstones may complicate the condition (Fig. 5.3) and some patients (particularly with sickle cell disease) develop ulcers around the ankle. Aplastic crises may occur, usually precipitated by infection with

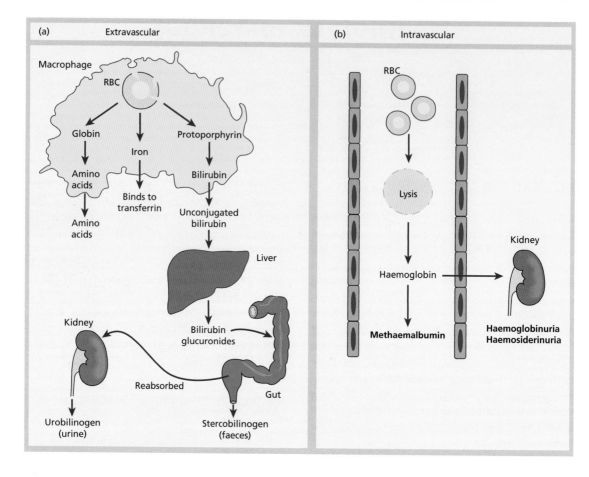

Fig. 5.1 (a) Normal red blood cell (RBC) breakdown. This takes place extravascularly in the macrophages of the reticuloendothelial system. (b) Intravascular haemolysis occurs in some pathological disorders.

parvovirus which 'switches off' erythropoiesis, and are characterized by a sudden increase in anaemia and drop in reticulocyte count (see Fig. 7.4).

Rarely folate deficiency may cause an aplastic crisis in which the bone marrow is megaloblastic.

Laboratory findings

The laboratory findings are conveniently divided into three groups.

1 Features of increased red cell breakdown:
(a) serum bilirubin raised, unconjugated and bound to albumin;
(b) urine urinobilinogen increased;
(c) faecal stercobilinogen increased;
(d) serum haptoglobins absent because the haptoglobins become saturated with haemoglobin and the complex is removed by RE cells.

2 Features of increased red cell production:
(a) reticulocytosis;
(b) bone marrow erythroid hyperplasia; the normal marrow myeloid : erythoid ratio of 2 : 1 to 12 : 1 is reduced to 1 : 1 or reversed.

3 Damaged red cells:
(a) morphology—microspherocytes, elliptocytes, fragments, etc.;
(b) osmotic fragility, autohaemolysis, etc.;
(c) red cell survival shortened; this is best shown by ^{51}Cr labelling with study of the sites of destruction (Fig. 5.2).

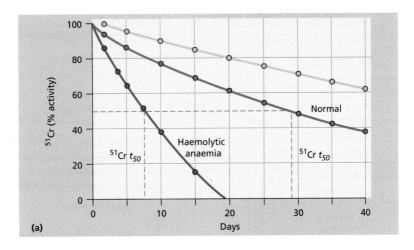

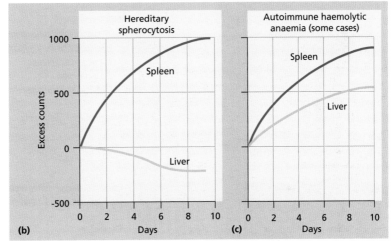

Fig. 5.2 (a) ^{51}Cr red cell survival studies. The ^{51}Cr t_{50} (half-life) in normal subjects is 30 ± 2 days. When data are corrected for elution of ^{51}Cr from red cells (yellow line), the mean cell life is 50 ± 5 days. In haemolytic anaemia, the ^{51}Cr t_{50} is usually less than 15 days. (b) Surface counting pattern in haemolytic anaemia during ^{51}Cr red cell survival studies showing dominant splenic destruction in hereditary spherocytosis and a combination of splenic and hepatic destruction in autoimmune haemolytic anaemia (some types).

INTRAVASCULAR AND EXTRAVASCULAR HAEMOLYSIS

There are two main mechanisms whereby red cells are destroyed in haemolytic anaemia. There may be excessive removal of red cells by cells of the RE system (extravascular haemolysis) or they may be broken down directly in the circulation in a process known as intravascular haemolysis (Fig. 5.1, Table 5.2). Whichever mechanism dominates will depend on the pathology involved. In intravascular haemolysis free haemoglobin is released which rapidly saturates plasma haptoglobins and the excess free haemoglobin is filtered by the glomerulus. If the rate of haemolysis saturates the renal tubular reabsorptive capacity, free haemoglobin enters urine (Fig. 5.4) and, as iron is released, the renal tubules become loaded with haemosiderin. Methaemalbumin and haemopexin are also formed from the process of intravascular haemolysis.

The main laboratory features of intravascular haemolysis are as follows.
1 Haemoglobinaemia and haemoglobinuria.
2 Haemosiderinuria (iron storage protein in the spun deposit of urine).
3 Methaemalbuminaemia (detected spectrophotometrically by Schumm's test).

Table 5.1 Classification of haemolytic anaemias

Hereditary	Acquired
Membrane Hereditary spherocytosis, hereditary elliptocytosis	**Immune** *Autoimmune* Warm antibody type Cold antibody type } see Table 5.5
Metabolism G6PD deficiency, pyruvate kinase deficiency	*Alloimmune* Haemolytic transfusion reactions Haemolytic disease of the newborn Allografts, especially marrow transplantation
Haemoglobin Abnormal (Hb S, Hb C, unstable); see Chapter 6	*Drug associated*
	Red cell fragmentation syndromes *Arterial grafts, cardiac valves*
	Microangiopathic Thrombotic thrombocytopenic purpura Haemolytic uraemic syndrome Meningococcal sepsis Pre-eclampsia Disseminated intravascular coagulation
	March haemoglobinuria
	Infections Malaria, clostridia
	Chemical and physical agents Especially drugs, industrial/domestic substances, burns
	Secondary Liver and renal disease
	Paroxysmal nocturnal haemoglobinuria

G6PD, glucose-6-phosphate dehydrogenase; Hb, haemoglobin.

Table 5.2 Causes of intravascular haemolysis

Mismatched blood transfusion (usually ABO)
G6PD deficiency with oxidant stress
Red cell fragmentation syndromes
Some autoimmune haemolytic anaemias
Some drug- and infection-induced haemolytic anaemias
Paroxysmal nocturnal haemoglobinuria
March haemoglobinuria
Unstable haemoglobin

G6PD, glucose-6-phosphate dehydrogenase.

HEREDITARY HAEMOLYTIC ANAEMIAS

Membrane defects

Hereditary spherocytosis

Hereditary spherocytosis (HS) is the most common hereditary haemolytic anaemia in North Europeans.

Pathogenesis

HS is usually caused by defects in the proteins

involved in the vertical interactions between the membrane skeleton and the lipid bilayer of the red cell (Table 5.3) (see Fig. 2.12). The loss of membrane may be caused by the release of parts of

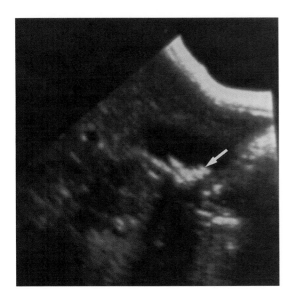

Fig. 5.3 Ultrasound of pigment gallstones (arrowed) in a 16-year-old male patient with hereditary spherocytosis. (Courtesy of L. Berger.)

Table 5.3 Molecular basis of hereditary spherocytosis and elliptocytosis

Hereditary spherocytosis
Ankyrin deficiency or abnormalities
Spectrin deficiency or abnormalities
Pallidin (protein 4.2) abnormalities

Hereditary elliptocytosis
α- or β-spectrin mutants leading to defective spectrin dimer formation
α- or β-spectrin mutants leading to defective spectrin–ankyrin associations
Protein 4.1 deficiency or abnormality
Band 3 abnormality
South-East Asian ovalocytosis band 3 deletion

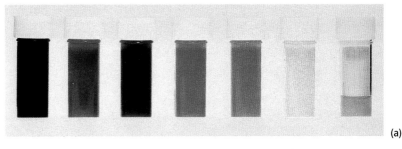

(a)

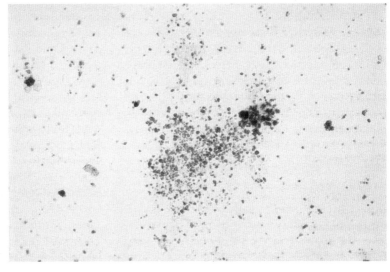

(b)

Fig. 5.4 (a) Progressive urine samples in an acute episode of intravascular haemolysis showing haemoglobinuria of decreasing severity. (b) Prussian blue-positive deposits of haemosiderin in a urine spun deposit (Perls' stain).

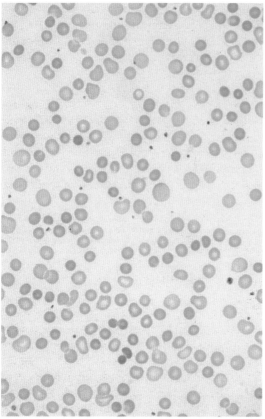

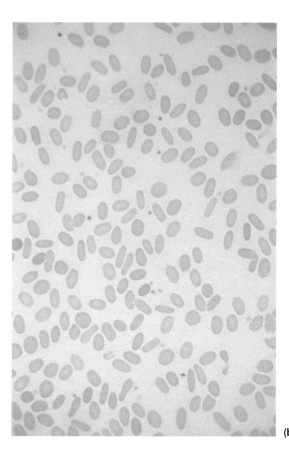

(a)   (b)

Fig. 5.5 (a) Blood film in hereditary spherocytosis. The spherocytes are deeply staining and of small diameter. Larger polychromatic cells are reticulocytes (confirmed by supravital staining). (b) Blood film in hereditary elliptocytosis.

the lipid bilayer that are not supported by the skeleton. The marrow produces red cells of normal biconcave shape but these lose membrane and become more and more spherical (loss of surface area relative to volume) as they circulate through the spleen and the rest of the RE system. Ultimately the spherocytes are unable to pass through the splenic microcirculation where they die prematurely.

Clinical features
The inheritance is autosomal dominant with variable expression. Rarely it may be autosomal recessive. The anaemia may present at any age from infancy to old age. Jaundice is typically fluctuat-

ing and is particularly marked if the haemolytic anaemia is associated with Gilbert's disease (a defect of hepatic conjugation of bilirubin); splenomegaly occurs in most patients. Pigment gallstones are frequent (Fig. 5.3); aplastic crises, usually precipitated by parvovirus infection, may cause a sudden increase in severity of anaemia (see Fig. 7.4).

Haematological findings
Anaemia is usual but not invariable; its severity tends to be similar in members of the same family. Reticulocytes are usually 5–20%. The blood film shows microspherocytes (Fig. 5.5a) which are densely staining with smaller diameters than normal red cells.

Investigation and treatment
The classic finding is that the osmotic fragility is increased (Fig. 5.6). The abnormality may require

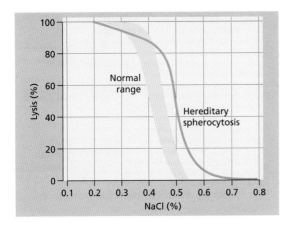

Fig. 5.6 The osmotic fragility in hereditary spherocytosis. The curve is shifted to the right of the normal range (in yellow), but a tail of more resistant cells (reticulocytes) is also present.

24-h incubation at 37°C to become obvious. Autohaemolysis is increased and corrected by glucose. The cells are incubated with their own plasma for 48 h with or without glucose. The direct antiglobulin (Coombs') test is normal, excluding an autoimmune cause of spherocytosis and haemolysis. [51]Cr studies may be used to document the dominant splenic destruction (Fig. 5.2).

The principal form of treatment is splenectomy although this should not be performed unless clinically indicated because of anaemia or gallstones because of the risk of post-splenectomy sepsis, particularly in early childhood (see p. 304). Splenectomy should always produce a rise in the haemoglobin level to normal, even though microspherocytes formed in the rest of the RE system will remain. Folic acid is given in severe cases to prevent folate deficiency.

Hereditary elliptocytosis

This has similar clinical and laboratory features to hereditary spherocytosis except for the appearance of the blood film (Fig. 5.5b), but it is usually a clinically milder disorder. Occasional patients require splenectomy. The basic defect is a failure of spectrin heterodimers to self-associate into heterotetramers. A number of genetic mutations affecting horizontal interactions have been detected (Table 5.3). Homozygous or doubly hetero-

zygous elliptocytosis presents with a severe haemolytic anaemia with microspherocytes, poikilocytes and splenomegaly (hereditary pyropoikilocytosis).

South-East Asian ovalocytosis

This is common in Melanesia, Malaysia, Indonesia and the Philippines and is caused by a nine amino acid deletion at the junction of the cytoplasmic and transmembrane domains of the band 3 protein. The cells are rigid and resist invasion by malarial parasites. Most cases are asymptomatic.

Defective red cell metabolism

Glucose-6-phosphate dehydrogenase deficiency

Glucose-6-phosphate dehydrogenase (G6PD) functions to reduce nicotinamide adenine dinucleotide phosphate (NADPH) while oxidizing glucose-6-phosphate. It is the only source of NADPH in red cells and as NADPH is needed for the production of reduced glutathione a deficiency renders the red cell susceptible to oxidant stress (Fig. 5.7). There are a wide variety of normal genetic variants of the enzyme G6PD, the most common being type B (Western) and type A in Africans. In addition, more than 400 variants due to point mutations or deletions of the enzyme G6PD have been characterized which show less activity than normal and worldwide over 400 million people are G6PD deficient in enzyme activity. Nevertheless, G6PD deficiency is usually asymptomatic. Although G6PD is present in all cells the main syndromes which occur are acute haemolytic anaemia in response to oxidant stress: drugs, fava beans or infections (Table 5.4). Neonatal jaundice and, rarely, a congenital non-spherocytic haemolytic anaemia may result from different types of enzyme deficiency.

The inheritance is sex-linked, affecting males, and carried by females who show approximately half normal red cell G6PD values. The female heterozygotes have an advantage of resistance to *Falciparum* malaria. The main races affected are in West Africa, the Mediterranean, the Middle East and South-East Asia. The degree of deficiency

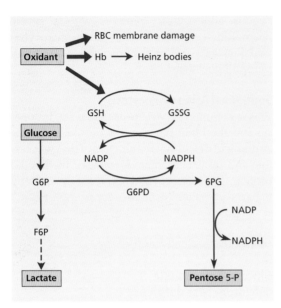

Fig. 5.7 Haemoglobin and red blood cell (RBC) membranes are usually protected from oxidant stress by reduced glutathione (GSH). In G6PD deficiency, NADPH and GSH synthesis is impaired. F6P, fructose-6-phosphate; G6P, glucose-6-phosphate; G6PD, glucose-6-phosphate dehydrogenase; GSSG, glutathione (oxidized form); NADP, NADPH, nicotinamide adenine dinucleotide phosphate.

Table 5.4 Agents which may cause haemolytic anaemia in glucose-6-phosphate dehydrogenase (G6PD) deficiency

Infections and other acute illnesses, e.g. diabetic ketoacidosis

Drugs
  Antimalarials, e.g. primaquine, pamaquine, chloroquine, Fansidar, Maloprim
  Sulphonamides and sulphones, e.g. co-trimoxazole, sulphanilamide, dapsone, salazopyrin
  Other antibacterial agents, e.g. nitrofurans, chloramphenicol
  Analgesics, e.g. aspirin (moderate doses are safe), phenacetin
  Antihelminths, e.g. β-naphthol, stibophen, nitrodazole
  Miscellaneous, e.g. vitamin K analogues, naphthalene (moth balls), probenecid

Fava beans (possibly other vegetables)

NB. Many common drugs have been reported to precipitate haemolysis in G6PD deficiency in some patients, e.g. aspirin, quinine and penicillin, but not at conventional dosage.

varies, often being mild (10–15% of normal activity) in black Africans, more severe in Orientals and most severe in Mediterraneans. Severe deficiency occurs occasionally in white people.

Clinical features

These are of rapidly developing intravascular haemolysis with haemoglobinuria, precipitated by infection and other acute illness, drugs or the ingestion of fava beans (Table 5.4). The anaemia may be self-limiting as new young red cells are made with near normal enzyme levels. Other clinical features of G6PD deficiency include neonatal jaundice and, rarely, a continuous congenital haemolytic anaemia.

Diagnosis

Between crises the blood count is normal. The enzyme deficiency is detected by one of a number of screening tests or by direct enzyme assay on red cells. During a crisis, the blood film may show

contracted and fragmented cells, 'bite' cells and 'blister' cells (Fig. 5.8) which have had Heinz bodies removed by the spleen. Heinz bodies (oxidized, denatured haemoglobin) may be seen in the reticulocyte preparation, particularly if the spleen is absent. There are also features of intravascular haemolysis. Because of the higher enzyme level in young red cells, red cell enzyme assay may give a 'false' normal level in the phase of acute haemolysis with a reticulocyte response. Subsequent assay after the acute phase reveals the low G6PD level when the red cell population is of normal age distribution.

Treatment

The offending drug is stopped, any underlying infection is treated, a high urine output is maintained and blood transfusion undertaken where necessary for severe anaemia. G6PD-deficient babies are prone to neonatal jaundice and in severe cases phototherapy and exchange transfusion may be needed. The jaundice is usually not caused by excess haemolysis but by deficiency of G6PD affecting neonatal liver function.

Glutathione deficiency and other syndromes

Other defects in the pentose phosphate pathway leading to similar syndromes to G6PD deficiency

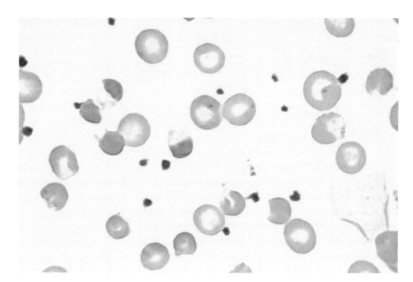

Fig. 5.8 Blood film in G6PD deficiency with acute haemolysis after an oxidant stress. Some of the cells show loss of cytoplasm with separation of remaining haemoglobin from the cell membrane ('blister' cells). There are also numerous contracted and deeply staining cells. Supravital staining (as for reticulocytes) showed the presence of Heinz bodies (see Fig. 2.16).

have been described—particularly glutathione deficiency.

Glycolytic (Embden–Meyerhof) pathway defects

These are all uncommon and lead to a congenital non-spherocytic haemolytic anaemia. The most frequently encountered is pyruvate kinase (PK) deficiency.

Pyruvate kinase deficiency

This is inherited as an autosomal recessive, the affected patients being homozygous or doubly heterozygous. The red cells become rigid as a result of reduced adenosine triphosphate (ATP) formation. The severity of the anaemia varies widely (haemoglobin 4–10 g/dl) and causes relatively mild symptoms because of a shift to the right in the oxygen (O_2) dissociation curve caused by a rise in intracellular 2,3-diphosphoglycerate (2,3-DPG). Clinically jaundice is usual and gallstones frequent. Frontal bossing may be present. The blood film shows poikilocytosis and distorted 'prickle' cells, particularly post-splenectomy. Laboratory tests show that autohaemolysis is increased but, in contrast to HS, it is not corrected by glucose; direct enzyme assay is needed to make the diagnosis. Splenectomy may alleviate the anaemia but does not cure it and is

indicated in those patients who need frequent transfusions.

Hereditary disorders of haemoglobin synthesis

Several of these cause clinical haemolysis. They are discussed in Chapter 6.

ACQUIRED HAEMOLYTIC ANAEMIAS

Immune haemolytic anaemias

Autoimmune haemolytic anaemias

Autoimmune haemolytic anaemias (AIHAs) are caused by antibody production by the body against its own red cells. They are characterized by a positive direct antiglobulin test (DAT) also known as the Coombs' test (see Fig. 23.4) and divided into 'warm' and 'cold' types (Table 5.5) according to whether the antibody reacts more strongly with red cells at 37°C or 4°C.

Warm autoimmune haemolytic anaemias

The red cells are usually coated with immunoglobulin (Ig), usually immunoglobulin G

Table 5.5 Autoimmune haemolytic anaemias: classification

Warm type	Cold type
Idiopathic	*Idiopathic*
Secondary	*Secondary*
SLE, other 'autoimmune' diseases	Infections — *Mycoplasma*
CLL, lymphomas	pneumonia, infectious
Drugs, e.g. methyldopa, fludarabine	mononucleosis
	Lymphoma
	Paroxysmal cold
	* haemoglobinuria*
	Rare, sometimes associated
	with infections, e.g. syphilis

CLL, chronic lymphocytic leukaemia; SLE, systemic lupus erythematosus.

(IgG) alone or with complement, and are therefore taken up by RE macrophages which have receptors for the Ig Fc fragment. Part of the coated membrane is lost so the cell becomes progressively more spherical to maintain the same volume and is ultimately prematurely destroyed, predominantly in the spleen. When the cells are coated with IgG and complement (C3d, the degraded fragment of C3) or complement alone, red cell destruction occurs more generally in the RE system.

Clinical features
The disease may occur at any age in either sex and presents as a haemolytic anaemia of varying severity. The spleen is often enlarged. The disease tends to remit and relapse. It may occur alone or in association with other diseases or arise in some patients as a result of methyldopa therapy (Table 5.5). When associated with idiopathic thrombocytopenic purpura (ITP), which is a similar condition affecting platelets (see p. 253), it is known as Evans' syndrome. When secondary to systemic lupus erythematosus, the cells typically are coated with immunoglobulin and complement.

Laboratory findings
The haematological and biochemical findings are typical of an extravascular haemolytic anaemia with spherocytosis prominent in the peripheral blood (Fig. 5.9a). The DAT is positive as a result of

IgG, IgG and complement or IgA on the cells and, in some cases, the autoantibody shows specificity within the rhesus system. The antibodies both on the cell surface and free in serum are best detected at 37°C.

Treatment
1 Remove the underlying cause (e.g. methyldopa, fludarabine).
2 Corticosteroids. Prednisolone is the usual first-line treatment; 60 mg daily is a typical starting dose in adults and should then be tapered down. Those with predominantly IgG on red cells do best whereas those with complement often respond poorly, both to corticosteroids or splenectomy.
3 Splenectomy may be of value in those who fail to respond well or fail to maintain a satisfactory haemoglobin level on an acceptably small steroid dosage. ^{51}Cr organ uptake studies may help to confirm whether or not the spleen is the dominant site of destruction (Fig. 5.2b) and thus may be used to predict the value of splenectomy.
4 Immunosuppression may be tried after other measures have failed but is not always of great value. Azathioprine, cyclophosphamide, chlorambucil, cyclosporin and mycophenolate mofetil have been tried.
5 Folic acid is given to severe cases.
6 Blood transfusion may be needed if anaemia is severe and causing symptoms. The blood should be the least incompatible and if the specificity of the autoantibody is known, donor blood is chosen which lacks the relevant antigen(s). The patients also readily make alloantibodies against donor red cells.
7 High-dose immunoglobulin has been used but with less success than in ITP (see p. 254).

Cold autoimmune haemolytic anaemias
In these syndromes the autoantibody, whether monoclonal (as in the idiopathic cold haemagglutinin syndrome or associated with lymphoproliferative disorders) or polyclonal (as following infection, e.g. infectious mononucleosis or *Mycoplasma* pneumonia) attaches to red cells mainly in the peripheral circulation where the blood temperature is cooled (Table 5.5). The antibody is usually IgM and binds to red cells best at 4°C. IgM

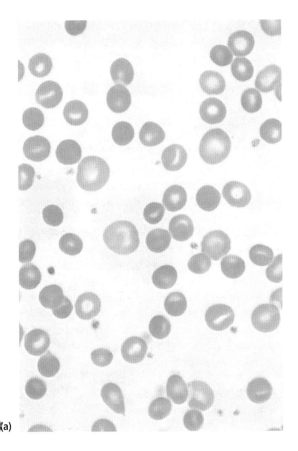

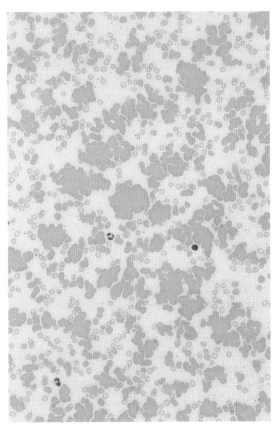

(a)

(b)

Fig. 5.9 (a) Blood film in warm autoimmune haemolytic anaemia. Numerous microspherocytes are present and larger polychromatic cells (reticulocytes). (b) Blood film in cold autoimmune haemolytic anaemia. Marked red cell agglutination is present in films made at room temperature. The background is caused by the raised plasma protein concentration.

antibodies are highly efficient at fixing complement and both intravascular and extravascular haemolysis can occur. Complement alone is usually detected on the red cells, the antibody having eluted off the cells in warmer parts of the circulation. Interestingly, in nearly all these cold AIHA syndromes, the antibody is directed against the 'I' antigen on the red cell surface. In infectious mononucleosis it is anti-i.

Clinical features

The patient may have a chronic haemolytic anaemia aggravated by the cold and often as-

sociated with intravascular haemolysis. Mild jaundice and splenomegaly may be present. The patient may develop acrocyanosis (purplish skin discoloration) at the tip of the nose, ears, fingers and toes caused by the agglutination of red cells in small vessels.

Laboratory findings are similar to those of warm AIHA, except that spherocytosis is less marked, red cells agglutinate in the cold (Fig. 5.9b) and the DAT reveals complement (C3d) only on the red cell surface.

Treatment consists of keeping the patient warm and treating the underlying cause, if present. Alkylating agents such as chlorambucil may be helpful in the chronic varieties. Splenectomy does not usually help unless massive splenomegaly is present, and steroids are not helpful. Underlying lymphoma should be excluded in 'idiopathic' cases.

Paroxysmal cold haemoglobinuria is a rare

syndrome of acute intravascular haemolysis after exposure to the cold. It is caused by the Donath–Landsteiner antibody, an IgG antibody with specificity for the P blood group antigens, which binds to red cells in the cold but causes lysis with complement in warm conditions. Viral infections and syphilis are predisposing causes and the condition is usually self-limiting.

Alloimmune haemolytic anaemias

In these anaemias, antibody produced by one individual reacts with red cells of another. Two important situations are transfusion of ABO-incompatible blood and rhesus disease of the newborn which are considered in Chapters 23 and 24. The increased use of allogeneic transplantation for renal, hepatic, cardiac and bone marrow diseases has led to the recognition of alloimmune haemolytic anaemia resulting from the production of red cell antibodies in the recipient by donor lymphocytes transferred in the allograft.

Drug-induced immune haemolytic anaemias

Drugs may cause immune haemolytic anaemias via three different mechanisms (Fig. 5.10):

1 antibody directed against a drug–red cell membrane complex (e.g. penicillin, ampicillin);

2 deposition of complement via a drug–protein (antigen)–antibody complex onto the red cell surface (e.g. quinidine, rifampicin); or

3 a true autoimmune haemolytic anaemia in which the role of the drug is unclear (e.g. methyldopa, fludarabine).

In each case, the haemolytic anaemia gradually disappears when the drug is discontinued but with methyldopa the autoantibody may persist for several months. The penicillin-induced immune haemolytic anaemias only occur with massive doses of the antibiotic.

Red cell fragmentation syndromes

These arise through physical damage to red cells either on abnormal surfaces (e.g. artificial heart valves or arterial grafts) or as a microangiopathic haemolytic anaemia caused by red cells passing through fibrin strands deposited in small vessels. The latter may be caused by disseminated intravascular coagulation (DIC; see p. 268), malignant hypertension, the haemolytic uraemic syndrome, thrombotic thrombocytopenic purpura, pre-eclampsia or meningococcal sepsis. The peripheral blood contains many deeply staining red cell fragments (Fig. 5.11). Clotting abnormalities typical of DIC (see p. 270) with a low platelet count are also present when DIC underlies the haemolysis.

March haemoglobinuria

This is caused by damage to red cells between the small bones of the feet, usually during prolonged marching or running. The blood film does not show fragments.

Infections

Infections may cause haemolysis in a variety of ways. They may precipitate an acute haemolytic crisis in G6PD deficiency or cause microangiopathic haemolytic anaemia, e.g. with meningo-

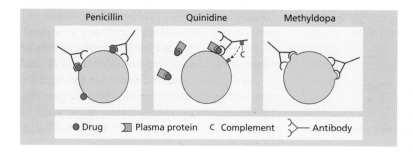

Fig. 5.10 Three different mechanisms of drug-induced immune haemolytic anaemia. In each case the coated (opsonized) cells are destroyed in the reticuloendothelial system.

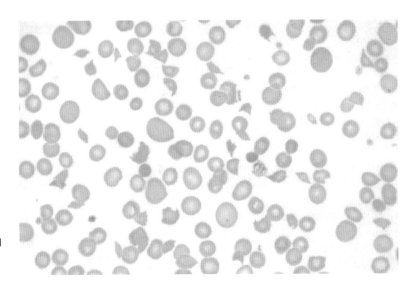

Fig. 5.11 Blood film in microangiopathic haemolytic anaemia (in this patient Gram-negative septicaemia). Numerous contracted and deeply staining cells and cell fragments are present.

coccal or pneumococcal septicaemia. Malaria causes haemolysis by extravascular destruction of parasitized red cells as well as by direct intravascular lysis. Blackwater fever is an acute intravascular haemolysis accompanied by acute renal failure caused by *Falciparum* malaria. *Clostridium perfringens* septicaemia may cause intravascular haemolysis with marked microspherocytosis.

Chemical and physical agents

Certain drugs, e.g. dapsone and salazopyrin, in high doses cause oxidative intravascular haemolysis with Heinz body formation in normal subjects. In Wilson's disease an acute haemolytic anaemia may occur as a result of high levels of copper in the blood. Chemical poisoning, e.g. with lead, chlorate or arsine, may cause severe haemolysis. Severe burns damage red cells causing acanthocytosis or spherocytosis.

Secondary haemolytic anaemias

In many systemic disorders red cell survival is shortened. This may contribute to anaemia (Chapter 20).

Paroxysmal nocturnal haemoglobinuria

PNH is a rare, acquired, clonal disorder of marrow stem cells in which there is deficient synthesis of the glycosylphosphatidylinositol (GPI) anchor, a structure that attaches several surface proteins to the cell membrane. It results from mutations in the X-chromosome gene coding for the protein, phosphatidylinositol glycan protein A (PIG-A) which is essential for the formation of the GPI anchor. The net result is that GPI-linked proteins (such as CD55 and CD59) are absent from the cell surface of all the cells derived from the abnormal stem cell (Fig. 5.12). The lack of surface molecules, decay-activating factor (DAF, CD55) and membrane inhibitor of reactive lysis (MIRL, CD59) render red cells sensitive to lysis by complement and the result is chronic intravascular haemolysis. Haemosiderinuria is a constant feature and can give rise to iron deficiency which may exacerbate the anaemia. CD55 and CD59 are also present on white cells and platelets. The other main clinical problem seen in PNH is thrombosis and patients may develop recurrent thromboses of large veins including portal and hepatic veins, as well as intermittent abnormal pain due to thrombosis of mesenteric veins.

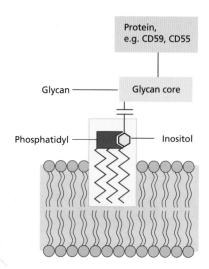

Fig. 5.12 Schematic representation of the phosphatidylinositol glycan which anchors many different proteins to the cell membrane, e.g. CD59 (MIRL, membrane inhibitor of reactive lysis).

PNH is almost invariably associated with some form of bone marrow hypoplasia, often frank aplastic anaemia. It appears that the PNH clone may expand as a result of a selective pressure, possibly immunologically mediated, against cells that have normal GPI-linked membrane proteins.

PNH may be diagnosed by demonstration of red cell lysis in serum at low pH—the Ham's test. Low pH activates complement by the alternative pathway. Flow cytometry to look for loss of expression of GPI-linked proteins such as CD55 (DAF) and CD59 (MIRL) is more sensitive.

Treatment is unsatisfactory. Iron therapy is used for iron deficiency and long-term anticoagulation with warfarin may be needed. Immunosuppression can be useful and allogeneic bone marrow transplantation is a definitive treatment. The disease occasionally remits but the median survival is around 10 years.

BIBLIOGRAPHY

Beutler E. (1996) Glucose-6-phosphate-dehydrogenase: population genetics and clinical manifestations. *Blood Rev.* **10**, 45–52.

Bolton-Maggs P.H.B. (2000) The diagnosis and management of hereditary spherocytosis. *Clin. Haematol.* **13**, 327–42.

Dacie J.V. (1988, 1999) *The Haemolytic Anaemias*; Vol. 2, *The Hereditary Haemolytic Anaemias*; Vol. 3, *The Haemolylic Anaemias of Immune Origin*; Vol. 4, *Secondary and Symptomatic Haemolytic Anaemias*; Vol. 5, *Drug and Chemical-induced Haemolytic Anaemias; PNH; Haemolytic Disease of the Newborn*, 3rd edn. Churchill Livingstone, Edinburgh.

Hillmen P. and Richards S. (2000) Paroxysmal nocturnal haemoglobinuria. *Rev. Clin. Exp. Hematol.* **4**, 216–235.

McMullin M.F. (1999) The molecular basis of disorders of red cell enzymes. *J. Clin. Pathol.* **52**, 241–4.

McMullin M.F. (1999) The molecular basis of disorders of the red cell membrane. *J. Clin. Pathol.* **52**, 245–8.

Tanner M.J.A. and Anstee D.J. (eds) (1999) Red cell membrane disorders. *Clin. Haematol.* **12**, 605–770.

Tse W.T. and Lux S.E. (1999) Red blood cell membrane disorders. *Br. J. Haematol.* **104**, 2–13.

Zanella A. (ed.) (2000) Inherited disorders of red cell metabolism. *Clin. Haematol.* **13**, 1–150.

Genetic disorders of haemoglobin

This chapter deals with inherited diseases caused by reduced or abnormal synthesis of globin. Mutations in the globin genes are the most prevalent monogenic disorders worldwide and affect around 7% of the world's population. The synthesis of normal haemoglobin both in the fetus and adult is described first.

HAEMOGLOBIN SYNTHESIS

Normal adult blood contains three types of haemoglobin (see Table 2.1). The major component is haemoglobin A with the molecular structure $\alpha_2\beta_2$. The minor haemoglobins contain γ (fetal Hb or Hb F) or δ (Hb A_2) chains instead of β chains. In the embryo and fetus, Gower 1, Portland, Gower 2 and fetal Hb dominate at different stages (Fig. 6.1). The genes for the globin chains occur in two clusters, ε, δ and β on chromosome 11 and ζ and α on chromosome 16. Two types of γ chain, G_γ and A_γ, occur which differ by a glycine or alanine amino acid at position 136 in the polypeptide chain. The α-chain gene is duplicated and both α genes (α_1 and α_2) on each chromosome are active (Fig. 6.1).

Molecular aspects

All the globin genes have three exons (coding regions) and two introns (non-coding regions whose DNA is not represented in the finished protein). The initial RNA is transcribed from both introns and exons, and from this transcript the RNA derived from introns is removed by a process known as splicing (Fig. 6.2) The introns always begin with a G-T dinucleotide and end with an A-G dinucleotide. The splicing machinery recognizes these sequences as well as neighbouring conserved sequences. The RNA in the nucleus is also 'capped' by addition of a structure at the 5' end which contains a seven methyl-guanosine group. The cap structure may be important for attachment of the mRNA to ribosomes. The newly formed mRNA is also polyadenylated at the 3' end (Fig. 6.2). This stabilizes it. Thalassaemia may arise from mutations or deletions of any of these sequences.

A number of other conserved sequences are important in globin synthesis and mutations at these sites may also give rise to thalassaemia. These sequences influence gene transcription, ensure its fidelity and specify sites for the initiation and termination of translation, and ensure the stability of newly synthesized mRNA. Promoters are found 5' of the gene, either close to the initiation site or more distally. They are the sites where RNA polymerases bind and catalyse gene transcription (see Fig. 1.11). Enhancers occur either 5' or 3' to the gene (Fig. 6.2). Enhancers are important in the tissue-specific regulation of globin gene expression, and in regulation of the synthesis of the various globin chains during fetal and postnatal life. The locus control region (LCR) is a genetic regulatory element situated a long way upstream of the β-globin cluster which controls the genetic activity of each domain, probably by physically interacting with the promoter region and opening up the chromatin to allow transcription factors to bind. The α-globin gene cluster also contains an LCR-like region termed HS40. GATA-1, FoG and NF-E2 transcription factors expressed mainly in erythroid precursors, are important in determining the expression of globin genes in erythroid cells.

Globin mRNA enters the cytoplasm and

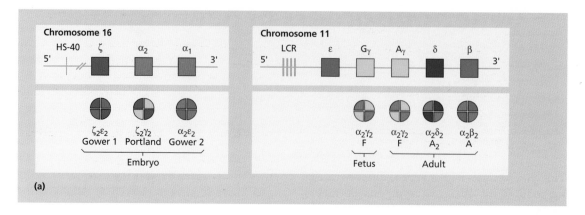

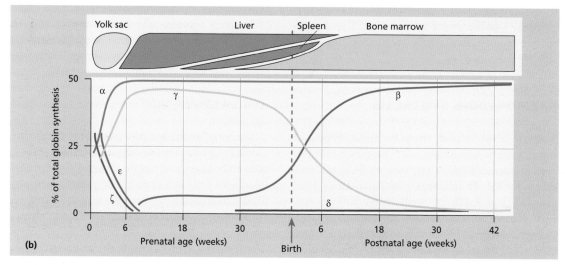

Fig. 6.1 (a) The globin gene clusters on chromosomes 16 and 11. In embryonic, fetal and adult life different genes are activated or suppressed. The different globin chains are synthesized independently and then combine with each other to produce the different haemoglobins. The γ gene may have two sequences, which code for either a glutamic acid or alanine residue at position 136 (G$_\gamma$ or A$_\gamma$ respectively). LCR, locus control region. (b) Synthesis of individual globin chains in prenatal and postnatal life.

attaches to ribosomes (translation) where the synthesis of globin chains takes place. This occurs by attachment of transfer RNAs, each with its individual amino acid, by codon/anticodon base pairing to an appropriate position on the mRNA template.

Switch from fetal to adult haemoglobin

The globin genes are arranged on chromosomes 11 and 16 in the order in which they are expressed (Fig. 6.1). Certain embryonic haemoglobins are usually only expressed in yolk sac erythroblasts. The β-globin gene is expressed at a low level in early fetal life, but the main switch to adult haemoglobin occurs 3–6 months after birth when synthesis of the γ chain is largely replaced by the β chain. How this switch comes about is largely unknown. It is clear, however, that the methylation state of the gene (expressed genes tend to be hypomethylated, non-expressed hypermethylated), the state of the chromosome packaging and various enhancer sequences all play a part in determining whether a particular gene will be transcribed.

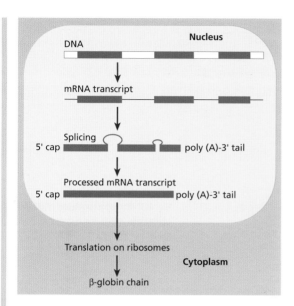

Fig. 6.2 The expression of a human globin gene from transcription, excision of introns, splicing of exons and translation to ribosomes. The primary transcript is cut 20 nucleotides downstream from this sequence, 'capped' at the 5′ end and a poly A tail is then added.

HAEMOGLOBIN ABNORMALITIES

These result from the following.
1 Synthesis of an abnormal haemoglobin.
2 Reduced rate of synthesis of normal α- or β-globin chains (the α- and β-thalassaemias).

Table 6.1 shows some of the first group of syndromes which arise from synthesis of an α or β chain with an amino acid substitution. In many cases, however, the abnormality is completely silent. The clinically most important abnormality is sickle cell anaemia. Haemoglobin (Hb) C, D and E are also common and, like Hb S, are substitutions in the β chain. Unstable haemoglobins are rare and cause a chronic haemolytic anaemia of varying severity with intravascular haemolysis (see Table 5.2). Abnormal haemoglobins may also cause (familial) polycythaemia (Chapter 17) or congenital methaemoglobinaemia (Chapter 2).

The genetic defects of haemoglobin are the most common genetic disorders worldwide. They occur in tropical and subtropical areas (Fig. 6.3) and most appear to have been selected because the carrier state affords some protection against

Table 6.1 The clinical syndromes produced by haemoglobin abnormalities

Syndrome	Abnormality
Haemolysis	Crystalline haemoglobins (Hb S, C, D, E, etc.)
	Unstable haemoglobin
Thalassaemia	α or β resulting from reduced globin chain synthesis
Familial polycythaemia	Altered oxygen affinity
Methaemoglobinaemia	Failure of reduction (Hb Ms)

malaria. β-thalassaemia is more common in the Mediterranean region while α-thalassaemia is more common in the Far East.

THALASSAEMIAS

These are a heterogeneous group of genetic disorders which result from a reduced rate of synthesis of α or β chains.

α-thalassaemia syndromes

These are usually caused by gene deletions and are listed in Table 6.2. As there are normally four copies of the α-globin gene the clinical severity can be classified according to the number of genes that are missing or inactive. Loss of all four genes completely suppresses α-chain synthesis (Fig. 6.4) and since the α chain is essential in fetal as well as in adult haemoglobin this is incompatible with life and leads to death *in utero* (hydrops fetalis, Fig. 6.5). Three α-gene deletions leads to a moderately severe (haemoglobin 7–11 g/dl) microcytic, hypochromic anaemia (Fig. 6.6) with splenomegaly. This is known as Hb H disease because haemoglobin H (β_4) can be detected in red cells of these patients by electrophoresis or in reticulocyte preparations (Fig. 6.6). In fetal life, Hb Barts (γ_4) occurs.

The α-thalassaemia traits are caused by loss of one or two genes and are usually not associated with anaemia, although the mean corpuscular

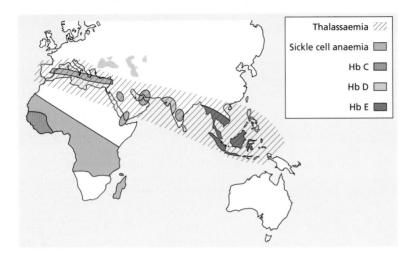

Fig. 6.3 The geographical distribution of the thalassaemias and the more common, inherited, structural haemoglobin abnormalities.

Table 6.2 Classification of thalassaemia

Clinical

Hydrops fetalis
   Four gene deletion α-thalassaemia

Thalassaemia major
   Transfusion dependent, homozygous
   β⁰-thalassaemia or other combinations of β-thalassaemia trait

Thalassaemia intermedia
   See Table 6.5

Thalassaemia minor
   β⁰-thalassaemia trait
   β⁺-thalassaemia trait
   Hereditary persistence of fetal haemoglobin
   δβ-thalassaemia trait
   α⁰-thalassaemia trait
   α⁺-thalassaemia trait

Genetic

Type	Haplotype	Heterozygous thalassaemia trait (minor)*	Homozygous
α-thalassaemias†			
α⁰	$--/$	MCV, MCH low	Hydrops fetalis
α⁺	$-\alpha/$	MCV, MCH minimally reduced	As heterozygous α⁰-thalassaemia
β-thalassaemias			
β⁰		MCV, MCH low (Hb A₂ > 3.5%)	Thalassaemia major (Hb F 98%, Hb A₂ 2%)
β⁺		MCV, MCH low (Hb A₂ > 3.5%)	Thalassaemia major or intermedia (Hb F 70–80%, Hb A 10–20%, Hb A₂ variable)
δβ-thalassaemia and hereditary persistence of fetal haemoglobin		MCV, MCH low (Hb F 5–20%, Hb A₂ normal)	Thalassaemia intermedia (Hb F 100%)
Hb Lepore		MCV, MCH low (Hb A 80–90%, Hb Lepore 10%, Hb A₂ reduced)	Thalassaemia major or intermedia (Hb F 80%, Hb Lepore 10–20%, Hb A, Hb A₂ absent)

* Occasionally, heterozygous β-thalassaemia is dominant (associated with the clinical picture of thalassaemia intermedia). There are several explanations.
† Compound heterozygote α⁰α⁺ ($--/-\alpha$) is haemoglobin H disease.
MCH, mean corpuscular haemoglobin; MCV, mean corpuscular volume.

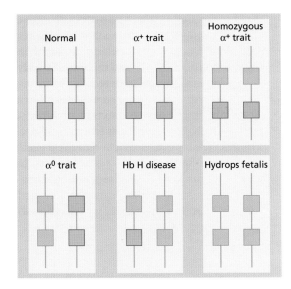

Fig. 6.4 The genetics of α-thalassaemia. Each α gene may be deleted or (less frequently) dysfunctional. The orange boxes represent normal genes, and the blue boxes represent gene deletions or dysfunctional genes.

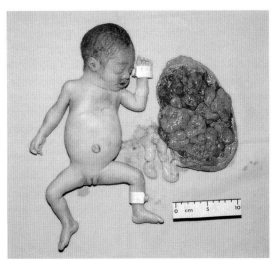

Fig. 6.5 α-thalassaemia: hydrops fetalis, the result of deletion of all four α-globin genes (homozygous α⁰-thalassaemia). The main haemoglobin present is Hb Barts (γ_4). The condition is incompatible with life beyond the fetal stage. (Courtesy of Professor D. Todd.)

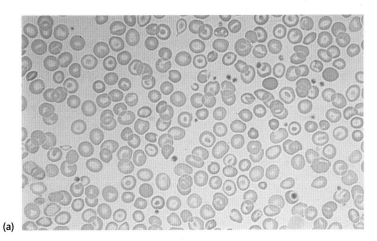

(a)

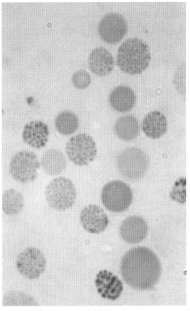

(b)

Fig. 6.6 (a) α-thalassaemia: haemoglobin H disease (three α-globin gene deletion). The blood film shows marked hypochromic, microcytic cells with target cells and poikilocytosis. (b) α-thalassaemia: haemoglobin H disease. Supravital staining with brilliant cresyl blue reveals multiple fine, deeply stained deposits ('golf ball' cells) caused by precipitation of aggregates of β-globin chains. Hb H can also be detected as a fast-moving band on haemoglobin electrophoresis (Fig. 6.13).

volume (MCV) and mean corpuscular haemoglobin (MCH) are low and the red cell count is over $5.5 \times 10^{12}/l$. Haemoglobin electrophoresis is normal and α/β-chain synthesis studies or DNA analyses are needed to be certain of the diagnosis. The normal α/β-synthesis ratio is $1:1$ and this is reduced in the α-thalassaemias and raised in β-thalassaemias. Uncommon non-deletional forms of α-thalassaemia are caused by point mutations producing dysfunction of the genes or rarely by mutations affecting termination of translation which give rise to an elongated but unstable chain, e.g. Hb Constant Spring.

β-thalassaemia syndromes

β-thalassaemia major

This condition occurs on average in one in four offspring if both parents are carriers of the β-thalassaemia trait. Either no β chain (β^0) or small amounts (β^+) are synthesized. Excess α chains precipitate in erythroblasts and in mature red cells causing the severe ineffective erythropoiesis and haemolysis that are typical of this disease. The greater the α-chain excess, the more severe the anaemia. Production of γ chains helps to 'mop up' excess α chains and to ameliorate the condition. Over 200 different genetic defects have now been detected (Figs 6.7 and 6.8).

Unlike α-thalassaemia, the majority of genetic lesions are point mutations rather than gene deletions. These mutations may be within the gene complex itself or in promoter or enhancer regions. Certain mutations are particularly frequent in some communities (Fig. 6.7) and this may simplify antenatal diagnosis aimed at detecting the mutations in fetal DNA. Thalassaemia major is often a result of inheritance of two different mutations, each affecting β-globin synthesis (compound heterozygotes). In some cases deletion of the β gene, δ and β genes or even δ, β and γ genes occurs. In others, unequal crossing-over has produced $\delta\beta$ fusion genes (so called Lepore syndrome named after the first family in which this was diagnosed) (see p. 82).

Clinical features

1 Severe anaemia becomes apparent at 3–6 months after birth when the switch from γ- to β-chain production should take place.

2 Enlargement of the liver and spleen occurs as a result of excessive red cell destruction, extramedullary haemopoiesis and later because of iron overload. The large spleen increases blood requirements by increasing red cell destruction and pooling, and by causing expansion of the plasma volume.

3 Expansion of bones caused by intense marrow hyperplasia leads to a thalassaemic facies (Fig. 6.9), and to thinning of the cortex of many bones with a tendency to fractures and bossing of the skull with a 'hair-on-end' appearance on X-ray (Fig. 6.10).

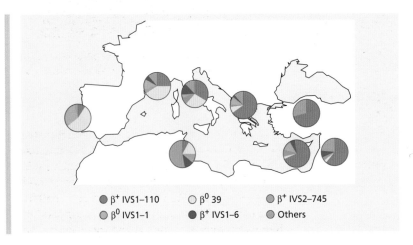

Fig. 6.7 Distribution of different mutations of β-thalassaemia major round the Mediterranean area. IVSI, IVS2 intervening sequences; 1, 6, 39, 110, 745 are mutations of corresponding codons. (Courtesy of Professor A. Cao.)

● β^+ IVS1–110   ○ β^0 39   ● β^+ IVS2–745
● β^0 IVS1–1   ● β^+ IVS1–6   ● Others

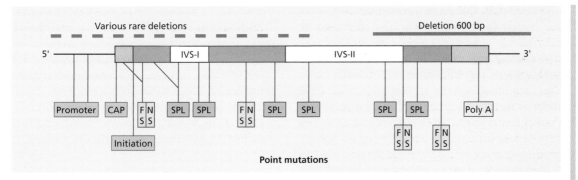

Fig. 6.8 Examples of mutations which produce β-thalassaemia. These include single base changes, small deletions and insertions of one or two bases affecting introns, exons or the flanking regions of the β-globin gene. FS, 'frameshifts': deletion of nucleotide(s) which places the reading frame out of phase downstream of the lesion; NS, 'nonsense': premature chain termination as a result of a new translational stop codon (e.g. UAA); SPL, 'splicing': inactivation of splicing or new splice sites generated (aberrant splicing) in exons or introns; promoter, CAP, initiation: reduction of transcription or translation as a result of lesion in promoter, CAP or initiation regions; Poly A: mutations on the poly A addition signal resulting in failure of poly A addition and an unstable mRNA.

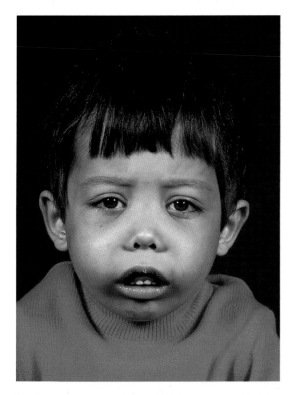

Fig. 6.9 The facial appearance of a child with β-thalassaemia major. The skull is bossed with prominent frontal and parietal bones; the maxilla is enlarged.

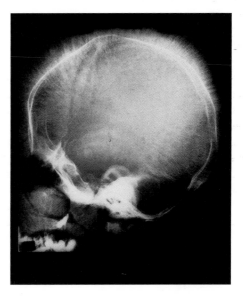

Fig. 6.10 The skull X-ray in β-thalassaemia major. There is a 'hair-on-end' appearance as a result of expansion of the bone marrow into cortical bone.

4 The patient can be sustained by blood transfusions but iron overload caused by repeated transfusions is inevitable unless chelation therapy is given (Table 6.3). Each 500 ml of transfused blood contains about 250 mg iron. To make matters worse, iron absorption from food is *increased* in β-thalassaemia, probably secondary to ineffective

erythropoiesis. Iron damages the liver (Fig. 6.11), the endocrine organs (with failure of growth, delayed or absent puberty, diabetes mellitus, hypothyroidism, hypoparathyroidism) and the myocardium. In the absence of intensive iron chelation death occurs in the second or third decade, usually from congestive heart failure or cardiac arrhythmias. Skin pigmentation as a result of excess melanin and haemosiderin gives a slatey grey appearance at an early stage of iron overload.

5 Infections may occur for a variety of reasons. In infancy, without adequate transfusion, the anaemic child is prone to bacterial infections. Pneumococcal, *Haemophilus* and meningococcal infections are likely if splenectomy has been carried out and prophylactic penicillin is not taken. *Yersinia enterocolitica* occurs particularly in iron-loaded patients being treated with desfer-

rioxamine; it may cause severe gastroenteritis. Transfusion of viruses by blood transfusion may occur. Liver disease in thalassaemia is most frequently a result of hepatitis C but hepatitis B is also common where the virus is endemic. Human immunodeficiency virus (HIV) has been transmitted to some patients by blood transfusion.

6 Osteoporosis may occur in well-transfused patients. It is more common in diabetic patients.

Table 6.3 Causes of refractory anaemia which may lead to transfusional iron overload

Congenital	Acquired
β-thalassaemia major	Myelodysplasia
β-thalassaemia/Hb E disease	Red cell aplasia
Sickle cell anaemia (some cases)	Aplastic anaemia
Red cell aplasia (Diamond–Blackfan)	Myelofibrosis
Sideroblastic anaemia	
Dyserythropoietic anaemia	

Fig. 6.11 β-thalassaemia major: needle biopsy of liver. (a) Grade IV siderosis with iron deposition in the hepatic parenchymal cells, bile duct epithelium, macrophages and fibroblasts (Perls' stain). (b) Reduction of iron excess in liver after intensive chelation therapy.

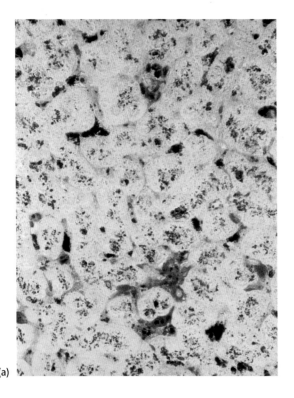

(a)

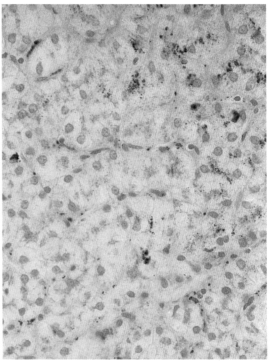

(b)

Laboratory diagnosis

1 There is a severe hypochromic, microcytic anaemia with raised reticulocyte percentage with normoblasts, target cells and basophilic stippling in the blood film (Fig. 6.12).

2 Haemoglobin electrophoresis reveals absence or almost complete absence of Hb A with almost all the circulating haemoglobin being Hb F. The Hb A_2 percentage is normal, low or slightly raised (Fig. 6.13). α/β-globin chain synthesis studies on reticulocytes show an increased $\alpha : \beta$ ratio with reduced or absent β-chain synthesis. DNA analysis can be used to identify the defect on each allele.

Assessment of iron status

The tests that may be performed to assess iron

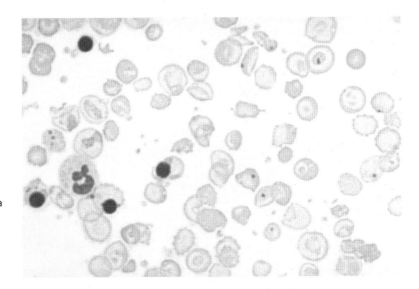

Fig. 6.12 Blood film in β-thalassaemia major post-splenectomy. These are hypochromic cells, target cells, many nucleated red cells (normoblasts). Howell–Jolly bodies are seen in same red cells.

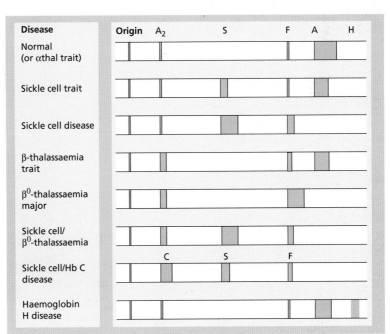

Fig. 6.13 Haemoglobin electrophoretic patterns in normal adult human blood and in subjects with sickle cell (Hb S) trait or disease, β-thalassaemia trait, β-thalassaemia major, Hb S/β-thalassaemia or Hb S/Hb C disease and Hb H disease.

overload are listed in Table 6.4. Tests may also be carried out to determine the degree of organ damage caused by iron. The serum ferritin is the most widely used test. It is usual in thalassaemia major to attempt to keep the level between 1000 and 1500 μg/l, when the body iron stores are about five to 10 times normal. However, the serum ferritin is raised in relation to iron status in viral hepatitis and other inflammatory disorders and should therefore be interpreted in conjunction with other tests such as liver biopsy, (Fig. 6.11) urine excretion of iron in response to desferrioxamine, skin pigmentation and function of the heart, liver and endocrine and the clinical picture.

Treatment

1 Regular blood transfusions are needed to maintain the haemoglobin over 10 g/dl at all times. This usually requires 2–3 units every 4–6 weeks. Fresh blood, filtered to remove white cells, gives the best red cell survival with the fewest reactions.

The patients should be genotyped at the start of the transfusion programme in case red cell antibodies against transfused red cells develop.

2 Regular folic acid (e.g. 5 mg daily) is given if the diet is poor.

3 Iron chelation therapy is used to treat iron overload. Unfortunately desferrioxamine is inactive orally. It may be given by a separate infusion bag 1–2 g with each unit of blood transfused and by subcutaneous infusion 20–40 mg/kg over 8–12 h, 5–7 days weekly (Fig. 6.14). It is commenced in infants after 10–15 units of blood have been transfused. Iron-chelated by desferrioxamine is mainly excreted in the urine but up to one-third is also excreted in the stools. If patients comply with this intensive iron chelation regime, life expectancy for patients with thalassaemia major and other chronic refractory anaemias receiving regular

Table 6.4 Assessment of iron overload

Assessment of iron stores

Serum ferritin

Serum iron and percentage saturation of transferrin (iron-binding capacity)

Bone marrow biopsy (Perls' stain) for reticuloendothelial stores

DNA test for mutation resulting in Cys282Tyr in the *HFE* gene

Liver biopsy (parenchymal and reticuloendothelial stores)

Liver CT scan or MRI

Cardiac MRI

Desferrioxamine iron excretion test (chelatable iron)

Repeated phlebotomy until iron deficiency occurs

Assessment of tissue damage caused by iron overload

Cardiac	Clinical; chest X-ray; ECG; 24-h monitor; echocardiography; radionuclide (MUGA) scan to check left ventricular ejection fraction at rest and with stress
Liver	Liver function tests; liver biopsy; CT scan
Endocrine	Clinical examination (growth and sexual development); glucose tolerance test; pituitary gonadotrophin release tests; thyroid, parathyroid, gonadal, adrenal function, growth hormone assays; radiology for bone age; isotopic bone density study

CT, computed tomography; ECG, electrocardiography; MRI, magnetic resonance imaging; MUGA, multiple gated acquisition.

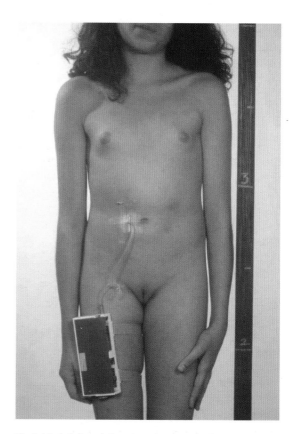

Fig. 6.14 β-thalassaemia major: subcutaneous infusion of desferrioxamine infusion in progress using a portable, battery-driven pump.

blood transfusion (Table 6.3) improves considerably. In some cases intensive continuous chelation therapy with intravenous desferrioxamine can reverse heart damage caused by iron overload. Lack of compliance, however, is frequent and the drug is costly. In addition, desferrioxamine is not without side-effects, especially in children with relatively low serum ferritin levels, including high tone deafness, retinal damage, bone abnormalities and growth retardation. Patients should have auditory and fundoscopic examinations at regular intervals. Desferiprone (L1), an orally active iron chelator, is now licensed in Europe and India and is used alone or in combination with desferrioxamine. The two drugs have an additive or even synergistic action on iron excretion. Alone it is less effective than desferrioxamine. Compliance is usually better. Side-effects include an arthropathy, agranulocytosis or severe neutropenia, gastrointestinal disturbance and zinc deficiency.

4 Vitamin C, 200 mg daily, increases excretion of iron produced by desferrioxamine.

5 Splenectomy may be needed to reduce blood requirements. This should be delayed until the patient is over 6 years old because of the high risk of dangerous infections post-splenectomy. The vaccinations and antibiotics to be given are described in Chapter 22.

6 Endocrine therapy is given either as replacement because of end-organ failure or to stimulate the pituitary if puberty is delayed. Diabetics will require insulin therapy. Patients with osteoporosis may need additional therapy with increased calcium and vitamin D in their diet, together with administration of a bisphosphonate.

7 Immunization against hepatitis B should be carried out in all non-immune patients. Treatment for transfusion-transmitted hepatitis C with α-interferon and ribavirin is needed if viral genomes are detected in plasma.

8 Allogeneic bone marrow transplantation offers the prospect of permanent cure. The success rate (long-term thalassaemia major-free survival) is over 80% in well-chelated younger patients without liver fibrosis or hepatomegaly. A human leucocyte antigen (HLA) matching sibling (or rarely other family member or matching unrelated donor) acts as donor. Failure is mainly a result of recurrence of thalassaemia, death (e.g.

from infection) or severe chronic graft-versus-host disease.

β-thalassaemia trait (minor)

This is a common, usually symptomless, abnormality characterized like α-thalassaemia trait by a hypochromic, microcytic blood picture (MCV and MCH very low) but high red cell count ($>5.5 \times 10^{12}/l$) and mild anaemia (haemoglobin 10–15 g/dl). It is usually more severe than α trait; a raised Hb A_2 ($>3.5\%$) confirms the diagnosis. One of the most important indications for making the diagnosis is that it allows the possibility of prenatal counselling to patients with a partner who also has a significant haemoglobin disorder. If both carry β-thalassaemia trait there is a 25% risk of a thalassaemia major child.

Thalassaemia intermedia

Cases of thalassaemia of moderate severity (haemoglobin 7.0–10.0 g/dl) who do not need regular transfusions are called thalassaemia intermedia (Table 6.5). This is a *clinical* syndrome which may be caused by a variety of genetic defects. It may be caused by homozygous β-thalassaemia with production of more Hb F than usual or with mild defects in β-chain synthesis, or by β-thalassaemia trait alone but of unusual severity ('dominant' β-thalassaemia) or β-thalassaemia trait in association with mild globin abnormalities

Table 6.5 Thalassaemia intermedia

Homozygous β-thalassaemia
Homozygous mild β^+-thalassaemia
Coinheritance of α-thalassaemia
Enhanced ability to make fetal haemoglobin (γ-chain production)

Heterozygous β-thalassaemia
Coinheritance of additional α-globin genes (ααα/αα or ααα/ααα)
Dominant β-thalassaemia trait

δβ-thalassaemia and hereditary persistence of fetal haemoglobin
Homozygous δβ-thalassaemia
Heterozygous δβ-thalassaemia/β-thalassaemia
Homozygous Hb Lepore (some cases)

Haemoglobin H disease

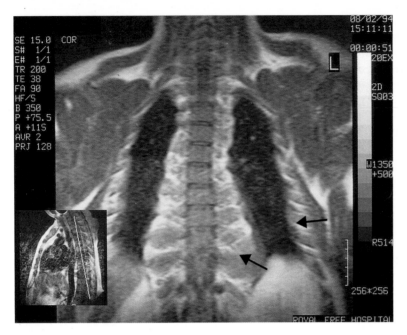

Fig. 6.15 β-thalassaemia intermedia: MRI scan showing masses of extramedullary haemopoietic tissue arising from the ribs and in the paravertebral region without encroachment of the spinal cord.

such as Hb Lepore. The coexistence of α-thalassaemia trait improves the haemoglobin level in homozygous β-thalassaemia by reducing the degree of chain imbalance and thus of α-chain precipitation and ineffective erythropoiesis. Conversely, patients with β-thalassaemia trait who also have excess (five or six) α genes tend to be more anaemic than usual. The patient with thalassaemia intermedia may show bone deformity, enlarged liver and spleen, extramedullary erythropoiesis (Fig. 6.15) and features of iron overload caused by increased iron absorption. Hb H disease, three-gene deletion α-thalassaemia, is a type of thalassaemia intermedia without iron overload or extramedullary haemopoiesis.

δβ-thalassaemia

This involves failure of production of both β and δ chains. Fetal haemoglobin production is increased to 5–20% in the heterozygous state which resembles thalassaemia minor haematologically. In the homozygous state only Hb F is present and haematologically the picture is of thalassaemia intermedia.

Haemoglobin Lepore

This is an abnormal haemoglobin caused by unequal crossing-over of the β and δ genes to produce a polypeptide chain consisting of the δ chain at its amino end and β chain at its carboxyl end. The δβ-fusion chain is synthesized inefficiently and normal δ- and β-chain production is abolished. The homozygotes show thalassaemia intermedia and the heterozygotes thalassaemia trait.

Hereditary persistence of fetal haemoglobin

These are a heterogeneous group of genetic conditions caused by deletions or cross-overs affecting the production of β and γ chains or, in non-deletion forms, by to point mutations upstream from the γ-globin genes.

Association of β-thalassaemia trait with other genetic disorders of haemoglobin

The combination of β-thalassaemia trait with Hb E

trait usually causes a transfusion-dependent tha-lassaemia major syndrome, but some cases are in-termediate. β-thalassaemia trait with Hb S trait produces the clinical picture of sickle cell anaemia rather than of thalassaemia (p. 87). β-thalassaemia trait with Hb D trait causes a hypochromic, micro-cytic anaemia of varying severity.

SICKLE CELL ANAEMIA

Sickle cell disease is a group of haemoglobin dis-orders in which the sickle β-globin gene is inher-ited. Homozygous sickle cell anaemia (Hb SS) is the most common whilst the doubly heterozygote conditions of Hb SC and Hb Sβthal also cause sick-ling disease. Hb S (Hb $\alpha_2\beta_2{}^S$) is insoluble and forms crystals when exposed to low oxygen ten-sion. Deoxygenated sickle haemoglobin poly-merizes into long fibres, each consisting of seven intertwined double strands with cross-linking. The red cells sickle and may block different areas of the microcirculation or large vessels causing infarcts of various organs. The sickle β-globin abnormality is caused by substitution of valine for glutamic acid at position 6 in the β chain (Fig. 6.16). It is very widespread and is found in up to one in four West Africans, maintained at this level because of the protection against malaria that is afforded by the carrier state.

Homozygous disease

Clinical features

Clinical features are of a severe haemolytic anaemia punctuated by crises. The symptoms of anaemia are often mild in relation to the severity of the anaemia because Hb S gives up oxygen (O_2) to tissues relatively easily compared with Hb A, its O_2 dissociation curve being shifted to the right (see Fig. 2.9). The clinical expression of Hb SS is very variable, some patients having an almost normal life, free of crises but others develop severe crises even as infants and may die in early childhood or as young adults. Crises may be vaso-occlusive, visceral, aplastic or haemolytic.

		pro	glu	glu
Normal β- chain	Amino acid	pro	glu	glu
	Base composition	CCT	G A G	GAG
Sickle β- chain	Base composition	CCT	G T G	GAG
	Amino acid	pro	val	glu

Fig. 6.16 Molecular pathology of sickle cell anaemia. There is a single base change in the DNA coding for the amino acid in the sixth position in the β-globin chain (adenine is replaced by thymine). This leads to an amino acid change from glutamic acid to valine. A, adenine; C, cytosine; G, guanine; glu, glutamic acid; pro, proline; T, thymine; val, valine.

Painful vaso-occlusive crises

These are the most frequent and are precipitated by such factors as infection, acidosis, dehydration or deoxygenation (e.g. altitude, operations, ob-stetric delivery, stasis of the circulation, exposure to cold, violent exercise, etc.). Infarcts may occur in a variety of organs including the bones (hips, shoulders and vertebrae are commonly affected) (Fig. 6.17), the lungs and the spleen. The most seri-ous vaso-occlusive crisis is of the brain (a stroke occurs in 7% of all patients) or spinal cord. The 'hand–foot' syndrome (painful dactylitis caused by infarcts of the small bones) is frequently the first presentation of the disease and may lead to digits of varying lengths (Fig. 6.18).

Visceral sequestration crises

These are caused by sickling within organs and pooling of blood, often with a severe exacerbation of anaemia. The acute sickle chest syndrome is a feared complication and the most common cause of death after puberty. It presents with dyspnoea, falling P_{O_2}, chest pain and pulmonary infiltrates on chest X-ray. Treatment is with analgesia, oxygen, exchange transfusion and ventilatory support if necessary. Hepatic and girdle seques-tration crises and splenic sequestration all may lead to severe illness requiring exchange transfu-sions. Splenic sequestration is typically seen in infants and presents with an enlarging spleen, falling haemoglobin and abdominal pain. Treat-ment is with transfusion and patients must be monitored at regular intervals as progression may be rapid. Attacks tend to be recurrent and splenec-tomy is often advised.

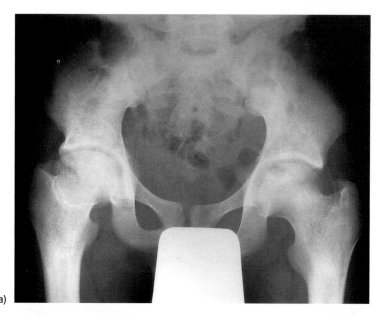

(a)

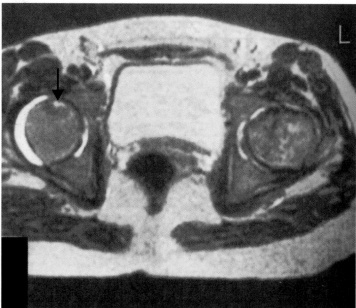

(b)

Fig. 6.17 Sickle cell anaemia. (a) Radiograph of the pelvis of a young man of West Indian origin which shows avascular necrosis with flattening of the femoral heads, more marked on the right, coarsening of the bone architecture and cystic areas in the right femoral neck caused by previous infarcts. (b) MRI scan of the hips of a 17 year-old female, showing a small area of high signal in the anterior portion of the right hip (arrowed) with a low intensity rim. This is typical of early avascular necrosis. The irregular outline and signal in the left hip results from more advanced avascular necrosis. Joint fluid is shown as a high signal (white rim) surrounding the femoral head. (Courtesy of Dr L. Berger.)

Aplastic crises

These may occur as a result of infection with parvovirus or folate deficiency and are characterized by a sudden fall in haemoglobin, usually requiring transfusion. They are characterized by a fall in reticulocytes as well as haemoglobin (see Fig. 7.4).

Haemolytic crises

These are characterized by an increased rate of haemolysis with a fall in haemoglobin but rise in reticulocytosis and usually accompany a painful crisis.

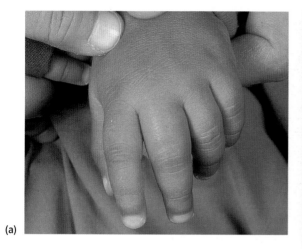

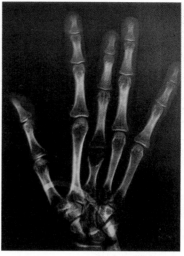

(a)

(b)

Fig. 6.18 Sickle cell anaemia: (a) painful swollen fingers (dactylitis) in a child and (b) the hand of an 18-year-old Nigerian boy with the 'hand–foot' syndrome. There is marked shortening of the right middle finger because of dactylitis in childhood affecting the growth of the epiphysis.

Other clinical features

Ulcers of the lower legs are common, as a result of vascular stasis and local ischaemia (Fig. 6.19). The spleen is enlarged in infancy and early childhood but later is often reduced in size as a result of infarcts (autosplenectomy). A proliferative retinopathy and priapism are other clinical complications. Chronic damage to the liver may occur through microinfarcts. Pigment (bilirubin) gallstones are frequent. The kidneys are vulnerable to infarctions of the medulla with papillary necrosis. Failure to concentrate urine aggravates the tendency to dehydration and crisis, and nocturnal enuresis is common. Osteomyelitis may also occur, usually from *Salmonella* spp. (Fig. 6.20).

Laboratory findings

1 The haemoglobin is usually 6–9 g/dl—low in comparison to symptoms of anaemia.
2 Sickle cells and target cells occur in the blood (Fig. 6.21a). Features of splenic atrophy (e.g. Howell–Jolly bodies) may also be present.
3 Screening tests for sickling are positive when

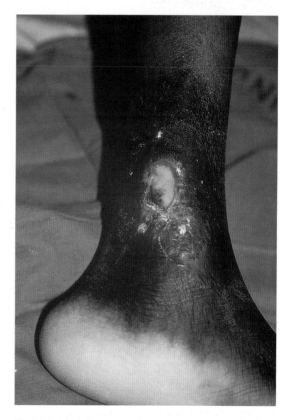

Fig. 6.19 Sickle cell anaemia: medial aspect of the ankle of a 15-year-old Nigerian boy showing necrosis and ulceration.

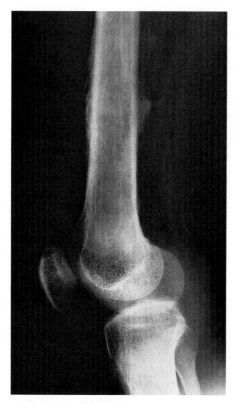

Fig. 6.20 *Salmonella* osteomyelitis: lateral radiograph of the lower femur and knee. The periosteum is irregularly raised in the lower third of the femur.

the blood is deoxygenated (e.g. with dithionate and Na_2HPO_4).

4 Haemoglobin electrophoresis (Fig. 6.13): in Hb SS, no Hb A is detected. The amount of Hb F is variable and is usually 5–15%, larger amounts are normally associated with a milder disorder.

Treatment

1 Prophylactic—avoid those factors known to precipitate crises, especially dehydration, anoxia, infections, stasis of the circulation and cooling of the skin surface.

2 Folic acid, e.g. 5 mg daily.

3 Good general nutrition and hygiene.

4 Pneumococcal, haemophilus and meningococcal vaccination and regular oral penicillin are effective at reducing the infection rate with these organisms and should be strongly encouraged. Oral penicillin should start at diagnosis and continue at least until puberty. Hepatitis B vaccination is also given as transfusions may be needed.

5 Crises—treat by rest, warmth, rehydration by oral fluids and/or intravenous normal saline (31 in 24 hours) and antibiotics if infection is present. Analgesia at the appropriate level

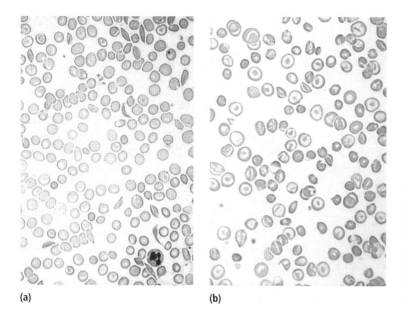

(a)   (b)

Fig. 6.21 (a) Sickle cell anaemia: peripheral blood film showing deeply staining sickle cells, target cells and polychromasia (a Howell–Jolly body is seen in a red cell in the top right portion of the field). (b) Homozygous Hb C disease: peripheral blood film showing many target cells, deeply staining rhomboidal and spherocytic cells.

should be given. Suitable drugs are paracetamol, a non-steroidal anti-inflammatory agent and opiates, e.g. continuous subcutaneous diamorphine. Blood transfusion is given only if there is very severe anaemia with symptoms. Exchange transfusion may be needed particularly if there is neurological damage, a visceral sequestration crisis or repeated painful crises. This is aimed at achieving an Hb S percentage of less than 30 in severe cases.

6 Particular care is needed in pregnancy and anaesthesia. There is debate as to whether or not patients need transfusions with normal blood to reduce Hb S levels during pregnancy or before delivery or for minor operations. Careful anaesthetic and recovery techniques must be used to avoid hypoxaemia or acidosis. Routine transfusions throughout pregnancy are given to those with a bad obstetric history or a history of frequent crises.

7 Transfusions—these are also sometimes given repeatedly as prophylaxis to patients having frequent crises or who have had major organ damage, e.g. of the brain. The aim is to suppress Hb S production over a period of several months or even years. Iron overload and alloimmunization against donated blood are common problems.

8 Hydroxyurea (15.0–20.0 mg/kg) can increase Hb F levels and has been shown to improve the clinical course of patients who are having three or more painful crises each year. It should not be used during pregnancy.

9 Stem cell transplantation can cure the disease and many patients have now been successfully treated. The mortality rate is less than 10%. Transplantation is only indicated in the severest of cases whose quality of life or life expectancy are substantially impaired.

10 Research into other drugs, e.g. butyrates, to enhance Hb F synthesis or to increase the solubility of Hb S is taking place. 'Gene therapy' is a distant prospect not yet available (Chapter 8).

Sickle cell trait

This is a benign condition with no anaemia and normal appearance of red cells on a blood film. Haematuria is the most common symptom and is thought to be caused by minor infarcts of the renal papillae. Hb S varies from 25 to 45% of the total haemoglobin (Fig. 6.13). Care must be taken with anaesthesia, pregnancy and at high altitudes.

Combination of Haemoglobin S with other genetic defects of haemoglobin

The most common of these are Hb S/β-thalassaemia, and sickle cell/C disease. In Hb S/β-thalassaemia, the MCV and MCH are lower than in homozygous Hb SS. The clinical picture is of sickle cell anaemia; splenomegaly is usual. Patients with Hb SC disease have a particular tendency to thrombosis and pulmonary embolism, especially in pregnancy. In general, when compared to Hb SS disease, they have a higher incidence of retinal abnormalities, milder anaemia, splenomegaly and generally a longer life expectancy. Diagnosis is made by haemoglobin electrophoresis, particularly with family studies.

Haemoglobin C disease

This genetic defect of haemoglobin is frequent in West Africa and is caused by substitution of lysine for glutamic acid in the β-globin chain at the same point as the substitution in Hb S. Hb C tends to form rhomboidal crystals and in the homozygous state there is a mild haemolytic anaemia with marked target cell formation, cells with rhomboidal shape and microspherocytes (Fig. 6.21b). The spleen is enlarged. The carriers show a few target cells only.

Haemoglobin D disease

This is a group of variants all with the same electrophoretic mobility. Heterozygotes show no haematological abnormality while homozygotes have a mild haemolytic anaemia.

Haemoglobin E disease

This is the most common haemoglobin variant in South-East Asia. In the homozygous state there is a mild microcytic, hypochromic anaemia. Haemoglobin E/β^0-thalassaemia, however, resembles homozygous β^0-thalassaemia both clinically and haematologically.

PRENATAL DIAGNOSIS OF GENETIC HAEMOGLOBIN DISORDERS

It is important to give genetic counselling to couples at risk of having a child with a major haemoglobin defect. If a pregnant woman is found to have a haemoglobin abnormality, her partner should be tested to determine whether he also carries a defect. When both partners show an abnormality and there is a risk of a serious defect in the offspring, particularly β-thalassaemia major, it is important to offer antenatal diagnosis. Several techniques are available, the choice depending on the stage of pregnancy and the potential nature of the defect.

DNA diagnosis

The majority of samples are obtained by chorionic villus biopsy although amniotic fluid cells are sometimes used. The DNA is then analysed using one of the following methods.

Polymerase chain reaction is the most commonly used technique (Fig. 6.22) and may be performed by using primer pairs that only amplify individual alleles ('allele-specific priming') (Fig. 6.23) or by using consensus primers that amplify all the alleles followed by restriction digestion to detect a particular allele. This is best illustrated by Hb S in which the enzyme Mst II detects the A-T change (Fig. 6.24).

Southern blot analysis is useful for detecting gene deletions in α-thalassaemia.

Restriction fragment length polymorphism (RFLP) linkage studies are used widely to diagnose many genetic disorders (Fig. 6.25). Scattered along each gene cluster are single base changes which may vary from one individual to the next, i.e. are polymorphic. These changes give rise to sites recognized by restriction enzymes or remove sites previously identified so that the size of the DNA fragment produced by that restriction en-

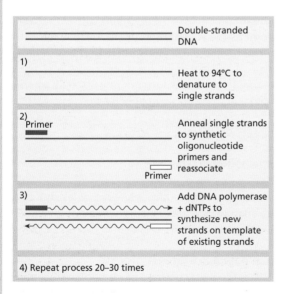

Fig. 6.22 Polymerase chain reaction. The primers hybridize to DNA on either side of the piece of DNA to be analysed. Repeated cycles of denaturation, association with the primers, incubation with a DNA polymerase and deoxyribonucleotides (dNTPs) results in amplification of the DNA over a million times within a few hours.

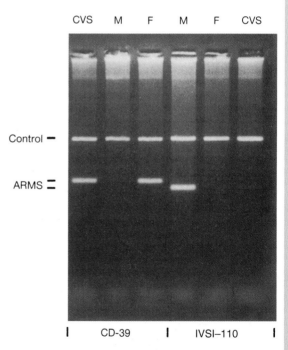

Fig. 6.23 The rapid prenatal diagnosis of β-thalassaemia by amplification refractory mutation system (ARMS). The father has the common Mediterranean codon 39 (CD39) mutation, the mother the IVS1–110 G → A mutation. The fetus is heterozygous for the CD39 mutation. CVS, fetal DNA from chorionic villus sampling; F, father; M, mother. (Courtesy of Dr J. Old and Professor D. J. Weatherall.)

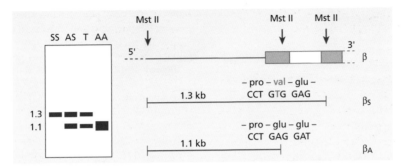

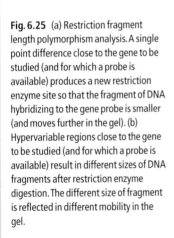

Fig. 6.24 Sickle cell anaemia: antenatal diagnosis. Direct DNA analysis. The DNA has been digested by the restriction enzyme Mst II. The replacement of an adenine base in the normal β-globin gene by thymine in the sickle cell gene removes a normal restriction site for Mst II, producing a larger 1.3-kb fragment than the normal 1.1-kb fragment to hybridize with the β-globin gene probe. In this case the trophoblast DNA (T) shows both normal (A) and sickle cell (S) restriction fragments and so is AS (sickle trait). (Courtesy of Dr J. Old and the Royal College of Obstetrics and Gynaecology.)

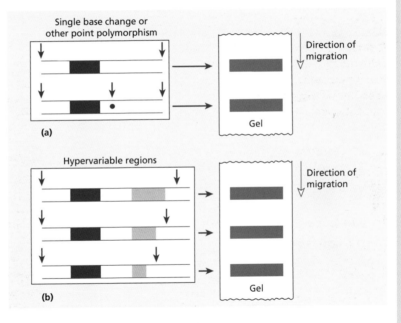

Fig. 6.25 (a) Restriction fragment length polymorphism analysis. A single point difference close to the gene to be studied (and for which a probe is available) produces a new restriction enzyme site so that the fragment of DNA hybridizing to the gene probe is smaller (and moves further in the gel). (b) Hypervariable regions close to the gene to be studied (and for which a probe is available) result in different sizes of DNA fragments after restriction enzyme digestion. The different size of fragment is reflected in different mobility in the gel.

zyme varies. A restriction site present is denoted as (+) and its absence as (−). The RFLPs caused by these sites are inherited in a Mendelian manner and can be used, provided they are sufficiently close to the gene of interest, as linkage markers to recognize a chromosome that carries a thalassaemia or other mutation. The combination of various RFLPs along one chromosome is called the 'haplotype'. If two sites along a chromosome are found to occur together more frequently than by chance, this is known as linkage disequilibrium. Family studies are first needed to establish the linkage of normal and abnormal globin genes to particular haplotypes. The haplotypes of the fetal DNA are then analysed. This technique therefore requires a previous child or grandparents to be studied as well as parents, and the parents must not be homozygous. Rarely cross-over between the markers studied and the globin gene may lead to false results.

Fetal blood sampling

Fetal blood sampling may be performed in mid-second trimester and allows DNA study and protein synthesis studies.

BIBLIOGRAPHY

Bain B. *et al.* (1998) Guideline: the laboratory diagnosis of haemoglobinopathies. *Br. J. Haematol.* **101**, 783–92.

Bunn H.F. (1997) Pathogenesis and treatment of sickle cell disease. *N. Engl. J. Med.* **337**, 762–9.

Charache S. *et al.* (1995) Effect of hydroxyurea on the frequency of painful crises in sickle cell anaemia. *N. Engl. J. Med.* **332**, 1317.

Embury S.H., Hebbel R.P., Mohandas N. and Steinberg M.H. (eds) (1994) *Sickle Cell Disease*, Raven Press, New York.

Hershko C. and Hoffbrand A.V. (2000) Iron chelation therapy. *Rev. Clin. Exp. Hematol.* **4**, 337–61.

Hillery C.A. (1998) Potential therapeutic approaches for the treatment of vaso-occlusion in sickle-cell disease. *Curr. Opin. Hematol.* **5**, 151–5.

Olivieri N. and Brittenham G. (1997) Iron-chelating therapy and the treatment of thalassemia. *Blood* **89**, 739–61.

Sergeant G.R. (2001) *Sickle Cell Anaemia*, 3rd edn. Oxford University Press, Oxford.

Steinberg M.H. (1999) Management of sickle cell disease *N. Engl. J. Med.* **340**, 1021–30.

Steinberg M.H., Forget B.G., Higgs D.R. and Nagel R.L. (eds) (2001) *Disorders of Hemoglobin*. Cambridge University Press, Cambridge.

Vermylen C. and Cornu G. (1997) Haematopoietic stem cell transplantation for sickle cell anaemia. *Curr. Opin. Haematol.* **4**, 377–80.

Weatherall D.J. and Clegg J.B. (2001) *The Thalassaemia Syndromes*, 4th edn. Blackwell Science, Oxford.

Wonke B. and De Sanctis V. (2000) Clinical aspects of transfusional iron overload. *Rev. Clin. Exp. Hematol.* **4**, 322–36.

Aplastic anaemia and bone marrow failure

PANCYTOPENIA

Pancytopenia describes a reduction in the blood count of all the major cell lines—red cells, white cells and platelets. It has several causes (Table 7.1) that can be broadly divided into decreased bone marrow production or increased peripheral destruction.

APLASTIC ANAEMIA

Aplastic (hypoplastic) anaemia is defined as pancytopenia resulting from aplasia of the bone marrow. It is classified into primary (congenital or acquired) or secondary types (Table 7.2).

Pathogenesis

The underlying defect in all cases appears to be a substantial reduction in the number of haemopoietic pluripotential stem cells, and a fault in the remaining stem cells or an immune reaction against them, which makes them unable to divide and differentiate sufficiently to populate the bone marrow (Fig. 7.1). A primary fault in the marrow microenvironment has also been suggested but the success of stem cell transplantation (SCT) shows this can only be a rare cause because normal donor stem cells are usually able to thrive in the recipient's marrow cavity.

Congenital

The Fanconi type has an autosomal recessive pattern of inheritance and is often associated with growth retardation and congenital defects of the skeleton (e.g. microcephaly, absent radii or thumbs), of the renal tract (e.g. pelvic or horseshoe kidney) (Fig. 7.2) or skin (areas of hyper- and hypopigmentation); sometimes there is mental retardation. The syndrome is genetically heterogeneous with seven different complimentation groups termed FAA to FAG and the genes for FAA, FAC, FAF and FAG have been identified. The underlying problem appears to be defective DNA repair. Cells from Fanconi's anaemia (FA) patients show an abnormally high frequency of spontaneous chromosomal breakage and the diagnostic test is elevated breakage after incubation of peripheral blood lymphocytes with diepoxybutane (DEB test). Dyskeratosis congenita is a rare sex-linked disorder with nail and skin atrophy and is associated with mutations in a gene associated with nucleolar function encoded at Xq28.

The usual age of presentation of FA is 5–10 years. About 10% of cases develop acute myeloid leukaemia. Treatment is usually with androgens and/or SCT. The blood count usually improves with androgens but side-effects, especially in children, are distressing (virilization and liver abnormalities); remission rarely lasts more than 2 years. SCT may cure the patient; because of the sensitivity of the patient's cells to DNA damage, conditioning regimes are mild.

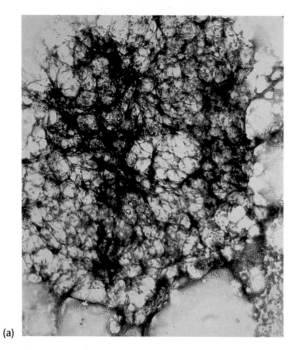

(a)

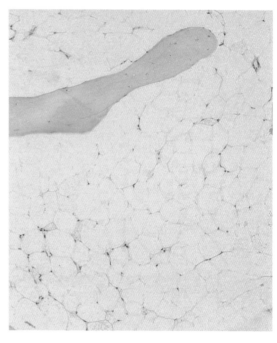

(b)

Fig. 7.1 Aplastic anaemia: low power views of bone marrow show severe reduction of haemopoietic cells with an increase in fat spaces. (a) Aspirated fragment. (b) Trephine biopsy.

Table 7.1 Causes of pancytopenia

Decreased bone marrow function
Aplasia
Acute leukaemia, myelodysplasia, myeloma
Infiltration with lymphoma, solid tumours, tuberculosis
Megaloblastic anaemia
Paroxysmal nocturnal haemoglobinuria
Myelofibrosis (rare)
Haemophagocytic syndrome

Increased peripheral destruction
Splenomegaly

Table 7.2 Causes of aplastic anaemia

Primary	Secondary
Congenital (Fanconi and non-Fanconi types)	**Ionizing radiations**: accidental exposure (radiotherapy, radioactive isotopes, nuclear power stations)
Idiopathic acquired	**Chemicals**: benzene and other organic solvents, TNT, insecticides, hair dyes, chlordane, DDT
	Drugs Those that regularly cause marrow depression (e.g. busulphan, cyclophosphamide, anthracyclines, nitrosoureas) Those that occasionally or rarely cause marrow depression (e.g. chloramphenicol, sulphonamides, gold and others)
	Infection: viral hepatitis (A or non-A, non-B)

DDT, dichloro-diphenyl-trichloro-ethane; TNT, trinitrotoluene.

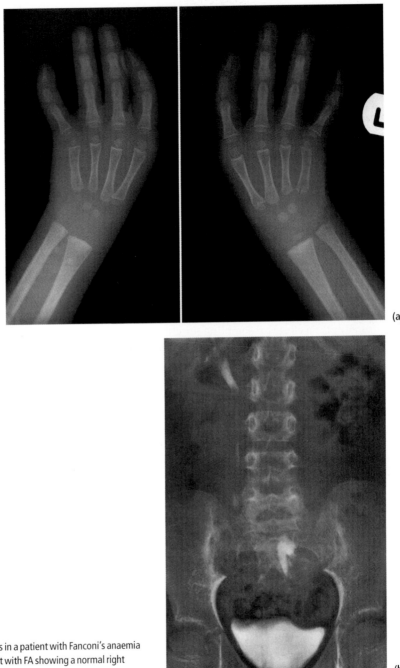

(a)

(b)

Fig. 7.2 (a) X-rays showing absent thumbs in a patient with Fanconi's anaemia (FA). (b) Intravenous pyelogram in a patient with FA showing a normal right kidney but a left kidney abnormally placed in the pelvis.

Idiopathic acquired

This is the most common type of aplastic anaemia. Although the mechanism is unknown, the favourable responses to antilymphocyte globulin (ALG) and cyclosporin A suggest that autoimmune T-cell mediated damage, possibly against functionally and structurally altered stem cells, is important.

Secondary

This is often caused by direct damage to the haemopoietic marrow by radiation or cytotoxic drugs. The antimetabolite drugs (e.g. methotrexate) and mitotic inhibitors (e.g. daunorubicin) cause only temporary aplasia but the alkylating agents, particularly busulphan, may cause chronic aplasia closely resembling the chronic idiopathic disease. Some individuals develop aplastic anaemia as a rare idiosyncratic side-effect of drugs such as chloramphenicol or gold which are not known to be cytotoxic (Table 7.2). They may also develop the disease during or within a few months of viral hepatitis (hepatitis A or non-A, non-B, non-C). Because the incidence of marrow toxicity is particularly high for chloramphenicol, this drug should be reserved for treatment of those infections which are life-threatening and for which it is the optimum antibiotic (e.g. typhoid). Chemicals such as benzene may be implicated and rarely aplastic anaemia may be the presenting feature of acute lymphoblastic or myeloid leukaemia, especially in childhood. Myelodysplasia (Chapter 13) may also present with a hypoplastic marrow.

Clinical features

The onset is at any age with a peak incidence around 30 years and a slight male predominance; it can be insidious or acute with symptoms and signs resulting from anaemia, neutropenia or thrombocytopenia. Infections, particularly of the mouth and throat, are common and generalized infections are frequently life-threatening; bruising, bleeding gums, epistaxes and menorrhagia are the most frequent haemorrhagic manifesta-

tions and the usual presenting features, often with symptoms of anaemia. The lymph nodes, liver and spleen are not enlarged.

Laboratory findings

1 Anaemia is normochromic, normocytic or macrocytic (mean corpuscular volume (MCV) often 95–110 fl). The reticulocyte count is usually extremely low in relation to the degree of anaemia.
2 Leucopenia. There is a selective fall in granulocytes, usually but not always to below $1.5 \times 10^9/l$. In severe cases, the lymphocyte count is also low. The neutrophils appear normal and their alkaline phosphatase score is high.
3 Thrombocytopenia is always present and, in severe cases, is less than $10 \times 10^9/l$.
4 There are no abnormal cells in the peripheral blood.
5 Bone marrow shows hypoplasia, with loss of haemopoietic tissue and replacement by fat which comprises over 75% of the marrow. Trephine biopsy is essential and may show patchy cellular areas in a hypocellular background (Fig. 7.1b). The main cells present are lymphocytes and plasma cells; megakaryocytes in particular are severely reduced or absent.

Diagnosis

The disease must be distinguished from other causes of pancytopenia (Table 7.1) and this is not usually difficult provided an adequate bone marrow sample is obtained. If the reticulocyte count is raised, paroxysmal nocturnal haemoglobinuria (PNH) must be excluded by the acid lysis test and testing the urine for haemosiderin. Flow-cytometric testing of red cells for CD55 and CD59 is also used. In older patients, hypoplastic myelodysplasia may show similar appearances. Qualitative abnormalities of the cells and clonal cytogenetic changes suggest myelodysplasia rather than aplastic anaemia. Some patients diagnosed as having aplastic anaemia develop PNH, myelodysplasia or acute myeloid leukaemia in subsequent years. This may occur even in patients who have responded well to immunosuppressive therapy.

Treatment

General

The cause, if known, is removed, e.g. radiation or drug therapy is discontinued. Initial management consists largely of supportive care with blood transfusions, platelet concentrates, and treatment and prevention of infection. All blood products should be filtered to reduce the risk of alloimmunization and irradiated to prevent grafting of live donor lymphocytes. In severely thrombocytopenic (platelet count $<10 \times 10^9/l$) and neutropenic (neutrophils $<0.5 \times 10^9/l$) patients, management is similar to the supportive care of patients receiving intensive chemotherapy for acute leukaemia. An antifibrinolytic agent (e.g. tranexamic acid) may be used in patients with severe prolonged thrombocytopenia. Oral antifungal agents and oral antibiotics are used prophylactically in some units to reduce the incidence of infection.

Specific

This must be tailored to the severity of the illness as well as the age of the patient and potential sibling stem cell donors. Severity is assessed by the reticulocyte, neutrophil and platelet counts and degree of marrow hypoplasia. Severe cases have a high mortality in the first 6–12 months, unless they respond to specific therapy. Less severe cases may have an acute transient course, or a chronic course with ultimate recovery, although the platelet count often remains subnormal for many years. Relapses, sometimes severe and occasionally fatal, may also occur and rarely the disease transforms into myelodysplasia, acute leukaemia or PNH (Chapter 5).

The following 'specific' treatments are used with varying success.

1 Antilymphocyte (thymocyte) globulin (ALG or ATG). This is prepared in animals (e.g. horse or rabbit) and is of benefit in about 50–60% of acquired cases. It is usually given with corticosteroids which also reduce the side-effects of ALG including the serum sickness of fever, rash and joint pains which may occur about 7 days after administration. Corticosteroids should not be used alone as they increase the risk of infection.

Typically, if there is no response to ALG after 4 months a second course may be tried, prepared from another species. Overall, up to 80% of patients respond to combined ALG, steroids and cyclosporin.

2 Cyclosporin. This is an effective agent which appears particularly valuable in combination with ALG and steroids.

3 Haemopoietic growth factors. Granulocyte–macrophage colony-stimulating factor (GM-CSF), granulocyte colony-stimulating factor (G-CSF), interleukin-3 (IL-3) and stem cell factor may produce minor responses but do not lead to sustained improvement.

4 Androgens. These are beneficial in some patients with FA and acquired aplastic anaemia although an overall improved survival in acquired aplastic anaemia has not been proven. Oxymetholone 2.5 mg/kg/day is usually tried but side-effects are marked including virilization, salt retention and liver damage with cholestatic jaundice or rarely hepatocellular carcinoma. If there is no response in 4–6 months, androgens should be stopped. If there is a response, the drug should be withdrawn gradually.

5 Stem cell transplantation. Allogeneic transplantation offers the chance of permanent cure and for aplastic anaemia conditioning with cyclophosphamide without irradiation is usually sufficient. The relative role of SCT versus immunosuppressive therapy in individual patients with aplastic anaemia is under constant review. In general terms SCT is favoured in younger patients with severe aplastic anaemia and a human leucocyte antigen (HLA) matching sibling donor. Cure rates of up to 80% are obtained. In older subjects and those with less severe disease, immunosuppression is usually tried first.

RED CELL APLASIA

Chronic form

This is a rare syndrome characterized by anaemia with normal leucocytes and platelets and grossly reduced or absent erythroblasts in the marrow

(Fig. 7.3). The congenital form is known as Diamond–Blackfan syndrome (Table 7.3) and is inherited as a recessive condition. It is associated with a varying number of somatic disorders, e.g. of the face or heart. Mutation of a gene on chromosome 19 that encodes a ribosomal protein underlies some cases.

The acquired chronic form may occur without

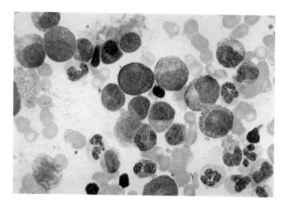

Fig. 7.3 The bone marrow in primary red cell aplasia. There is selective loss of erythropoiesis.

any obvious associated disease or precipitating factor (idiopathic), or may be seen with autoimmune diseases (especially systemic lupus erythematosus), with a thymoma, lymphoma or chronic lymphocytic leukaemia. In some cases immunosuppression with corticosteroids, cyclosporin, azathioprine or ALG is helpful. Corticosteroids are also the first line of therapy for congenital anaemia.

Androgens may also produce improvement in congenital anaemia but the side-effects on growth can be serious. If regular blood transfusions are needed iron chelation therapy will also be necessary. SCT has been carried out in some severe cases and stem cell factor is undergoing trials.

Transient form

Parvovirus B19 infects red cell precursors via the P antigen and causes a transient red cell aplasia with the rapid onset of severe anaemia in patients with pre-existing shortened red cell survival, e.g. sickle cell disease or hereditary spherocytosis (Fig. 7.4).

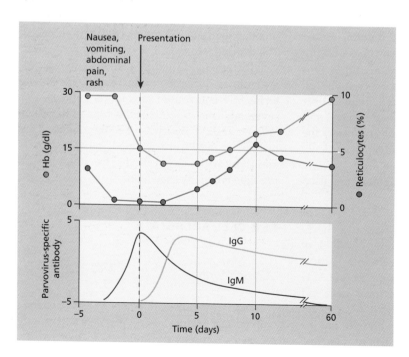

Fig. 7.4 Parvovirus infection: flow chart showing transient fall in haemoglobin and reticulocytes in a patient with hereditary spherocytosis.

Table 7.3 Classification of pure red cell aplasia

| Acute, transient | Chronic | |
	Congenital	Acquired

Parvovirus infection
Infancy and childhood
Drugs, e.g. azathioprine,
    co-trimoxazole
	Diamond–Blackfan
	    syndrome
		Idiopathic
		Associated with thymoma, lymphoma, systemic lupus erythematosus, chronic
		    B-cell lymphocytic leukaemia or large granular lymphocytic leukaemia
		    (T cell)

Transient red cell aplasia with anaemia may also occur in association with drug therapy (Table 7.3), and in normal infants or children, often with a history of a viral infection in the preceding 3 months.

CONGENITAL DYSERYTHROPOIETIC ANAEMIA

Congenital dyserythropoietic anaemias (CDAs) are a group of hereditary refractory anaemias characterized by ineffective erythropoiesis and erythroblast multinuclearity. The white cell and platelet counts are normal. The reticulocyte count is low for the degree of anaemia, despite increased marrow cellularity. The anaemia is of variable severity and is usually first noted in infancy or childhood. Iron overload may develop and splenomegaly is common. The CDAs have been classified into four types based on the degree to which megaloblastic changes, giant erythroblasts and dyserythropoietic changes are present. Type II is known as HEMPAS (hereditary erythroblast multinuclearity with a positive acidified serum lysis test). The basic lesion is a genetic defect in an enzyme N-acetylglucosaminyltransferase, which is concerned in glycosylation of several red cell membrane proteins. α-interferon has induced remission in some cases.

BIBLIOGRAPHY

Charles R.J. *et al.* (1996) The pathophysiology of pure red cell aplasia: implications for therapy. *Blood* **87**, 4831–8.

Clarke A.A. *et al.* (1998) Molecular genetics and Fanconi anaemia: new insights into old problems. *Br. J. Haematol.* **103**, 287–96.

Dokal I. (2000) The inherited bone marrow failure syndromes: Fanconi anemia, dyskeratosis congenita and Diamond Blackfan anemia. *Rev. Clin. Exp. Hematol.* **4**, 183–215.

Doney K. *et al.* for the Seattle Bone Marrow Transplant Team (1997) Primary treatment of aplastic anaemia: outcome of bone marrow transplantation and immunosuppressive therapy. *Ann. Intern. Med.* **126**, 107–15.

Faire L. *et al.* (2000) Association of complementation group and mutation type with clinical outcome in Fanconi anaemia. *Blood* **96**, 4064–70.

Freedman M.H. (2000) Diamond–Blackfan anemia. *Clin. Haematol.* **13**, 391–406.

Gordon-Smith E.C. and Marsh J.C.W. (eds) Management of acquired aplastic anemia. *Rev. Clin. Exp. Hematol.* **4**, 260–78.

Passweg J.R. *et al.* (1997) Bone marrow transplantation for severe aplastic anaemia: has outcome improved? *Blood* **90**, 858–64.

Wickramasinghe S.N. (1998) Dyserythropoiesis and congenital dyserythropoietic anaemias. *Br. J. Haematol.* **98**, 785–97.

Young N.S. (2000) *Bone Marrow Failure Syndrome.* W.B. Saunders, Philadelphia.

Young N.S. (2000) The aetiology of acquired aplastic anemia. *Rev. Clin. Exp. Hematol.* **4**, 236–59.

CHAPTER 8

Stem cell transplantation

PRINCIPLES OF STEM CELL TRANSPLANTATION

Stem cell transplantation (SCT) is a procedure which involves eliminating an individual's haemopoietic and immune system by chemotherapy and/or radiotherapy and replacing it with stem cells either from another individual or with a previously harvested portion of the individual's own haemopoietic stem cells (Fig. 8.1). The term encompasses both bone marrow transplantation (BMT) which refers to collection of stem cells from bone marrow and peripheral blood stem cell (PBSC) transplantation in which stem cells are collected from peripheral blood.

SCT may be syngeneic (from an identical twin), allogeneic (from another person) or autologous (from the patient's own stem cells) (Table 8.1).

The principal diseases for which SCTs are performed are listed in Table 8.2. However, the exact role of SCT in the management of each disease is complex and depends on factors such as disease severity and subtype, remission status, age and, for allogeneic transplantation, availability of donors.

Conditioning

Prior to infusion of haemopoietic stem cells patients receive high doses of chemotherapy, sometimes in combination with total-body irradiation (TBI) (Fig. 8.1). This procedure is called conditioning and is designed to eradicate the recipient's haemopoietic and immune system and, if present, malignancy. In addition it has a critical role in the recipients of allogeneic stem cells by suppressing the host immune system thereby preventing rejection of the 'foreign' stem cells. TBI is usually used in patients with malignant disease and is administered as a single dose or in smaller doses over several days (fractionated). The most commonly used drug is cyclophosphamide but busulphan, melphalan, cytosine arabinoside, etoposide or nitrosoureas are given in some protocols. Following the last dose of chemotherapy, at least 36 h are allowed for the elimination of the drugs from the circulation before donor stem cells are infused. The patient is given antiemetics and, if high doses of cyclophosphamide are used, the drug mesna is given to reduce the risk of haemorrhagic cystitis caused by renal excretion of cyclophosphamide metabolites. Conditioning therapy is often complicated by mucositis and patients sometimes need parenteral nutrition. Conditioning is also myelotoxic and patients also receive prophylactic oral antibiotics, antifungals and antivirals during the period of neutropenia.

Collection of stem cells

Stem cells may be collected from bone marrow or from peripheral blood.

Bone marrow collection

The donor is given a general anaesthetic and 500–1200 ml of marrow is harvested from the pelvis. The marrow is heparinized and a mononuclear cell count is taken to assess the yield which should be around 2–4×10^8 nucleated cells/kg body weight of the recipient.

Peripheral blood stem cell collection

PBSCs are taken using a cell-separator machine connected to the patient or donor via peripheral cannulae (Fig. 8.2). Blood is taken through one cannula and pumped around the machine where

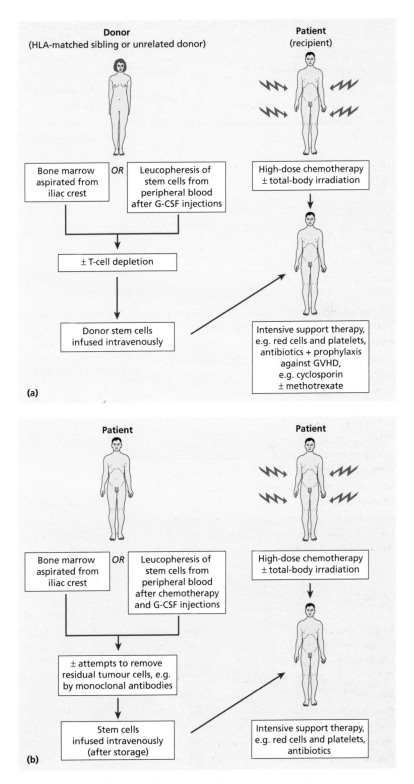

Fig. 8.1 Procedures for (a) allogeneic, and (b) autologous stem cell transplantation. G-CSF, granulocyte colony-stimulating factor; GVHD, graft-versus-host disease.

Table 8.1 Stem cell transplantation: potential donors

HLA-matching sibling		
Unrelated HLA-matching volunteer	}	Allogeneic
Umbilical cord blood		
Identical twin		Syngeneic
Self		Autologous

HLA, human leucocyte antigen.

mononuclear cells are collected by centrifugation before the red cells are returned to the patient. This continuous process may take a few hours before enough mononuclear cells are collected.

Peripheral blood normally contains a small number of circulating haemopoietic stem cells. The number is far too small to allow collection of peripheral blood stem cells on its own to be useful

Table 8.2 Stem cell transplantation: indications

Allogeneic (or syngeneic)	Autologous
Acute lymphoblastic or myeloid leukaemia	Hodgkin's disease and non-Hodgkin's lymphoma
Chronic myeloid leukaemia	Multiple myeloma
Other malignant disorders of the marrow, e.g. myelodysplasia, multiple myeloma, lymphoma, chronic lymphocytic leukaemia	Acute and chronic leukaemias
	Severe autoimmune disease
	Amyloidosis
Severe aplastic anaemia including Fanconi's anaemia	For 'gene therapy' of genetic disease, e.g. adenosine deaminase deficiency
Inherited disorders: thalassaemia major, sickle cell anaemia, immunodeficiencies, inborn errors of metabolism in the haemopoietic and mesenchymal system, e.g. osteopetrosis	
Other acquired severe marrow diseases, e.g. paroxysmal nocturnal haemoglobinuria, red cell aplasia, myelofibrosis	

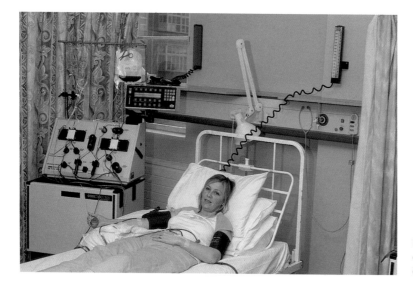

Fig. 8.2 Peripheral blood stem cell collection: a donor undergoing collection of PBSCs on a cell separator.

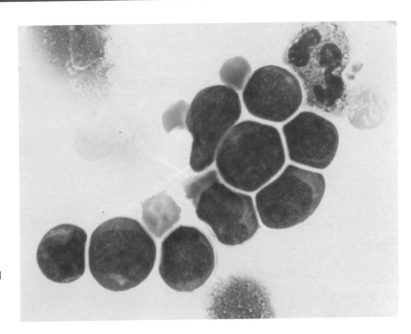

Fig. 8.3 Peripheral blood stem cell collection: enriched CD34+ cells stained by May–Grunwald–Giemsa. The cells have the appearance of small and medium-sized lymphocytes.

for transplantation. Experimental work has shown that two procedures, administration of prior chemotherapy and use of growth factors, can each increase the number of circulating progenitor cells by around 100 times. In future it is likely that stem cell populations will be expanded *in vitro*.

Chemotherapy is used in patients undergoing autologous stem cell collection but not in healthy donors. PBSCs are usually collected during the recovery phase from a cycle of chemotherapy such as $1.5\,g/m^2$ of cyclophosphamide which is incorporated into the patient's treatment programme.

The most commonly used growth factor for stem cell mobilization is granulocyte colony-stimulating factor (G-CSF) which can be given to patients or donors as a course of injections (typically $10\,\mu g/kg/day$ for 4–6 days) until the white cell count starts to rise. The donor's white cell count is monitored and CD34+ counts performed. PBSC collections are taken and, depending on the efficiency of stem cell mobilization, collections may be needed for up to 3 days. The adequacy of the collection may be assessed by:

1 CD34+ cell count using fluorescence-activated cell sorter (FACS) analysis. Generally $>2.5\times 10^6/kg$ are needed for autologous transplantation.

2 Colony assays, particularly granulocyte–macrophage colony-forming unit (CFU-GM), of which $1-5\times 10^5/kg$ would be considered adequate for transplantation.

Stem cell processing

After collection the stem cell harvest is processed. This usually involves removal of red cells and concentration of the mononuclear collection. Autologous collections may be 'purged' by chemotherapy or antibodies in an attempt to remove residual malignant cells. Allogeneic collections may be treated with antibodies to remove T cells. CD34+ stem cells may be selected from both types of harvest (Fig. 8.3). Autologous stem cells are generally frozen until needed whereas allogeneic collections are usually given to the patient immediately after processing.

Post-transplant engraftment

After a period of typically 1–3 weeks of severe pancytopenia, the first signs of successful engraftment are monocytes and neutrophils in the blood with a subsequent increase in platelet count (Fig. 8.4). A reticulocytosis also begins and natural killer (NK) cells are among the earliest

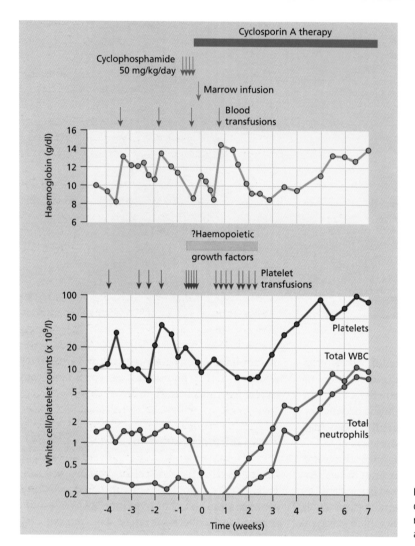

Fig. 8.4 Typical haematological chart of a patient undergoing allogeneic marrow transplantation for aplastic anaemia. WBC, white blood cells.

donor-derived lymphocytes to appear. Growth factors such as G-CSF or GM-CSF may be used to reduce the period of neutropenia. Engraftment, particularly of platelets, is usually quicker following PBSC transplantation compared to BMT.

AUTOLOGOUS STEM CELL TRANSPLANTATION

This allows the delivery of a high dose of chemotherapy with or without radiotherapy which otherwise would result in prolonged bone marrow aplasia. Stem cells are harvested

and stored before the treatment is given and are then reinfused to 'rescue' the patient from the myeloablative effects of the treatment (Fig. 8.1). A limitation with the procedure is that tumour cells contaminating the stem cell harvest may be reintroduced into the patient. Nevertheless, autografting has a major role in the treatment of haematological diseases such as lymphoma and myeloma. It also has a role in acute myeloid leukaemia and is under investigation in many other malignancies including acute lymphoblastic leukaemia, and in severe autoimmune diseases.

The major problems associated with autografting are the conditioning regime and recurrence of the original disease. Graft-versus-host disease (GVHD) is not an issue and although procedure-related mortality depends on patient selection it is generally well below 5%.

ALLOGENEIC STEM CELL TRANSPLANTATION

In this procedure stem cells harvested from another person are infused into the patient in order to reconstitute the haemopoietic and immune systems. The procedure has a significant morbidity and mortality and one of the major reasons is the immunological incompatibility, despite human leucocyte antigen (HLA) matching, between donor and patient. This may manifest as immunodeficiency, GVHD and graft failure. Paradoxically there is also a graft-versus-leukaemia (GVL) effect which probably underlies much of the success of the procedure.

Allografting would be impossible without the ability to perform HLA typing.

The human leucocyte antigen system

The short arm of chromosome 6 contains a cluster of genes known as the major histocompatibility complex (MHC) or the HLA region (Fig. 8.5). Genes in this region encode the HLA antigens and

several other molecules including complement components, tumour necrosis factor (TNF) and proteins associated with antigen processing. HLA proteins are divided into two types (Table 8.3) — class I and II. Their role is to bind intracellular peptides and 'present' these to T lymphocytes for antigen recognition. Class I molecules (HLA-A, -B and -C) present antigen to CD8+ T cells and class II molecules (HLA-DR, -DQ and -DP) present to CD4+ T cells (Chapter 10).

Class I antigens are present on most nucleated cells and on the cell surface they are associated with β_2-microglobulin. Class II antigens have a more restricted tissue distribution and comprise α and β chains both encoded by genes in the MHC locus.

The inheritance of the four loci (HLA-A, -B, -C and -DR) is closely linked, one set of loci is inherited from each parent so that there is approximately a one in four chance of two siblings having identical HLA antigens (Fig. 8.6). Crossing-over of genes during meiosis accounts for occasional unexpected disparities.

The nomenclature for HLA alleles can be confusing but is now standardized. Molecular typing has greatly increased the number of HLA alleles that have been identified and different alleles may carry the same serological antigen. As an example, alleles at the HLA-A loci are written as HLA-A*0101 to HLA-A*8001, where the first two digits after the asterisk indicate the type of the allele and

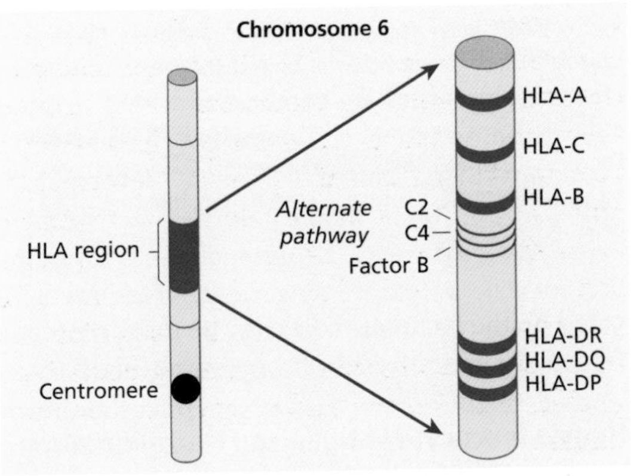

Fig. 8.5 The human leucocyte antigen (HLA) complex.

Table 8.3 The human leucocyte antigens

	Class I	Class II
Antigens	HLA-A, -B, -C	HLA-DR, -DP, -DQ
Distribution	All nucleated cells, platelets	B lymphocytes Monocytes Macrophages Activated T cells
Structure	Large polypeptide chain (MHC coded) and a β_2-microglobulin	Two polypeptide chains (α and β) both MHC coded
Interacts with	CD8 lymphocytes	CD4 lymphocytes

HLA, human leucocyte antigen; MHC, major histocompatibility complex.

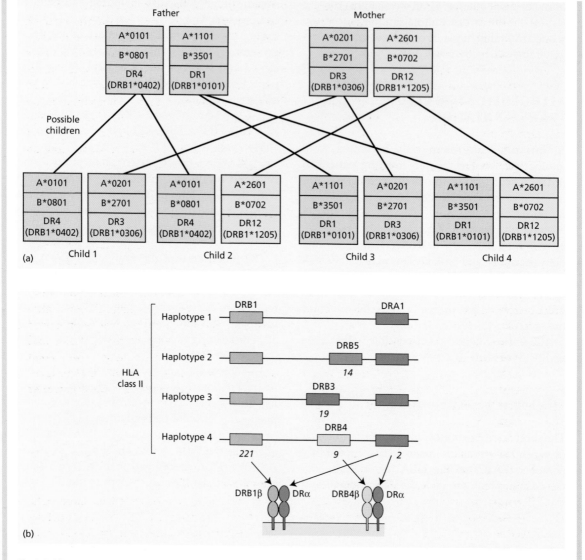

Fig. 8.6 (a) An example of the possible pattern of inheritance of the A, B and DR (DRB1) series alleles of the human leucocyte antigen (HLA) complex. (b) Molecular genetics of the HLA class II gene complex. There are four major haplotypes of MHC class II genes in the population and each individual may have up to two (one on each chromosome). The DRA1 gene codes for the DRα protein and the DRB1, DRB3, DRB4 and DRB5 genes encode DRβ chains. Expression from the DRB1 gene is higher than from the other genes. The number of alleles at each gene is shown underneath the gene in italics. Alleles at each locus have a standard nomenclature, for example the alleles at the DRB1 gene are termed DRB1*0101 to DRB1*1608. It is now known that the DR51, DR52 and DR53 antigens, which are defined by serological testing, are encoded from the DRB5, DRB4 and DRB3 genes, respectively.

the last two digits indicate the subtype. The type often corresponds to the serological antigen carried by the alleles — for example HLA-A2 for the HLA-A*0201 to HLA-A*0230 alleles. The nomenclature for the class II genes is similar but compli-

cated by the fact that there may be more than one *HLA-DRB* gene on each chromosome (Fig. 8.6b).

Human leucocyte antigen and transplantation

The MHC (called HLA in humans, H-2 in mice)

was originally identified in mice because a genetic mismatch at this region had a major influence on the outcome of organ transplants. When the HLA system was characterized this was shown to be similarly important in humans. The natural role of MHC molecules is in directing T-lymphocyte responses and the greater the MHC mismatch the more severe is the immune response between transplanted cells. HLA typing therefore remains a critical issue in donor selection for SCT.

Minor histocompatibility antigens are peptides that are presented by HLA molecules and are able to act as antigens in SCT either because they are polymorphic in the population or because they are encoded on the Y chromosome and therefore represent novel antigens when a female immune system engrafts in a male. They are likely to be important antigens in GVHD and the GVL reaction (see below).

HLA typing may be carried out by serological or molecular techniques. Serological testing involves the use of antibodies which are specific for individual HLA alleles or small families of alleles. Positivity may be detected by direct binding of a labelled antibody or by the use of complement to kill target cells that bind antibody (the two-stage lymphocytotoxicity test).

Molecular testing is done on DNA and may involve: polymerase chain reaction (PCR) amplification of individual alleles using large panels of unique oligonucleotide primers; PCR amplification of HLA subgroups followed by hybridization with allele-specific oligonucleotides; or heteroduplex analysis or restriction fragment length polymorphism (RFLP) analysis to determine haplotype patterns that are associated with specific class II alleles.

Further cellular tests of histocompatibility that are sometimes employed, particularly in unrelated donor SCT, are limiting dilution analyses of cytotoxic T-lymphocyte or helper T-lymphocyte precursors (CTLp and HTLp). A higher value indicates greater mismatch and appears to correlate with increased GVHD.

The chance of a sibling being HLA matched with a patient is theoretically 25% although, because of cross-overs during meiosis, the true incidence is slightly less. HLA matching is independent of sex or blood group. When searching for an unrelated donor for SCT the aim is to match HLA-A, -B and -DR between recipient and donor and this is then a 6/6 match. Occasionally a single mismatch (5/6) can be tolerated but it is rare to accept a donor with a greater mismatch than this. There are now over 4 million volunteer donors on the international registries and the chance of identifing a matched unrelated donor for a patient lacking an HLA identical sibling (depending on the ethnic group) is greater than 50%.

Post-transplant immunity

The marrow cellularity gradually returns to normal but the marrow reserve remains impaired for 1–2 years. There is profound immune deficiency for 3–12 months with a low level of CD4 helper cells and a raised CD8 : CD4 ratio for 6 months or more. Immune recovery is quicker after autologous and syngeneic SCT than following allogeneic SCT. Specific immunity can be enhanced post-SCT by immunizing both the donor and recipient beforehand. The patient's own blood group changes to that of the donor and antigen-specific immunity becomes that of the donor after about 60 days.

Complications (Table 8.4)

Graft-versus-host disease

This is caused by donor-derived immune cells, particularly T lymphocytes, reacting against recipient tissues. Its incidence is increased with increasing age of donor and recipient and if there is any degree of HLA mismatch between them. Without any prophylactic treatment it would be virtually inevitable in all allogeneic transplants except those from a syngeneic donor and HLA compatibility does not necessarily prevent it.

GVHD prophylaxis is usually given as cyclosporin (intravenously or orally for 6–12 months) and methotrexate (three or four injections). An alternative is to remove T cells from the donor stem cell infusion. In addition, anti-T-cell antibodies may be given to the patient. Mycophenolate mofetil is a newer immunosuppressive drug currently under trial.

Table 8.4 Complications of bone marrow transplantation

Early (usually < 100 days)	Late (usually > 100 days)
Infections, especially bacterial, fungal, herpes simplex virus, CMV	Infections, especially varicella-zoster, capsulate bacteria
Haemorrhage	Chronic GVHD (arthritis, malabsorption, hepatitis, scleroderma, sicca syndrome, lichen planus, pulmonary disease, serous effusions)
Acute GVHD (skin, liver, gut)	
Graft failure, especially aplastic anaemia	Chronic pulmonary disease
Haemorrhagic cystitis	Autoimmune disorders
Interstitial pneumonitis	Cataract
Others: veno-occlusive disease, cardiac failure	Infertility
	Second malignancies

CMV, cytomegalovirus; GVHD, graft-versus-host disease.

Table 8.5 Acute graft-versus-host disease: clinical staging (Seattle system)

Stage	Skin	Liver (bilirubin, μmol/l)	Gut (diarrhoea, l/day)
I	Rash < 25%	20–35	0.5–1.0
II	Rash 25–50%	35–80	1.0–1.5
III	Erythroderma	80–150	1.5–2.5
IV	Bullae, desquamation	> 150	> 2.5; severe pain, ileus

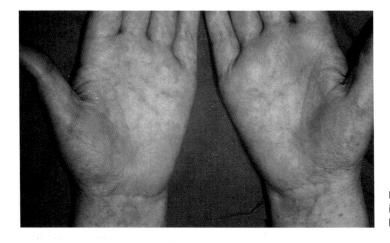

Fig. 8.7 Widespread erythematous skin rash in acute graft-versus-host disease following bone marrow transplantation.

In acute GVHD, occurring in the first 100 days, the skin, gastrointestinal tract or liver are affected (Table 8.5). The skin rash typically affects the face, palms, soles and ears but may in severe cases affect the whole body (Fig. 8.7). The diagnosis is usually confirmed by skin biopsy which shows initially single cell necrosis in the basal layer of the epidermis; lymphocyte infiltration may be scanty. Typically bilirubin and alkaline phosphatase are raised but the other hepatic enzymes are relatively

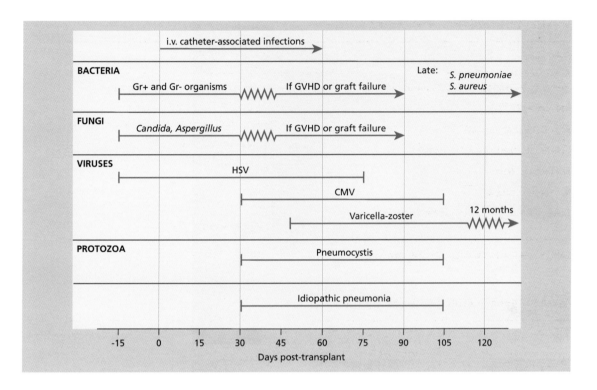

Fig. 8.8 Time sequence for development of different types of infection following allogeneic bone marrow transplantation. CMV, cytomegalovirus; Gr+, Gr−, Gram-positive or -negative; GVHD, graft-versus-host disease; HSV, herpes simplex virus.

normal. Acute GVHD is usually treated by high doses of corticosteroids which are effective in the majority of cases.

In chronic GVHD, occurring after 100 days and usually evolving from acute GVHD, these tissues are involved but also the joints and other serosal surfaces, the oral mucosa and lacrimal glands. Features of scleroderma, Sjögren's syndrome and lichen planus may develop. The immune system is impaired (including hyposplenism) with risk of infection. Malabsorption and pulmonary abnormalities are frequent. Drugs such as cyclosporin, azathioprine or corticosteroids are used although responses may be poor. Thalidomide is helpful in some cases.

Infections

In the early post-transplant period bacterial or fungal infections are frequent (Fig. 8.8). These may be reduced by reverse barrier nursing with laminar or positive pressure air flow and the use of skin and mouth antiseptics. In addition, prophylactic therapy with aciclovir, antifungal agents and oral antibiotics is often added. If a fever or other evidence of an infection occurs, broad-spectrum intravenous antibiotics are commenced immediately after blood cultures and other appropriate microbiological specimens have been taken. Failure of response to antibacterial agents is usually an indication to commence systemic antifungal therapy with amphotericin B. Fungal infections, especially *Candida* and *Aspergillus* species (Fig. 8.9), are a particular problem because of the prolonged neutropenia. Fluconazole is effective in reducing the risk of *Candida* infection and itraconazole may provide some prophylaxis against both organisms. Amphotericin B should be given relatively early for any fever of unknown origin. The standard formulation is nephrotoxic and the newer preparations such as liposomal amphotericin are better tolerated. Viral infections, par-

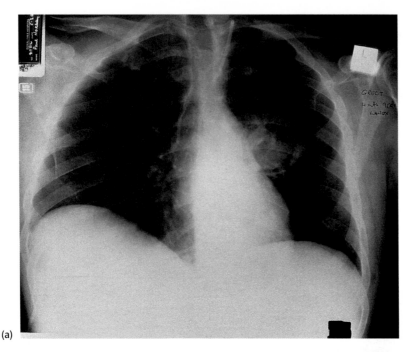

(a)

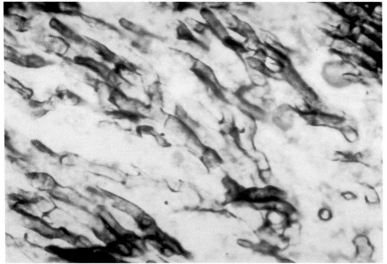

(b)

Fig. 8.9 (a) Chest radiograph showing an aspergilloma in a patient following stem cell transplantation. (b) Cytology of sputum illustrates the branching septate hyphae of *Aspergillus* (Methenamine silver stain).

ticularly with the herpes group of viruses, are frequent, with herpes simplex, cytomegalovirus (CMV) and varicella-zoster virus (VZV) occurring at different peak intervals (Fig. 8.8).

CMV presents a particular threat and is associated with a potentially fatal interstitial pneumonitis as well as with hepatitis and falling blood counts. The infection may be caused by reactiva-

tion of CMV in the recipient or a new infection transmitted by the donor. In CMV-seronegative patients with CMV-seronegative donors, CMV-negative blood products or filtered blood must be given. Aciclovir may be useful in prophylaxis. Most centres screen patients regularly for evidence of CMV reactivation following allogeneic transplantation using PCR or antibody-based tests. If these tests become positive ganciclovir may suppress the virus before disease occurs. Ganciclovir, foscarnet and CMV immunoglobulin may be tried for established CMV infection.

Pneumocystis carinii is another cause of pneumonitis but may be prevented by prophylactic co-trimoxazole. VZV infection is also frequent post-SCT but occurs later with a median onset at 4–5 months. Rarely, disseminated VZV infection occurs. Intravenous aciclovir is indicated. Epstein–Barr virus (EBV) infections and EBV-associated lymphoproliferative disease are less frequent after SCT than after solid organ transplants.

Interstitial pneumonitis

This is one of the most frequent causes of death post-SCT (Fig. 8.10). CMV is a frequent agent but other herpes viruses and *P. carinii* account for other cases; in many, no cause other than the previous radiation and chemotherapy can be implicated. Bronchoalveolar lavage or open lung biopsy may be needed to establish the diagnosis.

Blood product support

Platelet concentrates are given to maintain a count of $10 \times 10^9/l$ or more. Platelets and blood transfusions given in the post-transplant period are ir-

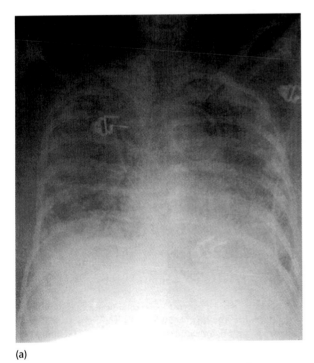

(a)

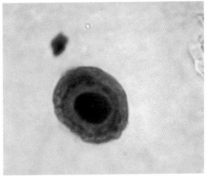

(b)

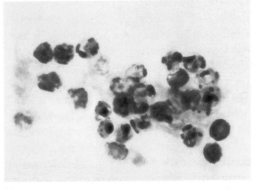

(c)

Fig. 8.10 (a) Chest radiograph showing interstitial pneumonitis following bone marrow transplantation. Widespread diffuse mottling can be seen. The patient had received total-body irradiation and had grade III graft-versus-host disease. No infective cause of the pneumonitis was identified. Possible causes include pneumocystis, cytomegalovirus, herpes, fungal infection or a combination of these. (b) Sputum cytology: intranuclear CMV inclusion body in a pulmonary cell. Papanicolaou stain. (c) *Pneumocystis carinii* in bronchial washings, Gram Weigert stain.

radiated to kill lymphocytes which might cause GVHD.

Other complications of allogeneic transplantation

Graft failure
The risk of graft failure is increased if the patient has aplastic anaemia or if T-cell depletion of donor marrow is used as GVHD prophylaxis. This suggests that donor T cells are needed to overcome host resistance to engraftment of stem cells.

Haemorrhagic cystitis
This is usually caused by the cyclophosphamide metabolite acrolein. Mesna is given in an attempt to prevent this. Certain viruses, e.g. adenovirus or polyomavirus, may also cause this complication.

Other complications
These include veno-occlusive disease of the liver (manifest as jaundice, hepatomegaly and ascites or weight gain) and cardiac failure as a result of the conditioning regime (especially high doses of cyclophosphamide) and previous chemotherapy on the heart. Haemolysis because of ABO incompatibility between donor and recipient may cause problems in the first weeks. Microangiopathic haemolytic anaemia may also occur.

Late complications
Relapse of the original disease, e.g. acute or chronic leukaemia, may occur. Bacterial infections are frequent, especially with Gram-negative or encapsulated organisms affecting the respiratory tract. VZV and fungal infections are also frequent. The use of prophylactic co-trimoxazole and oral aciclovir for 3–6 months reduces the risk of Pneumocystis and herpes infections, respectively.

Delayed pulmonary complications include restrictive pneumonitis and bronchiolitis obliterans. Endocrine complications include hypothyroidism, growth failure with low growth hormone levels in children, impaired sexual development and infertility. These endocrine problems are more marked if TBI has been used. Clinically apparent autoimmune disorders are infrequent and include myasthenia, rheumatoid

arthritis, anaemia, thrombocytopenia or neutropenia. Autoantibodies are frequently detected in the absence of symptoms. Second malignancies (especially non-Hodgkin's lymphoma) occur with a six- or sevenfold incidence compared with controls.

Other late complications include central nervous system (CNS) disturbances, neuropathies and eye problems caused by chronic GVHD (sicca syndrome) or cataracts, radiation nephritis, and late bladder problems because of previous haemorrhagic cystitis.

Umbilical cord transplants

Fetal blood contains a large number of haemopoietic stem cells and umbilical cord blood has been used successfully as a source of donor stem cells. The main problem is the small amount of blood and therefore limited number of stem cells that can be collected from each sample and this is limiting the application of umbilical blood transplants to children or small adults. Ex vivo expansion of progenitor cells may be of value in the future. The immunological properties of cord blood cells are under investigation.

Graft-versus-leukaemia effect and donor leucocyte infusions

Several observations suggest that during allogeneic transplantation the donor immune system can help to eradicate the patient's leukaemia, a phenomenon known as the GVL effect. These include the decreased relapse rate in patients with severe GVHD, the increased relapse rate in identical twins and, most convincingly, the ability of donor leucocyte infusions (DLI) to cure relapsed leukaemia in some patients. Graft-versus-lymphoma and myeloma effects also exist.

The principle of DLI is that peripheral blood mononuclear cells are collected from the original allograft donor and directly infused into the patient at the time of leukaemia relapse (Fig. 8.11). The DLI dose is counted as the number of donor T cells per kilogram of recipient—5×10^7/kg is a

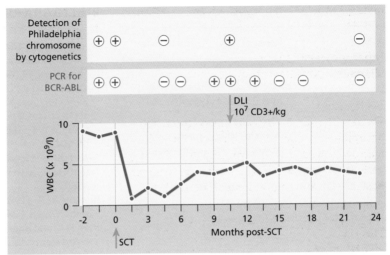

Detection of Philadelphia chromosome by cytogenetics

PCR for BCR-ABL

DLI
10^7 CD3+/kg

WBC (x 10^9/l)

Months post-SCT

SCT

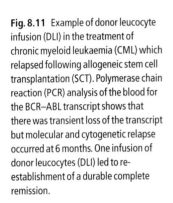

Fig. 8.11 Example of donor leucocyte infusion (DLI) in the treatment of chronic myeloid leukaemia (CML) which relapsed following allogeneic stem cell transplantation (SCT). Polymerase chain reaction (PCR) analysis of the blood for the BCR–ABL transcript shows that there was transient loss of the transcript but molecular and cytogenetic relapse occurred at 6 months. One infusion of donor leucocytes (DLI) led to re-establishment of a durable complete remission.

typical dose. There is a large difference in the outcome of various leukaemias treated by DLI. Chronic myeloid leukaemia (CML) is most sensitive whereas acute lymphoblastic leukaemia rarely responds. In CML the response to DLI is better in cases of early relapse and it is now possible to use PCR to monitor serial blood samples for evidence of recurrence of the BCR–ABL transcript before karyotypic or clinical relapse occurs. DLI can then be used in such cases of molecular relapse.

The response to DLI may take several weeks but usually results in a permanent cure. The mechanism is unclear but a T-cell mediated alloreactive immune response is likely to be a major component. The GVL effect offers the prospect of cure in several diseases in which this has not been previously possible and and is currently being investigated in association with low-intensity conditioning regimes.

Non-myeloablative transplants

In order to reduce the morbidity and mortality of allogeneic transplantation a number of low-intensity, non-myeloablative conditioning regimes are being introduced which do not completely destroy the host bone marrow. These can include fludarabine, low-dose irradiation, antilymphocyte globulin and low doses of busulphan

or cyclophosphamide. The aim in these 'minitransplants' is to use enough immunosuppression to allow donor stem cells to engraft. Donor leucocyte infusions are commonly used at a late stage in order to encourage complete donor engraftment. Such regimes rely heavily on the ability of the GVL effect to cure the underlying malignant disease (Fig. 8.11) and are likely to extend the age range and increase the treatment indications for allogeneic transplantation.

Targeted myeloablative therapy

Trials are taking place in which monoclonal antibodies directed against specific antigens, e.g. CD45, on recipient myeloid cells are attached to toxins or radioactive isotopes in an attempt to selectively eliminate the donor's haemopoietic and immune system.

Gene therapy

The ability to introduce novel genes into cells using appropriate vectors offers the opportunity to manipulate stem cells before reinfusion. Gene therapy vectors may be viral or non-viral and their relative properties are shown in Table 8.6.

Many different genes are being investigated for

Table 8.6 Vectors used in gene therapy

Vector	Properties
Viral vectors	
Retroviral	Integrate into DNA; infect variety of cell types. Only infect dividing cells
Adenovirus	Do not integrate, therefore transient expression. Infect dividing and non-dividing cells. Often provoke immune response
Adeno-associated virus	Limited integration sites
Herpes virus	Can carry large genes; no integration; can infect resting cells
Non-viral vectors	
Liposomal	Relatively simple and cheap to make
Naked DNA	Low efficiency of entry into cells
Ballistic (gene gun)	

possible expression in cells such as haemopoietic stem cells and specific differentiated populations such as T lymphocytes. These include genes to correct specific inborn errors of metabolism, genes such as neomycin to 'mark' specific populations for subsequent analysis, 'suicide' genes such as thymidine kinase that render cells susceptible to ganciclovir and resistance genes to protect normal stem cells from high-dose chemotherapy. Unfortunately haemopoietic stem cells are difficult to transfect because they are relatively rare and few are in cell cycle at any particular time. Therefore the sustained correction of metabolic disorders following the introduction of transduced autologous haemopoietic progenitors remains a difficult problem.

BIBLIOGRAPHY

Appelbaum E.F. (1999) Choosing the source of stem cells for allogeneic transplantation: no longer a peripheral issue. *Blood* **94**, 381–3.

Arkinson K. (ed.) (2000) *Clinical Bone Marrow and Blood Stem Cell Transplantation*, 2nd edn. Cambridge University Press, Cambridge.

Bensinger W.I., Martin P.J., Storer B. *et al.* (2001) Transplantation of bone marrow as compared with peripheral-blood cells from HLA-identical relatives in patients with hematologic cancers. *N. Engl. J. Med.* **344**, 175–81.

Brenner M.K. (1996) Gene transfer to haematopoietic cells. *N. Engl. J. Med.* **335**, 337–9.

Byrne J.L. and Russell N.H. (1999) The use of peripheral blood stem cells for allografting. *CME Bull. Haematol.* **2**, 90–3.

Craddock C. (2000) Haemopoietic stem cell transplantation: recent progress and future promise. *Lancet Oncol.* **1**, 227–34.

Gluckman E., Rocha V. and Chastang C. (1999) Cord blood stem-cell transplantation. *Clin. Haematol.* **12**, 279–92.

Gratwohl A. *et al.* (1996) Indications for haemopoietic precursor cell transplants in Europe. *Br. J. Haematol.* **92**, 35–43.

Ho A.D., Haas R. and Champlin R.E. (eds) (2000) *Hematopoietic Stem Cell Transplantation*. Marcel Dekker, New York.

Klein J. and Sato A. (2000) The HLA system. *N. Engl. J. Med.* **343**(1), 702–9.

McSweeny P. and Storb R. (1999) Establishing mixed chimerism with immunosuppressive, minimally myelosuppressive conditioning: preclinical and clinical studies. In: *Hematology*. American Society of Hematology Education Program Book, pp. 396–404.

Rubinstein P. and Stevens C.E. (2000) Placental blood for bone marrow replacement: the New York Blood Center's program and clinical results. *Clin. Haematol.* **13**, 565–84.

Thomas E.D., Blume K.G. and Forman S.J. (eds) (1999) *Hematopoietic Cell Transplantation*, 2nd edn. Blackwell Science, Boston.

The white cells 1: granulocytes, monocytes and their benign disorders

The white blood cells (leucocytes) may be divided into two broad groups—the phagocytes and the immunocytes. Granulocytes, which include three types of cell—neutrophils (polymorphs), eosinophils and basophils—together with monocytes comprise the phagocytes. Their normal development and function, and benign disorders of white blood cells, are dealt with in this chapter. Only mature phagocytic cells and lymphocytes are found in normal peripheral blood (Table 9.1 and Fig. 9.1). The lymphocytes, their precursor cells and plasma cells, which make up the immunocyte population, are considered in Chapter 10.

The function of phagocytes and immunocytes in protecting the body against infection is closely connected with two soluble protein systems of the body, immunoglobulins and complement. These proteins, which may also be involved in blood cell destruction in a number of diseases, are discussed together with the lymphocytes in Chapter 10.

GRANULOCYTES

Neutrophil (polymorph)

This cell has a characteristic dense nucleus consisting of between two and five lobes, and a pale cytoplasm with an irregular outline containing many fine pink–blue (azurophilic) or grey–blue granules (Fig. 9.1a). The granules are divided into primary, which appear at the promyelocyte stage, and secondary (specific) which appear at the myelocyte stage and predominate in the mature neutrophil. Both types of granule are lysosomal

in origin; the primary contains myeloperoxidase, acid phosphatase and other acid hydrolases, the secondary contains collagenase, lactoferrin and lysozyme (Fig. 9.6). The lifespan of neutrophils in the blood is only about 10 h.

Neutrophil precursors

These do not normally appear in normal peripheral blood but are present in the marrow (Fig. 9.2). The earliest recognizable precursor is the myeloblast, a cell of variable size which has a large nucleus with fine chromatin and usually two to five nucleoli. The cytoplasm is basophilic and no cytoplasmic granules are present. The normal bone marrow contains up to 4% of myeloblasts. Myeloblasts give rise by cell division to promyelocytes which are slightly larger cells and have developed primary granules in the cytoplasm. These cells then produce myelocytes which have specific or secondary granules. The nuclear chromatin is now more condensed and nucleoli are not visible. Separate myelocytes of the neutrophil, eosinophil and basophil series can be indentified. The myelocytes give rise by cell division to metamyelocytes, non-dividing cells, which have an indented or horseshoe-shaped nucleus and a cytoplasm filled with primary and secondary granules. Neutrophil forms between the metamyelocyte and fully mature neutrophil are termed 'band', 'stab' or 'juvenile'. These cells may occur in normal peripheral blood. They do not contain the clear fine filamentous distinction between nuclear lobes which is seen in mature neutrophils.

Table 9.1 White cells: normal blood counts

Adults	Blood count	Children	Blood count
Total leucocytes	$4.00–11.0 \times 10^9/l$*	*Total leucocytes*	
Neutrophils	$2.5–7.5 \times 10^9/l$*	Neonates	$10.0–25.0 \times 10^9/l$
Eosinophils	$0.04–0.4 \times 10^9/l$	1 year	$6.0–18.0 \times 10^9/l$
Monocytes	$0.2–0.8 \times 10^9/l$	4–7 years	$6.0–15.0 \times 10^9/l$
Basophils	$0.01–0.1 \times 10^9/l$	8–12 years	$4.5–13.5 \times 10^9/l$
Lymphocytes	$1.5–3.5 \times 10^9/l$		

* Normal black and Middle Eastern subjects may have lower counts. In normal pregnancy the upper limits are: total leucocytes $14.5 \times 10^9/l$, neutrophils $11 \times 10^9/l$.

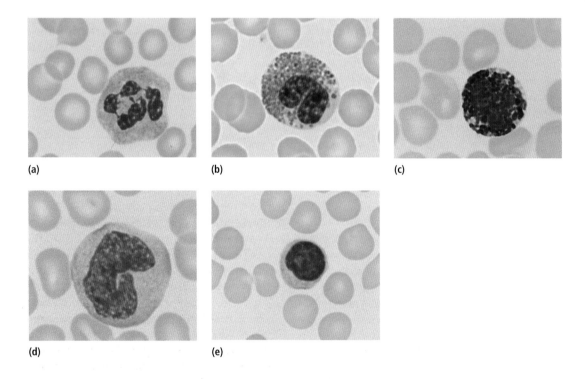

(a)   (b)   (c)

(d)   (e)

Fig. 9.1 White blood cells (leucocytes): (a) neutrophil (polymorph); (b) eosinophil; (c) basophil; (d) monocyte; (e) lymphocyte.

Monocytes

These are usually larger than other peripheral blood leucocytes and possess a large central oval or indented nucleus with clumped chromatin (Fig. 9.1d). The abundant cytoplasm stains blue and contains many fine vacuoles, giving a ground-glass appearance. Cytoplasmic granules are also often present. The monocyte precursors in the marrow (monoblasts and promonocytes) are difficult to distinguish from myeloblasts and monocytes.

Eosinophils

These cells are similar to neutrophils, except that the cytoplasmic granules are coarser and more deeply red staining and there are rarely more than three nuclear lobes (Fig. 9.1b). Eosinophil myelocytes can be recognized but earlier stages are in-

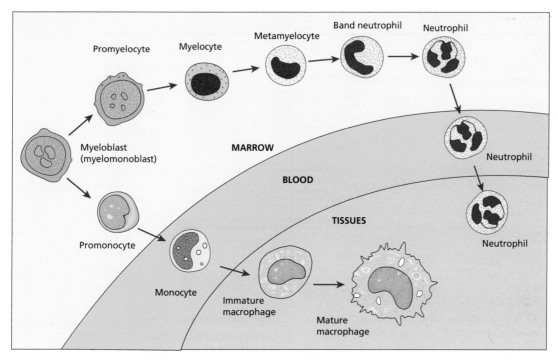

Fig. 9.2 The formation of the neutrophil and monocyte phagocytes. Eosinophils and basophils are also formed in the marrow in a process similar to that for neutrophils.

distinguishable from neutrophil precursors. The blood transit time for eosinophils is longer than for neutrophils. They enter inflammatory exudates and have a special role in allergic responses, defence against parasites and removal of fibrin formed during inflammation.

Basophils

These are only occasionally seen in normal peripheral blood. They have many dark cytoplasmic granules which overlie the nucleus and contain heparin and histamine (Fig. 9.1c). In the tissues they become mast cells. They have immunoglobulin E (IgE) attachment sites and their degranulation is associated with histamine release.

GRANULOPOIESIS

The blood granulocytes and monocytes are formed in the bone marrow from a common precursor cell (see Fig. 1.2). In the granulopoietic se-

ries progenitor cells, myeloblasts, promyelocytes and myelocytes form a proliferative or mitotic pool of cells while the metamyelocytes, band and segmented granulocytes, make up a postmitotic maturation compartment (Fig. 9.3). Large numbers of band and segmented neutrophils are held in the marrow as a 'reserve pool' or storage compartment. The bone marrow normally contains more myeloid cells than erythroid cells in the ratio of 2:1 to 12:1, the largest proportion being neutrophils and metamyelocytes. In the stable or normal state, the bone marrow storage compartment contains 10–15 times the number of granulocytes found in the peripheral blood. Following their release from the bone marrow, granulocytes spend only 6–10 h in the circulation before moving into the tissues where they perform their phagocytic function. In the bloodstream there are two pools usually of about equal size—the circulating pool (included in the blood count) and the marginating pool (not included in the blood count). It has been estimated that they spend on aver-

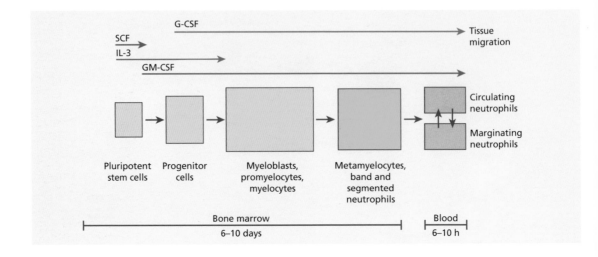

Fig. 9.3 Neutrophil kinetics. CSF, colony-stimulating factor; G, granulocyte; IL, interleukin; M, monocyte; SCF, stem cell factor.

age 4–5 days in the tissues before they are destroyed during defensive action or as the result of senescence.

Control of granulopoiesis: myeloid growth factors

The granulocyte series arises from bone marrow progenitor cells which are increasingly specialized. Many growth factors are involved in this maturation process including interleukin-1 (IL-1), IL-3, IL-5 (for eosinophils), IL-6, IL-11, granulocyte–macrophage colony-stimulating factor (GM-CSF), granulocyte CSF (G-CSF) and monocyte CSF (M-CSF) (see Fig. 1.6). The growth factors stimulate proliferation and differentiation and also affect the function of the mature cells on which they act (e.g. phagocytosis, superoxide generation and cytotoxicity in the case of neutrophils; phagocytosis, cytotoxicity and production of other cytokines by monocytes).

Increased granulocyte and monocyte production in response to an infection is induced by increased production of growth factors from stromal cells and T lymphocytes, stimulated by endotoxin, IL-1 or tumour necrosis factor (TNF) (see Fig. 1.5).

CLINICAL APPLICATIONS OF MYELOID GROWTH FACTORS

Clinical administration of G-CSF intravenously or subcutaneously has been found to produce a rise of neutrophils whereas administration of GM-CSF increases neutrophils, eosinophils and monocytes. These agents have become widely used in clinical practice and some of the indications are as follows.

Postchemotherapy, radiotherapy or bone marrow transplantation In these situations GM-CSF and G-CSF accelerate haemopoietic recovery and shorten the period of neutropenia (Fig. 9.4). This may translate into a reduction in length of time in hospital, antibiotic usage and frequency of infection but periods of extreme neutropenia after intensive chemotherapy cannot be prevented or shortened.

Acute myeloid leukaemia G-CSF is used in some protocols to stimulate myeloid blast cells into cell cycle enhancing their sensitivity to chemotherapy.

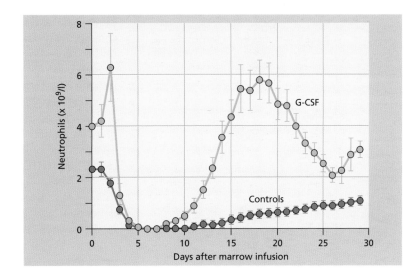

Fig. 9.4 Typical effect of granulocyte colony-stimulating factor (G-CSF) on recovery of neutrophils following autologous bone marrow transplantation.

Myelodysplasia Granulocyte growth factors have been given alone or in conjunction with agents such as erythropoietin in an attempt to improve bone marrow function without accelerating leukaemic transformation.

Severe neutropenia Both congenital and acquired neutropenia including cyclical and drug-induced neutropenia have been found to respond well to G-CSF.

Severe infection GM-CSF and G-CSF have been used as adjuvants to antimicrobial therapy and the former may be particularly valuable in invasive fungal disease.

Peripheral blood stem cell transplants G-CSF is used to increase the number of circulating multipotent progenitors, improving the harvest of sufficient peripheral blood stem cells for transplantation.

MONOCYTES

Monocytes spend only a short time in the marrow and, after circulating for 20–40 h, leave the blood to enter the tissues where they mature and carry out their principal functions. Their extravascular lifespan after their transformation to macrophages may be as long as several months or even

years. They may assume specific functions in different tissues, e.g. skin, gut, liver, etc. (Fig. 9.5). One particularly important lineage is that of dendritic cells which are involved in antigen presentation to T cells (Chapter 10). GM-CSF and M-CSF are involved in their production and activation.

DISORDERS OF NEUTROPHIL AND MONOCYTE FUNCTION

The normal function of neutrophils and monocytes may be divided into three phases.

Chemotaxis (cell mobilization and migration) The phagocyte is attracted to bacteria or the site of inflammation by chemotactic substances released from damaged tissues or by complement components and also by the interaction of leucocyte adhesion molecules with ligands on the damaged tissues.

Phagocytosis The foreign material (bacteria, fungi, etc.) or dead or damaged cells of the host are phagocytosed (Fig. 9.6). Recognition of a foreign particle is aided by opsonization with immunoglobulin or complement because both neutrophils and monocytes have Fc and C3b receptors. Opsonization of normal body cells (e.g. red cells or platelets) also makes them

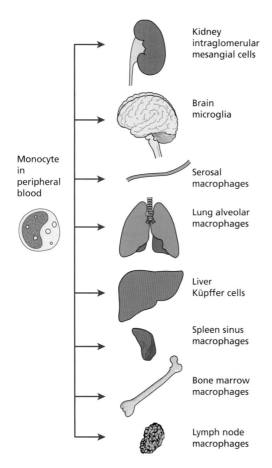

Kidney intraglomerular mesangial cells

Brain microglia

Monocyte in peripheral blood

Serosal macrophages

Lung alveolar macrophages

Liver Küpffer cells

Spleen sinus macrophages

Bone marrow macrophages

Lymph node macrophages

Fig. 9.5 Reticuloendothelial system: distribution of macrophages.

liable to destruction by macrophages of the reticuloendothelial system, as in autoimmune haemolysis, idiopathic (autoimmune) thrombocytopenic purpura or many of the drug-induced cytopenias.

Macrophages have a central role in antigen presentation — processing and presenting foreign antigens on human leucocyte antigen (HLA) molecules to the immune system. They also secrete a large number of growth factors which regulate inflammation and immune responses.

Chemokines are chemotactic cytokines of which there are two main classes — CXC (α) chemokines, small (8–10 000 MW) pro-inflammatory cytokines which mainly act on neutrophils, and CC (β) chemokines such as macrophage inflammatory protein (MIP)-1α and RANTES which act on monocytes, basophils, eosinophils and natural

killer (NK) cells. Chemokines may be produced constitutively and control lymphocyte traffic under physiological conditions; inflammatory chemokines are induced or up-regulated by inflammatory stimuli. They bind to and activate cells via chemokine receptors and play an important part in recruiting appropriate cells to the sites of inflammation. Chemokine receptors have been identified as coreceptors for human immunodeficiency virus (HIV) entry into cells (p. 141).

Killing and digestion This occurs by oxygen-dependent and oxygen-independent pathways. In the oxygen-dependent reactions, superoxide (O_2^-), hydrogen peroxide (H_2O_2) and other activated oxygen (O_2) species, are generated from O_2 and reduced nicotinamide adenine dinucleotide phosphate (NADPH). In neutrophils, H_2O_2 reacts with myeloperoxidase and intracellular halide to kill bacteria; activated oxygen may also be involved. The non-oxidative microbicidal mechanism involves a fall in pH within phagocytic vacuoles into which lysosomal enzymes are released. An additional factor, lactoferrin — an iron-binding protein present in neutrophil granules — is bacteriostatic by depriving bacteria of iron (Fig. 9.6).

Defects of phagocytic cell function

Chemotaxis These defects occur in rare congenital abnormalities (e.g. 'lazy leucocyte' syndrome) and in more common acquired abnormalities either of the environment, e.g. corticosteroid therapy, or of the leucocytes themselves, e.g. in acute or chronic myeloid leukaemia, myelodysplasia and the myeloproliferative syndromes.

Phagocytosis These defects usually arise because of a lack of opsonization which may be caused by congenital or acquired causes of hypogammaglobulinaemia or lack of complement components.

Killing This abnormality is clearly illustrated by the rare X-linked or autosomal recessive chronic granulomatous disease which results from abnormal leucocyte oxidative metabolism. There is an

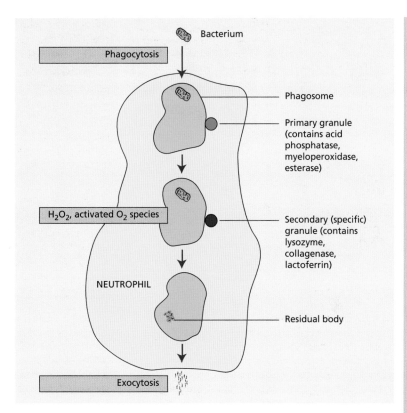

Fig. 9.6 Phagocytosis and bacterial destruction. On entering the neutrophil, the bacterium is surrounded by an invaginated surface membrane and fuses with a primary lysosome to form a phagosome. Enzymes from the lysosome attack the bacterium. Secondary granules also fuse with the phagosomes, and new enzymes from these granules including lactoferrin attack the organism. Various types of activated oxygen, generated by glucose metabolism, also help to kill bacteria. Undigested residual bacterial products are excreted by exocytosis.

abnormality affecting different elements of the respiratory burst oxidase or its activating mechanism. The patients have recurring infections, usually bacterial but sometimes fungal, which present in infancy or early childhood in most cases.

Other rare congenital abnormalities may also result in defects of bacterial killing, e.g. myeloperoxidase deficiency and the Chediak–Higashi syndrome (see below). Acute or chronic myeloid leukaemia and myelodysplastic syndromes may also be associated with defective killing of ingested microorganisms.

Benign disorders

A number of the hereditary conditions may give rise to changes in granulocyte morphology.

Pelger–Hüet anomaly In this uncommon condition bilobed neutrophils are found in the peripheral blood. Occasional unsegmented neu-

trophils are also seen. Inheritance is autosomal dominant.

May–Hegglin anomaly In this rare condition the neutrophils contain basophilic inclusions of RNA (resembling Doehle bodies) in the cytoplasm. There is an associated mild thrombocytopenia with giant platelets. Inheritance is autosomal dominant.

Other rare disorders In contrast to these two relatively benign anomalies, other rare congenital leucocyte disorders may be associated with severe disease. The Chediak–Higashi syndrome is inherited in an autosomal recessive manner, and there are giant granules in the neutrophils, eosinophils, monocytes and lymphocytes accompanied by neutropenia, thrombocytopenia and marked hepatosplenomegaly. Abnormal leucocyte granulation or vacuolation is also seen in patients with rare mucopolysaccharide disorders, e.g. Hurler's syndrome.

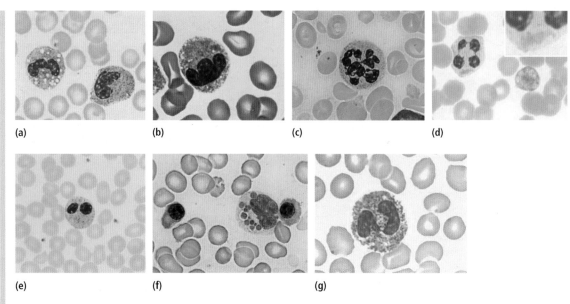

(a)   (b)   (c)   (d)

(e)   (f)   (g)

Fig. 9.7 Abnormal white blood cells. (a) Neutrophil leucocytosis: toxic changes shown by the presence of red–purple granules in the band-form neutrophils. (b) Neutrophil leucocytosis: a Doehle body can be seen in the cytoplasm of the neutrophil. (c) Megaloblastic anaemia: hypersegmented oversized neutrophil in peripheral blood. (d) May–Hegglin anomaly: the neutrophils contain basophilic inclusions 2–5 μm in diameter; there is an associated mild thrombocytopenia with giant platelets. (e) Pelger–Hüet anomaly: coarse clumping of the chromatin in pince-nez configuration. (f) Chediak–Higashi syndrome: bizarre giant granules in the cytoplasm of a monocyte. (g) Alder's anomaly: coarse violet granules in the cytoplasm of a neutrophil.

Common morphological abnormalities Figure 9.7 shows some of the more common abnormalities of neutrophil morphology which can be seen in peripheral blood. Hypersegmented forms occur in megaloblastic anaemia, Doehle bodies and toxic changes in infection. The 'drumstick' appears on the nucleus of a proportion of the neutrophils in normal females and is caused by the presence of two X chromosomes. Pelger cells are seen in the benign congenital abnormality but also in patients with acute myeloid leukaemia or myelodysplasia.

Table 9.2 Causes of neutrophil leucocytosis

Bacterial infections (especially pyogenic bacterial, localized or generalized)
Inflammation and tissue necrosis, e.g. myositis, vasculitis, cardiac infarct, trauma
Metabolic disorders, e.g. uraemia, eclampsia, acidosis, gout
Neoplasms of all types, e.g. carcinoma, lymphoma, melanoma
Acute haemorrhage or haemolysis
Corticosteroid therapy (inhibits margination)
Myeloproliferative disease, e.g. chronic myeloid leukaemia, polycythaemia vera, myelosclerosis
Treatment with myeloid growth factors, e.g. G-CSF, GM-CSF

G- and GM-CSF, granulocyte and granulocyte–macrophage colony-stimulating factor.

CAUSES OF LEUCOCYTOSIS AND MONOCYTOSIS

Neutrophil leucocytosis

An increase in circulating neutrophils to levels greater than 7.5×10^9/l is one of the most frequently observed blood count changes. The causes of neutrophil leucocytosis are given in Table 9.2. Neutrophil leucocytosis is sometimes accompanied by fever as a result of the release of leucocyte pyrogens. Other characteristic features of reactive neutrophilia may include: (a) a 'shift to the left' in the peripheral blood differential white cell count, i.e. an increase in the number of band forms and the occasional presence of more primitive cells such as metamyelocytes and myelocytes; (b) the presence of cytoplasmic toxic granulation and Doehle bodies (Fig. 9.7a, b); and (c) an elevated neutrophil alkaline phosphatase (NAP) score. For this the strength of the staining of each of 100 neutrophils is scored between 0 and 4. The maximum score is therefore 400; a normal score is between 20 and 100.

The leukaemoid reaction

The leukaemoid reaction is a reactive and excessive leucocytosis usually characterized by the presence of immature cells (e.g. myeloblasts, promyelocytes and myelocytes) in the peripheral blood. Occasionally lymphocytic reactions occur. Associated disorders include severe or chronic infections, severe haemolysis or metastatic cancer. Leukaemoid reactions are often particularly marked in children. Granulocyte changes such as toxic granulation and Doehle bodies and a high NAP score help to differentiate the leukaemoid reaction from chronic myeloid leukaemia (in which the NAP score is low).

Eosinophilic leucocytosis (eosinophilia)

The causes of an increase in blood eosinophils (Fig. 9.8) above $0.4 \times 10^9/l$ are listed in Table 9.3. Sometimes no underlying cause is found and if the eosinophil count is elevated ($> 1.5 \times 10^9/l$) for over 6 months and associated with tissue damage then the hypereosinophilic syndrome is diagnosed.

Table 9.3 Causes of eosinophilia

Allergic diseases, especially hypersensitivity of the atopic type, e.g. bronchial asthma, hay fever, urticaria and food sensitivity
Parasitic diseases, e.g. amoebiasis, hookworm, ascariasis, tapeworm infestation, filariasis, schistosomiasis and trichinosis
Recovery from acute infection
Certain skin diseases, e.g. psoriasis, pemphigus and dermatitis herpetiformis
Pulmonary eosinophilia and the hypereosinophilic syndrome
Drug sensitivity
Polyarteritis nodosa
Hodgkin's disease and some other tumours
Metastatic malignancy with tumour necrosis
Eosinophilic leukaemia (rare)
Treatment with GM-CSF

GM-CSF, granulocyte–macrophage colony-stimulating factor.

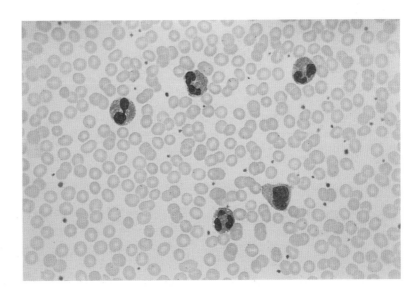

Fig. 9.8 Eosinophilia.

The heart valves, skin and lungs may be affected and treatment is usually with steroids or cytotoxic drugs. Increased production of cytokines such as IL-5 from CD4+ T cells may underlie a proportion of cases.

Basophil leucocytosis (basophilia)

An increase in blood basophils above $0.1 \times 10^9/l$ is uncommon. The usual cause is a myeloproliferative disorder such as chronic myeloid leukaemia or polycythaemia vera. Reactive basophil increases are sometimes seen in myxoedema, during smallpox or chickenpox infection, and in ulcerative colitis.

Monocytosis

A rise in blood monocyte count above $0.8 \times 10^9/l$ is infrequent. The conditions listed in Table 9.4 may be responsible.

CONGENITAL NEUTROPENIA

The lower limit of the normal neutrophil count is $2.5 \times 10^9/l$ except in black people and in the Middle East where $1.5 \times 10^9/l$ is normal. When the absolute neutrophil level falls below $0.5 \times 10^9/l$ the patient is likely to have recurrent infections and when the count falls to less than $0.2 \times 10^9/l$ the risks are very serious, particularly if there is also a

Table 9.4 Causes of monocytosis

Chronic bacterial infections: tuberculosis, brucellosis, bacterial endocarditis, typhoid
Protozoan infections
Chronic neutropenia
Hodgkin's disease and other malignancies
Myelodysplasia (especially chronic myelomonocytic leukaemia)
Treatment with GM-CSF or M-CSF

GM- and M-CSF, granulocyte–macrophage and macrophage colony-stimulating factor.

functional defect. Neutropenia may be selective or part of a general pancytopenia (Table 9.5).

Congenital neutropenia

Kostmann's syndrome is an autosomal recessive disease presenting in the first year of life with life-threatening infections. Most cases are due to mutation of the gene coding for neutrophil elastase. G-CSF produces a clinical response although marrow fibrosis and acute myeloid leukaemia may supervene.

Table 9.5 Causes of neutropenia

Selective neutropenia
Congenital
  Kostmann's syndrome

Acquired

Drug-induced
  Anti-inflammatory drugs (aminopyrine, phenylbutazone)
  Antibacterial drugs (chloramphenicol, co-trimoxazole, sulfasalazine, salazopyrine, imipenem)
  Anticonvulsants (phenytoin, carbamazepine)
  Antithyroids (carbimazole)
  Hypoglycaemics (tolbutamide)
  Phenothiazines (chlorpromazine, thioridazine)
  Psychotropics and antidepressants (clozapine, mianserin, imipramine)
  Bark derivatives, e.g. paclitaxil
  Miscellaneous (gold, penicillamine, mepacrine, amodiaquine, ticlopidine, frusemide, etc.)

Benign (racial or familial)

Cyclical

Immune
  Autoimmune
  Systemic lupus erythematosus
  Felty's syndrome
  Hypersensitivity and anaphylaxis

Large granular lymphocytic leukaemia (p. 197)

Infections
  Viral, e.g. hepatitis, influenza, HIV
  Fulminant bacterial infection, e.g. typhoid, miliary tuberculosis

Part of general pancytopenia (see Table 7.1)
Bone marrow failure

Splenomegaly

HIV, human immunodeficiency virus.

Drug-induced neutropenia

A large number of drugs have been implicated (Table 9.5) and may induce neutropenia either by direct toxicity or immune-mediated damage.

Cyclical neutropenia

This is a rare syndrome with 3–4-week periodicity. Severe but temporary neutropenia occurs. Monocytes tend to rise as the neutrophils fall. Mutation of the gene for neutrophil elastase underlies some cases.

Autoimmune neutropenia

In some cases of chronic neutropenia an autoimmune mechanism can be demonstrated. The antibody may be directed against one of the neutrophil-specific antigens (NA, NB, etc.).

Idiopathic benign neutropenia

An increase in the marginating fraction of blood neutrophils and a corresponding reduction in the circulating fraction is one cause of benign neutropenia. Many normal Africans and other races, especially in the Middle East, have a low peripheral blood neutrophil count. These subjects have no increased susceptibility to infection and the bone marrow appears normal although there is diminished neutrophil production.

Clinical features

Severe neutropenia is particularly associated with infections of the mouth and throat. Painful and often intractable ulceration may occur at these sites (Fig. 9.9), on the skin or at the anus. Septicaemia rapidly supervenes. Organisms carried as commensals by normal individuals, such as *Staphylococcus epidermidis* or Gram-negative organisms in the bowel, may become pathogens. Other features of infections associated with severe neutropenia are described on p. 170.

Diagnosis

Bone marrow examination is useful in determining the level of damage in granulopoiesis, i.e.

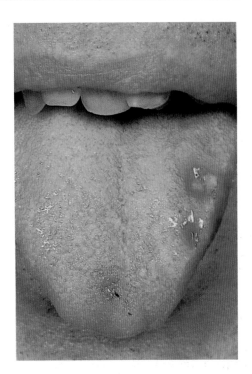

Fig. 9.9 Ulceration of the tongue in severe neutropenia.

whether there is reduction in early precursors or whether there is reduction only of circulating and marrow neutrophils with late precursors remaining in the marrow. Marrow aspiration and trephine biopsy may also provide evidence of leukaemia, myelodysplasia or other infiltration.

Management

The treatment of patients with acute severe neutropenia is described on p. 170. In many patients with drug-induced neutropenia spontaneous recovery occurs within 1 or 2 weeks after stopping the drug. Patients with chronic neutropenia have recurrent infections which are mainly bacterial in origin although fungal and viral infections (especially herpes) also occur. Early recognition and vigorous treatment with antibiotics, antifungal or antiviral agents, as appropriate, is essential. Prophylactic antibacterial agents, e.g. oral co-trimoxazole or ciprofloxacin and colistin, and antifungal agents, e.g. oral amphotericin and fluconazole or itraconazole, may be of value in reducing the incidence and severity of infections caused by severe neutropenia. The haemopoietic growth factor G-CSF may be used to stimulate neutrophil production and is effective in a variety of benign chronic neutropenic states. Corticosteroid therapy or splenectomy has been associated with good results in some patients with autoimmune neutropenia. Conversely, corticosteroids impair neutrophil function and should not be used indiscriminately in patients with neutropenia.

HISTIOCYTIC DISORDERS

A classification of the histiocytic disorders is given in Table 9.6.

Dendritic cells

There are specialized antigen-presenting cells found mainly in the skin, lymph nodes, spleen and thymus. They comprise myeloid- and monocyte-derived cells including Langerhans' cells and

a lymphocyte-derived subset. Their primary role is in antigen presentation to T and B lymphocytes (p. 133).

Langerhans' cell histiocytosis

Langerhans' cell histiocytosis (LCH) includes diseases previously called histiocytosis X, Letterer–Siwe disease, Hand–Schuller–Christian disease and eosinophilic granuloma. The disease may be single or multisystem. The multisystem disease affects children in the first 3 years of life with hepatosplenomegaly, lymphadenopathy and

Table 9.6 Classification of histiocytic disorders

Dendritic cell-related
Langerhans' cell histiocytosis

Macrophage-related
Haemophagocytic lymphohistiocytosis
   primary (genetic)
   secondary

Malignancies
AML FAB type M4 and M5 (see p. 163)
Chronic myelomonocytic leukaemia (see p. 186)
Dendritic cell and macrophage-related sarcomas

Fig. 9.10 Haemophagocytic lymphohistiocytosis: bone marrow aspirates showing histiocytes that have ingested red cells, erythroblasts and neutrophils.

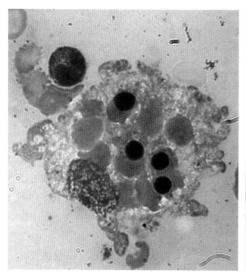
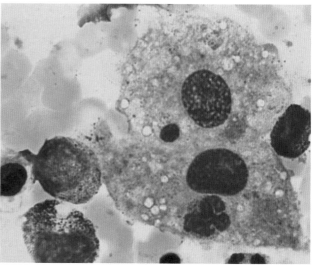

eczematous skin symptoms. Localized lesions may occur especially in the skull, ribs and long bones, the posterior pituitary causing diabetes insipidus, the central nervous system, gastrointestinal tract and lungs. The lesions include Langerhans' cells (characterized by the presence of tennis racquet-shaped Birbeck granules in electron-microscopy sections), eosinophils, lymphocytes, neutrophils and macrophages.

Haemophagocytic lymphohistiocytosis (haemophagocytic syndrome)

This is a rare recessively inherited or more frequently acquired disease, usually precipitated by a viral, bacterial or fungal infection or occuring in association with tumours. It presents with fever and pancytopenia, often with splenomegaly and liver dysfunction. There are increased numbers of histiocytes in the bone marrow which ingest red cells, white cells and platelets (Fig. 9.10). Clinical features are fever, pancytopenia and multi-organ dysfunction. Treatment is of the underlying infection, if known, with support care. T-cell activation is implicated in the aetiology and chemotherapy or cyclosporin may be tried. The condition is often fatal.

BIBLIOGRAPHY

Dale D.C., Person R.E., Bolyard A.A. *et al.* (2000) Mutations in the gene encoding neutrophil elastase in congenital and cyclic neutropenia. *Blood* **96**, 2317–22.

Gordon S. (1995) The macrophage. *Bioessays* **7**, 977–86.

Metcalf D. (1993) The hematopoietic regulators: redundancy or subtlety. *Blood* **82**, 3515–23.

Rothenberg M.E. (1998) Eosinophilia. *N. Engl. J. Med.* **338**, 1592–600.

Stock W. and Hoffman R. (2000) White blood cells 1: non-malignant disorders. *Lancet* **355**, 1351–7.

Welte K. and Boxer L.A. (1997) Severe chronic neutropenia: pathophysiology and therapy. *Semin. Hematol.* **34**, 267–78.

CHAPTER 10

The white cells 2: lymphocytes and their benign disorders

Lymphocytes (Fig. 10.1) are the immunologically competent cells which assist the phagocytes in the defence of the body against infection and other foreign invasion. Two unique features characteristic of the immune system are the ability to generate antigenic specificity and the phenomenon of immunological memory. A complete description of the functions of lymphocytes is beyond the scope of this book, but information essential to an understanding of the diseases of the lymphoid system, and of the role of lymphocytes in haematological diseases is included here.

LYMPHOCYTES

Primary lymphocyte formation

In postnatal life the bone marrow and thymus are the primary lymphoid organs in which lymphocytes develop (Fig. 10.2). The secondary lymphoid organs in which specific immune responses are generated are the lymph nodes, spleen and lymphoid tissues of the alimentary and respiratory tracts.

B and T lymphocytes

The immune response depends upon two types of lymphocytes, B and T cells (Table 10.1). In humans, B cells are derived from bone marrow stem cells. Whether any of the cells are processed out-

side the bone marrow to become mature B lymphocytes is uncertain. In birds, this process takes place in the bursa of Fabricius but an equivalent organ has not been identified in humans.

T cells also initially derive from bone marrow stem cells but migrate to the thymus where they differentiate into mature T cells during passage from the cortex to the medulla. During this process self-reactive T cells are deleted (negative selection) whereas T cells with some specificity for host human leucocyte antigen (HLA) molecules are selected (positive selection). The mature helper cells express CD4 and cytotoxic cells express CD8 (Table 10.1). The cells also express one of two T-cell antigen receptor heterodimers, $\alpha\beta$ ($>90\%$) or $\gamma\delta$ ($<10\%$).

Natural killer cells

Natural killer (NK) cells are cytotoxic CD8+ cells that lack the T-cell receptor (TCR). They are large cells with cytoplasmic granules and typically express surface molecules CD16 (Fc receptor), CD56 and CD57. NK cells are designed to kill target cells that have a low level of expression of HLA class I molecules such as may occur during viral infection or on a malignant cell. NK cells do this by displaying a number of receptors for HLA molecules on their surface. When HLA is expressed on the target cell these deliver an inhibitory signal into the NK cell. When HLA molecules are absent on the target cell this inhibitory signal is lost and the NK cell can then kill its target. In addition NK cells

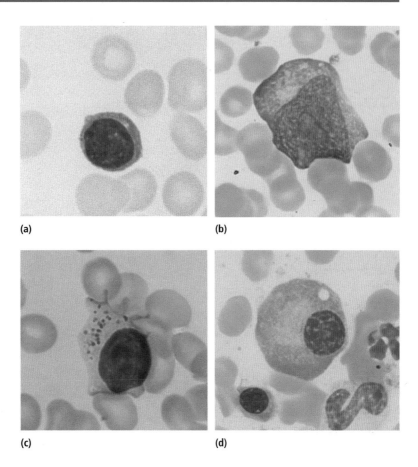

Fig. 10.1 Lymphocytes: (a) small lymphocyte; (b) activated lymphocyte; (c) large granular lymphocyte; (d) plasma cell.

(a)

(b)

(c)

(d)

display antibody-dependent cell-mediated cyto-toxicity (ADCC). In this, antibody binds to antigen on the cell surface and then NK cells bind to the Fc portion of the bound antibody and kill the target cell.

Lymphocyte circulation

Lymphocytes in the peripheral blood migrate through postcapillary venules into the substance of the lymph nodes or into the spleen. T cells home to the perifollicular zones of the cortical areas of lymph nodes (paracortical areas) (Fig. 10.2) and to the periarteriolar sheaths surrounding the central arterioles of the spleen. B cells selectively accumulate in follicles of the lymph nodes and spleen and also at the subcapsular periphery of the cortex and in the medullary cords of the lymph nodes. Lymphocytes return to the peripheral blood via the efferent lymphatic stream and the thoracic duct. In normal peripheral blood and germinal centres CD4 helper cells predominate, but in the marrow and gut the major T-cell subpopulation is CD8 positive.

IMMUNOGLOBULINS

These are a heterogeneous group of proteins produced by plasma cells and B lymphocytes which react with antigens. They are divided into five subclasses or isotypes: immunoglobulin G (IgG), IgA, IgM, IgD and IgE. IgG, the most common, contributes about 80% of normal serum immunoglobulin, and is further subdivided into four subclasses: IgG_1, IgG_2, IgG_3 and IgG_4. IgA is subdivided into two types. IgM is usually pro-

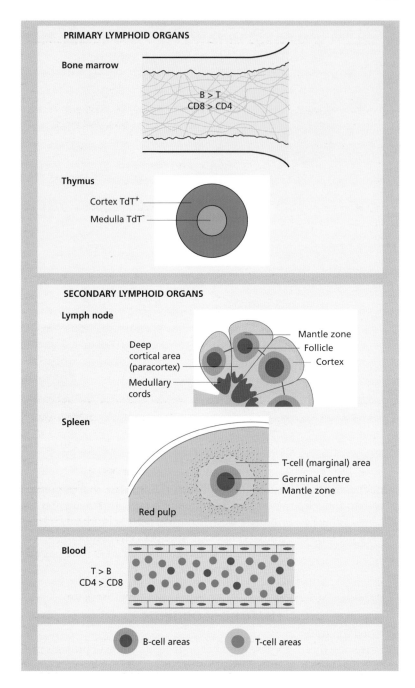

Fig. 10.2 Primary and secondary lymphoid organs and blood.

duced first in response to antigen, IgG subsequently and for a more prolonged period. The same cell can switch from IgM to IgG, or to IgA or IgE synthesis. IgA is the main immunoglobulin in secretions, particularly of the gastrointestinal tract. IgD and IgE (involved in delayed hypersensitivity reactions) are minor fractions. Some important biochemical and biological properties of the three main immunoglobulin subclasses are summarized in Table 10.2.

Table 10.1 Functional aspects of T and B cells

	T cells	B cells
Origin	Thymus	Bone marrow
Tissue distribution	Parafollicular areas of cortex in nodes, peri-arteriolar in spleen	Germinal centres of lymph nodes, spleen, gut, respiratory tract; also subcapsular and medullary cords of lymph nodes
Blood	80% of lymphocytes; CD4 > CD8	20% of lymphocytes
Membrane receptors	TCR for antigen	BCR (= immunoglobulin) for antigen
Bone marrow	CD8 > CD4	
Function	CD8+: CMI against intracellular organisms CD4+: T-cell help for antibody production and generation of CMI	Humoral immunity by generation of antibodies
Characteristic surface markers	CD1 CD2 CD3 CD4 or 8 CD5 CD6 CD7 MHC class I MHC class II when activated	CD19 CD20 CD22 CD9 (pre B cells) CD10 (precursor B cells) MHC class I and II
Genes rearranged	TCR $\alpha, \beta, \gamma, \delta$	IgH, Igκ, Igλ

BCR, B-cell receptor; C, complement; CMI, cell-mediated immunity; IFN, interferon; Ig, immunoglobulin; MHC, major histocompatibility complex; TCR, T-cell receptor; TNF, tumour necrosis factor.

Table 10.2 Some properties of the three main classes of immunoglobulin

	IgG	IgA	IgM
Molecular weight	140 000	140 000	900 000
Sedimentation constant	7S	7S	19S
Normal serum level (g/l)	6.0–16.0	1.5–4.5	0.5–1.5
Present in	Serum and extracellular fluid	Serum and other body fluids, e.g. of bronchi and gut	Serum only
Complement fixation	Usual	Yes (alternative pathway)	Usual and very efficient
Placental transfer	Yes	No	No
Heavy chain	(γ_{1-4})	α $(\alpha_1$ or $\alpha_2)$	μ

The immunoglobulins are all made up of the same basic structure (Fig. 10.3) consisting of two heavy chains which are called gamma (γ) in IgG, alpha (α) in IgA, mu (μ) in IgM, delta (δ) in IgD and epsilon (ε) in IgE and two light chains—kappa (κ) or lambda (λ)—which are common to all five immunoglobulins. The heavy and light chains each have highly variable regions which give the immunoglobulin specificity, and constant regions in which there is virtual complete correspondence in

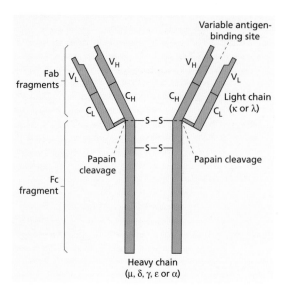

Fig. 10.3 Basic structure of an immunoglobulin molecule. Each molecule is made up of two light (κ or λ) (blue areas) and two heavy (purple) chains, and each chain is made up of variable (V) and constant (C) portions, the V portions including the antigen-binding site. The heavy chain (μ, δ, γ, ε or α) varies according to the immunoglobulin class. IgA molecules form dimers, while IgM forms a ring of five molecules. Papain cleaves the molecules into an Fc fragment and two Fab fragments.

amino acid sequence in all antibodies of a given isotype (e.g. IgA, IgG, etc.) or isotype subclass (e.g. IgG_1, IgG_2, etc.). In the variable regions of both the heavy and light chains there are hypervariable or complementarity-determining regions and framework regions with less variability. They can be broken into a constant Fc fragment and two highly variable Fab fragments. IgM molecules are much larger because they consist of five subunits.

The main role of immunoglobulins is defence of the body against foreign organisms. However, they also have a vital role in the pathogenesis of a number of haematological disorders. Secretion of a specific immunoglobulin from a monoclonal population of lymphocytes or plasma cells occurs in macroglobulinaemia, most cases of multiple myeloma and in other disorders (p. 216). Bence-Jones protein found in the urine in some cases of myeloma consists of a monoclonal secretion of light chains or light chain fragments (either κ or λ).

Immunoglobulins may bind to blood cells in a variety of immune disorders and cause agglutination (e.g. in cold agglutinin disease, p. 66) or destruction following direct complement lysis or after elimination by the reticuloendothelial system.

ANTIGEN–RECEPTOR GENE ARRANGEMENTS

Immunoglobulin gene rearrangements

The immunoglobulin heavy-chain and κ and λ light-chain genes occur on chromosomes 14, 2 and 22, respectively, in humans. In the embryonic germline state the heavy-chain gene occur as separate segments for variable (V), diversity (D), joining (J) and constant (C) regions. Each of the V, D and J regions contain a number (*n*) of different gene segments (Fig. 10.4). In cells not committed to immunoglobulin synthesis, these gene segments remain in their separate germline state. During early differentiation of B cells, there is rearrangement of heavy-chain genes so that one of the V heavy-chain segments combines with one of the D segments already combined with one of the J segments. They thus form a transcriptionally active gene for the heavy chain. The protein-coding segments of the C region mRNA are joined after splicing out intervening RNA. The class of immunoglobulin secreted depends on which of the nine (4γ, 2α, 1μ, 1δ and 1ε) constant regions is used. Diversity is introduced by the variability of which V segment joins with which D and with which J segment. In the arbitrary example shown in Fig. 10.4, V_2 joins with D_1 and J_2. Additional diversity is generated by the enzyme terminal deoxynucleotidyl transferase (TdT) which inserts a variable number of new bases into the DNA of the D region at the time of gene rearrangement.

For the light chains similar rearrangements occur within the light-chain gene segments. Enzymes called recombinases are needed both in B and T cells to join up the adjacent pieces of DNA after excision of intervening sequences.

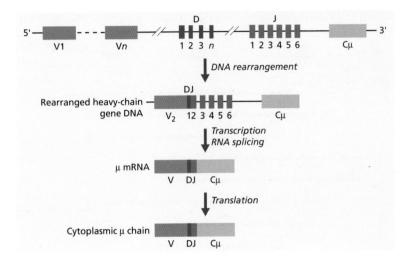

Fig. 10.4 Rearrangement of a heavy-chain immunoglobulin gene. One of the V segments is brought into contact with a D, a J and a C (in this case Cμ) segment, forming an active transcriptional gene from which the corresponding mRNA is produced. The DJ rearrangement precedes VDJ joining. The class of immunoglobin depends on which of the nine constant regions (1μ, 1δ, 4γ, 2α, 1ε) is used.

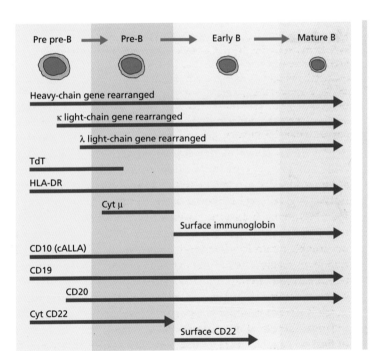

Fig. 10.5 The sequence of immunoglobulin gene rearrangement, antigen and immunoglobulin expression during early B-cell development. Intracytoplasmic CD22 is a feature of very early B cells. HLA, human leucocyte antigen; TdT, terminal deoxynucleotidyl transferase.

These recognize certain heptamer- and nonamer-conserved sequences flanking the various gene segments. Rearrangement occurs during the ontogeny of B cells in the sequence heavy, κ and λ genes (Fig. 10.5). Mistakes in recombinase activity play an important part in the chromosome translocations of B- or T-cell malignancy.

T-cell receptor rearrangements

The vast majority of T cells contain a TCR composed of a heterodimer of α and β chain. In a minority of T cells, the TCR is composed of γ and δ chains. The α, β, γ and δ genes of the TCRs

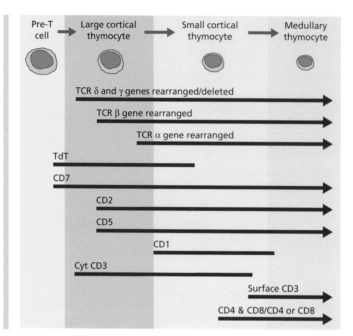

Fig. 10.6 The sequence of events during early T-cell development. The earliest events appear to be the expression of surface CD7, intranuclear terminal deoxynucleotidyl transferase (TdT) and intracytoplasmic CD3 followed by T-cell receptor (TCR) gene rearrangement. Early medullary thymocytes may express both CD4 and CD8, but they then lose one or other of these structures.

each include V, D, J and C regions. During T-cell ontogeny, rearrangements of these gene segments occur in a similar fashion to those for immunoglobulin genes in developing B cells, so creating T cells expressing a wide variety (10^8 or more) of TCR structures (Fig. 10.6). TdT is involved in creating additional diversity and the same recombinase enzymes used in B cells are involved in joining up TCR gene segments.

COMPLEMENT

This consists of a series of plasma proteins constituting an amplification enzyme system which is capable of lysis of bacteria (or of blood cells) or can 'opsonize' (coat) bacteria or cells so that they are phagocytosed. The complement sequence consists of nine major components—C1, C2, etc.— which are activated in turn (denoted thus $\overline{C1}$) and form a cascade, resembling the coagulation sequence (Fig. 10.7). The most abundant and pivotal protein is C3 which is present in plasma at a level of about 1.2 g/l. The early (opsonizing) stages leading to coating the cells with C3b can occur by two different pathways:

1 the classical pathway usually activated by IgG or IgM coating of cells; or
2 the alternate, more rapid, pathway activated by IgA, endotoxin (from Gram-negative bacteria) and other factors (Fig. 10.7).

Macrophages and neutrophils have C3b receptors and they phagocytose C3b-coated cells. C3b is degraded to C3d which is detected in the antiglobulin (Coombs) test using an anticomplement agent (p. 310). If the complement sequence goes to completion, there is generation of an active phospholipase that punches holes in the cell membrane (e.g. of the red cell or bacterium), causing direct lysis. The complement pathway also generates biologically active fragments C3a and C5a which act directly on phagocytes, especially neutrophils, to stimulate the respiratory burst associated with production of oxygen metabolites. Both may trigger anaphylaxis by release of mediators from tissue mast cells and basophils which may cause vasodilation and increased permeability.

THE IMMUNE RESPONSE

One of the most striking features of the immune

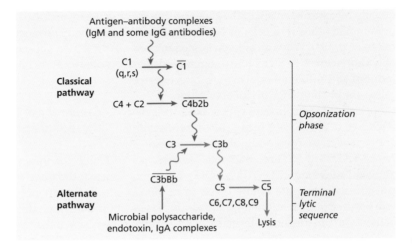

Fig. 10.7 The complement (C) sequence. The activated factors are denoted by a bar over the number. Both pathways generate a C3 convertase. In the classical pathway, the convertase is the major (b) component of C4 and C2 (C4b2b). In the alternate pathway, it is the combination of C3b and the major fragment (b) of factor B (C3bBb).

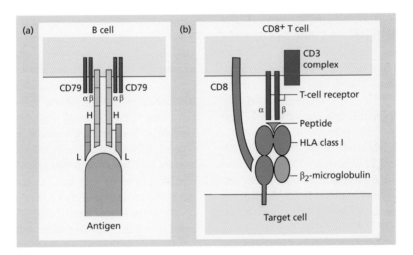

Fig. 10.8 Antigen receptors on lymphocytes and their interaction with antigen. (a) The B-cell antigen receptor is membrane-bound immunoglobulin. Two heavy chains (H) are covalently bonded to two light chains (L). This antigen-binding unit is associated with the CD79 heterodimer which acts as a signal transduction unit. (b) The T-cell receptor consists of a number of components which together constitute the CD3 complex. Two antigen-binding chains (α, β) are associated with several proteins (γ, δ, ε, ζ) that mediate signal transduction. Antigen is recognized in the form of short peptides held on the surface of HLA molecules. CD8+ T cells interact with peptide on a class I HLA molecule and the CD8 heterodimer interacts with the α3 domain of the class I protein.

system is its capacity to produce a highly *specific* response. For both T and B cells this specificity is achieved by the presence of a particular receptor on the lymphocyte surface (Fig. 10.8). The immune system contains many clones of lymphocytes. Each of these clones has a receptor which shows differences in structure from that of any other clone, and consequently will only bind to a restricted number of antigens. The B-cell receptor is membrane-bound immunoglobulin and after activation this is secreted as free, soluble immunoglobulin. The TCR is more complex. The portion that recognizes antigen is structurally analogous to immunoglobulin, and has either α and β chains or, in a small minority, γ and δ chains. Variability is produced during B- or T-cell development by rearrangement of the genes coding for immunoglobulins in B cells or for the TCR in T cells (see p. 131). When an antigen is encountered only those clones to which the antigen binds are induced to proliferate and mature into effector cells — the phenomenon of clonal selection.

Specialized macrophages called dendritic cells (DCs, see p. 124) have a major role in processing antigens before presenting them to B and T lymphocytes — they are therefore known as antigen-presenting cells (APCs). DC precursors constitutively migrate at low levels from blood into tissues but their rate of migration is increased at the site of inflammation. Immature DCs are efficient at macropinocytosis which allows them to capture antigens from the environment. DCs can be matured by a variety of stimuli such as inflammatory cytokines — tumour necrosis factor (TNF)-α and interleukin (IL)-1 — and viral and bacterial products such as lipopolysaccharide (LPS) or double-stranded (ds) RNA. CD4+ T cells also activate DCs through a CD40–CD40 ligand (L) interaction. Mature DCs express high levels of costimulatory molecules and can efficiently present antigen to naïve antigen-specific T cells.

T cells are unable to bind antigen free in solution and require it to be presented on APCs in the form of peptides held on the surface of major histocompatibility complex molecules (MHC, also known as the HLA system in humans) (Fig. 10.8a). T cells therefore recognize not only the antigen, but also 'self' MHC molecules and are therefore known as MHC-restricted. The CD4 molecule on helper cells recognizes class II (HLA-DP, -DQ and -DR) molecules whereas the CD8 molecule recognizes class I (HLA-A, -B and -C) molecules. The antigen recognition site of the TCR is joined to several other subunits in the CD3 complex which together mediate signal transduction. During these structural interactions the cells release cytokines such as IL-1, -2, -4 and -10 which act to modify expansion of activated cells. Depending on their cytokine production CD4+ T cells can be broadly subdivided into T helper type 1 (Th1) and Th2 cells. Th1 cells produce mainly IL-2, TNF-β and interferon-γ (IFN-γ), and are important in boosting cell-mediated immunity (and granuloma formation) whereas Th2 cells produce IL-4 and IL-10

and are mainly responsible for providing help for antibody production. An imbalance in the ratio of these two subsets may be partly responsible for some forms of immune deficiency.

Generation of specific immune responses in the secondary lymphoid organs

Naïve (or virgin) B and T lymphocytes which leave the bone marrow and thymus are resting cells that are not in cell division. They recirculate in the lymphatic system and undergo clonal expansion if they meet an APC that is presenting an antigen that can trigger their antigen receptor molecules. At this stage lymphocytes may develop into effector cells (such as plasma cells or cytotoxic T cells) or memory cells.

Antigen-specific immune responses are generated in secondary lymphoid organs and as an example it is useful to review how such a process occurs in a lymph node. Antigen is carried into the node on Langerhans' cells which differentiate into interdigitating cells by the time they reach the T zone in the node. Here T cells are screened for recognition of antigen and if a T cell makes an interaction it can activate B cells and in addition migrate into the follicle. In the follicle, germinal centres arise as a result of continuing response to antigenic stimulation (Fig. 10.10). These consist of follicular dendritic cells (FDC), which are loaded with antigen, and activated T and B cells which have migrated up from the T zone. Proliferating B cells move to the dark zone of the germinal centre as centroblasts where they undergo somatic mutation of their immunoglobulin variable-region genes. Their progeny are known as centrocytes and these must be selected by antigen on FDCs otherwise they will undergo apoptosis. If selected they become memory cells and plasma cells (Fig. 10.10).

Plasma cells

Plasma cells are larger than lymphocytes. Typically, they have an eccentric round nucleus with a 'clock-face' chromatin pattern. With the excep-

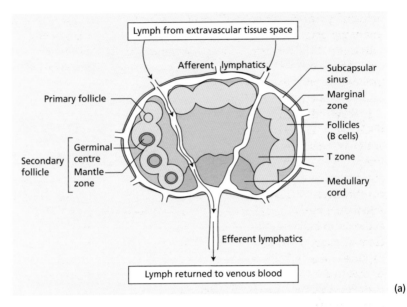

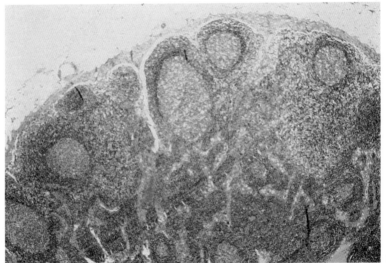

Fig. 10.9 (a) Structure of a lymph node. (b) Lymph node showing germinal follicles surrounded by a darker mantle zone rim and lighter, more diffuse marginal and T zone areas.

tion of a perinuclear light-staining Golgi body, the cytoplasm is strongly basophilic (Fig. 10.1d). They contain intracellular immunoglobulin but not surface immunoglobulin.

LYMPHOCYTOSIS

Lymphocytosis often occurs in infants and young children in response to infections which produce a neutrophil reaction in adults. Conditions particu-

larly associated with lymphocytosis are listed in Table 10.3.

Frequently there is a disease characterized by fever, sore throat, lymphadenopathy and atypical lymphocytes in the blood. It may be caused by primary infection with Epstein–Barr virus (EBV), cytomegalovirus, human immunodeficiency virus (HIV) or toxoplasmosis. EBV infection, otherwise known as infectious mononucleosis (or glandular fever), is the most common cause.

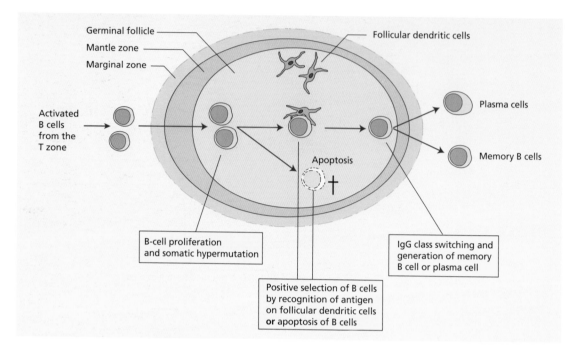

Germinal follicle
Mantle zone
Marginal zone
Follicular dendritic cells

Activated
B cells
from the
T zone

Plasma cells

Memory B cells

Apoptosis

B-cell proliferation
and somatic hypermutation

IgG class switching and
generation of memory
B cell or plasma cell

Positive selection of B cells
by recognition of antigen
on follicular dendritic cells
or apoptosis of B cells

Fig. 10.10 Generation of a germinal centre. B cells activated by antigen migrate from the T zone to the follicle where they undergo massive proliferation. Cells enter the dark zone as centroblasts and accumulate mutations in their immunoglobulin V genes. Cells then pass back into the light zone as centrocytes. Only those cells that can interact with antigen on follicular dendritic cells and receive signals from antigen-specific T cells (Fig. 10.8) are selected and migrate out as plasma cells and memory cells. Cells not selected die by apoptosis.

Table 10.3 Causes of lymphocytosis

Infections
    acute: infectious mononucleosis, rubella, pertussis, mumps, acute
    infectious lymphocytosis, infectious hepatitis, cytomegalovirus,
    HIV, herpes simplex or zoster
    chronic: tuberculosis, toxoplasmosis, brucellosis, syphilis
Chronic lymphoid leukaemias (Chapter 14)
Acute lymphoblastic leukaemia
Non-Hodgkin's lymphoma (some)
Thyrotoxicosis

HIV, human immunodeficiency virus.

Infectious mononucleosis

This is caused by primary infection with EBV and only occurs in a minority of infected individuals — in most cases infection is subclinical. The disease is characterized by a lymphocytosis caused by clonal expansions of T cells reacting against B lymphocytes infected with EBV. There is a low infec-

tivity rate. The disease is associated with a high titre of heterophile (reacting with cells of another species) antibody which reacts with sheep, horse or beef red cells.

Clinical features

The majority of patients are between the ages of 15 and 40 years. A prodromal period of a few days occurs with lethargy, malaise, headaches, stiff neck and a dry cough. In established disease the following features may be found.

1 Bilateral cervical lymphadenopathy is present in 75% of cases. Symmetrical generalized lymphadenopathy occurs in 50% of cases. The nodes are discrete and may be tender.

2 Over half the patients have a sore throat with inflamed oral and pharyngeal surfaces. Follicular tonsillitis is frequently seen.

3 Fever may be mild or severe.

4 A morbilliform rash, severe headache and eye signs, e.g. photophobia, conjunctivitis and peri-

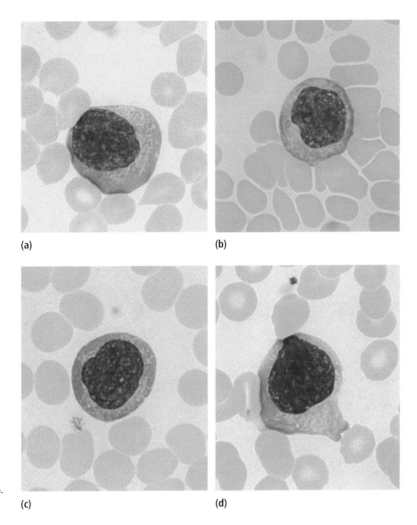

(a)   (b)

(c)   (d)

Fig. 10.11 Infectious mononucleosis: representative 'reactive' T lymphocytes in the peripheral blood film of a 21-year-old man (see also Fig. 10.1b).

orbital oedema are not uncommon. The rash may follow therapy with amoxycillin or ampicillin.

5 Palpable splenomegaly occurs in over half the patients and hepatomegaly in about 15%. About 5% of patients are jaundiced.

6 Peripheral neuropathy, severe anaemia (caused by autoimmune haemolysis) or purpura (caused by thrombocytopenia) are less frequent complications.

Diagnosis

Pleomorphic atypical lymphocytosis. A moderate rise in white cell count (e.g. 10×20 $10^9/l$) with an absolute lymphocytosis is usual, and some patients have even higher counts. Large numbers of atypical lymphocytes are seen in the peripheral blood film (Fig. 10.11). These T cells are variable in appearance but most have nuclear and cytoplasmic features similar to those seen during reactive lymphocyte transformation. The greatest number of atypical lymphocytes are usually found between the seventh and 10th day of the illness.

Heterophile antibodies. Heterophile antibodies against sheep red cells may be found in the serum at high titres. These form the basis of the Paul–Bunnell test—the antibodies are not absorbed by guinea-pig kidney cells but are absorbed by ox red cells (Fig. 10.12). Modern slide

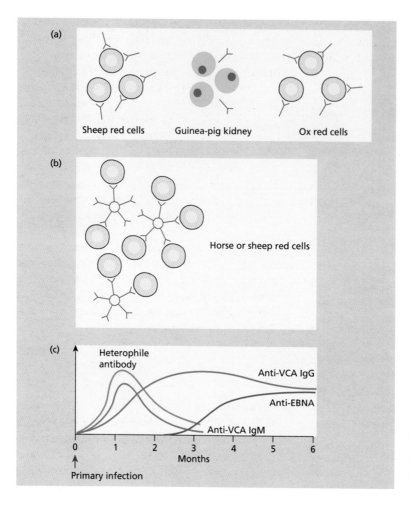

(a)

Sheep red cells   Guinea-pig kidney   Ox red cells

(b)

Horse or sheep red cells

(c)

Heterophile antibody

Anti-VCA IgG

Anti-EBNA

Anti-VCA IgM

0   1   2   3   4   5   6

Months

↑ Primary infection

Fig. 10.12 Serological diagnosis of acute Epstein–Barr virus (EBV) infection. (a) IgM heterophile antibodies (shown here as antibody monomers for ease of illustration) against sheep red cells are used in the Paul–Bunnell test. These are not absorbed out by guinea-pig kidney but do react with ox red cells. A positive Paul–Bunnell test should show a titre of sheep red cell agglutination that is at least fourfold lower after absorption with ox red cells but not greater than threefold lower after absorption with guinea-pig kidney. (b) The commonly used monospot test detects agglutination of sheep red cells or formolized horse red cells only. (c) After acute infection heterophile and EBV-specific IgM are present for about 3 months. IgG antibodies to viral capsid antigen (VCA) and EBV nucleur antigen (EBNA) remain elevated for years.

screening tests, such as the monospot test, substitute formalized horse red cells for the sheep cells used in the Paul–Bunnell test. Highest titres occur during the second and third week and the antibody persists in most patients for 6 weeks.

EBV antibody. If viral diagnostic facilities are available a rise in the titre of antibody against the EBV capsid antigen may be demonstrated during the first 2–3 weeks. Specific antibody to the EBV nuclear antigen develops later and persists for life.

Haematological abnormalities other than the atypical lymphocytosis are frequent. Occasional patients develop an autoimmune haemolytic anaemia. The IgM autoantibody is typically of the 'cold' type and usually shows 'i' blood group specificity. Thrombocytopenia is frequent and an

autoimmune thrombocytopenic purpura occurs in a smaller number of patients.

Differential diagnosis

The differential diagnosis of infectious mononucleosis includes cytomegalovirus, HIV or toxoplasmosis infection; acute leukaemia; influenza; rubella; bacterial tonsillitis; and infectious hepatitis.

Treatment

In the great majority of patients only symptomatic treatment is required. Corticosteroids are sometimes given to those with severe systemic symptoms. Patients characteristically develop an erythematous rash if given ampicillin therapy.

Most patients recover fully 4–6 weeks after initial symptoms. However, convalescence may be slow and associated with severe malaise and lethargy.

Lymphopenia

Lymphopenia may occur in severe bone marrow failure, with corticosteroid and other immunosuppressive therapy, in Hodgkin's disease and with widespread irradiation. It also occurs in a variety of immune deficiency syndromes, the most important of which is acquired immune deficiency syndrome (AIDS).

IMMUNE DEFICIENCY

A large number of inherited or acquired deficits in any of the components of the immune system may cause an impaired immune response with increased susceptibility to infection (Table 10.4). A primary lack of T cells (as in AIDS) leads not only to bacterial infections but also to viral, protozoal, fungal and mycobacterial infections. In some cases, however, lack of specific subsets of T cells which control B-cell maturation may lead to a secondary lack of B-cell function as in many cases of common variable immune deficiency which may develop in children or adults of either sex. In others, a primary defect of B cells or APCs is pre-sent. X-linked agammaglobulinaemia is caused by a failure of B-cell development. Pyogenic bacterial infections dominate the clinical course. Rare syndromes include aplasia of the thymus, severe combined (T and B) immune deficiency as a result of adenosine deaminase deficiency and selective deficiencies of IgA or IgM. Acquired immune deficiency occurs after cytotoxic chemotherapy or radiotherapy and is particularly pronounced after stem cell transplantation where dysregulation of the immune system persists for 1 year or more and is responsible for a high incidence of serious viral infections, e.g. with cytomegalovirus or herpes zoster. Immune deficiency is also frequently associated with tumours of the lymphoid system including chronic lymphocytic leukaemia, Hodgkin's disease and myeloma. A major cause of acquired immune deficiency is HIV infection and the clinical and haematological aspects of this disease are considered next.

HIV infection

Aetiology
Infection with HIV, a retrovirus of the lentivirus subgroup, is a frequent cause of immune deficiency, giving rise to a wide range of symptoms, opportunistic infections and malignancies. HIV-1 is thought to have originated in chimpanzees in Central Africa, where the greatest diversity of

Table 10.4 Classification of immune deficiencies

Primary	B cell (antibody deficiency)	X-linked agammaglobulinaemia, acquired common variable hypogammaglobulinaemia, selective IgA or IgG subclass deficiencies
	T cell	Thymic aplasia (di George syndrome), PNP deficiency
	Mixed B and T cell	Severe combined immune deficiency (as a result of ADA deficiency or other causes); Bloom's syndrome; ataxia-telangiectasia; Wiskott–Aldrich syndrome
Secondary	B cell (antibody deficiency)	Myeloma; nephrotic syndrome, protein-losing enteropathy
	T cell	AIDS; Hodgkin's disease, non-Hodgkin's lymphoma; drugs: steroids, cyclosporine, azathioprine, fludarabine, etc.
	T and B cell	Chronic lymphocytic leukaemia, post-bone marrow transplantation and post-chemotherapy/radiotherapy

ADA, adenosine deaminase; AIDS, acquired immune deficiency syndrome; Ig, immunoglobulin; PNP, purine nucleoside phosphorylase.

viral subgroups is now found. Most infections in the West result from the B clade of HIV-1, but different clades (HIV families distinguished on the basis of viral sequence) predominate in other parts of the world, such as the E clade in Thailand and A and C clades in sub-Saharan Africa. It is probable that the natural history associated with infection with different clades will vary. Infection with the related retrovirus, HIV-2, which is found predominantly in West Africa, gives rise to a more protracted disease course, such that the majority of HIV-2-infected people have few signs of immune deficiency.

Epidemiology

The virus is transmitted in semen, blood and other body fluids, including breast milk. On a worldwide basis, the vast majority of infections occur during heterosexual intercourse. As many as 40% of children born to infected mothers may become infected either at birth or through breast-feeding, but vertical transmission can be significantly reduced in the West by antiretroviral drug use in late pregnancy and at the time of delivery, and formula feeding. Infection from blood or blood products is now rare in countries where screening of donations is routine, but the sharing of contaminated needles by intravenous drug users remains a potent source of infection.

Pathogenesis

HIV produces its main effects through infection of T-helper (CD4) cells and cells of the monocyte lineage, and damage to the immune system can be demonstrated from the very earliest stages of infection. Entry into cells requires both the presence of the CD4 molecule and a member of the chemokine receptor family: in early infection this is usually the receptor CCR-5, but in late disease the virus often evolves to use another chemokine receptor, CXCR-4. As CXCR-4 is more widely expressed on CD4+ T cells, particularly cells of a naïve phenotype, this chemokine receptor switch is often associated with an acceleration in the rate of decline of CD4+ T cells. A cardinal feature of HIV infection is the rapid mutation rate of the virus in an infected person: this is a consequence of both the error-prone nature of the enzyme re-

verse transcriptase and the high rate of viral replication. As a consequence the virus can readily adapt to become resistant to antiretroviral therapy and the immune response directed against it.

Clinical features

The median time to AIDS in Western cohorts before the advent of highly active antiretroviral therapy (HAART) was between 10 and 12 years. A number of factors are known to influence the rate of disease progression: these include host factors such as HLA haplotype together with polymorphisms in the genes encoding some of the chemokine receptors and their ligands, and viral factors such as infection with replication-defective virus. Intercurrent infections are also believed to accelerate disease progression.

A prodromal period of about 6 weeks follows initial infection. Symptoms resembling infectious mononucleosis with transient lymphadenopathy and occasionally meningoencephalitis may occur, which coincide with the peak of viraemia and subsequent control by the immune response, following which the antibody test becomes positive. Plasma viral load may be extremely high during acute infection (up to 10^7 RNA copies/ml). Most infected people then experience a protracted asymptomatic period: however, the virus continues to replicate and the CD4+ T-cell count gradually falls. A number of HIV-related symptoms may develop, including generalized lymphadenopathy with persistent fever, weight loss, unexplained diarrhoea, skin changes, central nervous system (CNS) manifestations and haematological abnormalities including thrombocytopenia, leucopenia, neutropenia, hypergammaglobulinaemia and anaemia. Infections may occur with organisms not always associated with immunosuppression, such as herpes simplex or zoster, *Pneumococcus* and *Salmonella*. During this period HIV may be detectable in plasma, but the viral load is usually low. When the CD4+ T-cell count falls below $200 \times 10^9/l$, the patient becomes vulnerable to a wide spectrum of opportunistic infections including *Pneumocystis carinii* (Fig. 10.13), malignancies and CNS disease such as dementia may also develop, and this stage of infection is classified as fully developed AIDS. Many staging

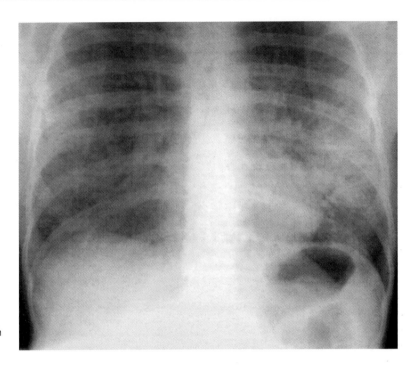

Fig. 10.13 *Pneumocystitis carinii* infection: a chest radiograph showing the typical 'bat wing' shadowing of both lung fields.

systems for HIV infection have been proposed and subsequently revised: in practice most clinicians determine the stage of infection according to the patient's symptoms and CD4+ T-cell count (Table 10.5). The plasma viral load is increasingly being used to predict outcome and determine the response to therapy.

AIDS has been defined by the Centers for Disease Control (CDC) in the USA as a CD4+ T-cell count below $0.2 \times 10^9/l$ or the development of opportunistic infections such as recurrent bacterial pneumonia (caused by *Streptococcus pneumoniae* and *Haemophilus influenzae*), *Pneumocystis carinii*, toxoplasmosis, *Cryptococcus*, cryptosporidiosis, atypical mycobacteria, *Mycobacterium tuberculosis* (both pulmonary and extrapulmonary), oral hairy leucoplakia (caused by EBV), histoplasmosis, candidiasis of the oesophagus or lungs, JC virus causing progressive multifocal leucoencephalopathy and cytomegalovirus infections of the gastrointestinal tract and retina. In addition a number of secondary cancers may develop such as Kaposi's sarcoma (Fig. 10.14), a vascular skin tumour of endothelial cell origin associated with infection by Kaposi's sarcoma herpes virus (KSHV or HHV-8),

Table 10.5 Clinical staging of HIV infection

CD4+ cell count ($\times 10^9/l$)	Stage	Clinical features
>0.5	Early	Low risk of disease Normal responses to immunization
0.2–0.5	Middle	Minor signs and symptoms common Moderate risk of opportunistic disease
0.05–0.2	Late	High risk of opportunistic disease Benefit from *Pneumocystis* prophylaxis and antiretroviral therapy
<0.05	Advanced	High risk of opportunistic diseases and death

non-Hodgkin's lymphoma (often brain primary, high grade and expressing markers of EBV infection), squamous carcinoma of the mouth or rectum, and invasive cervical cancer. Neurological diseases may also occur in late infection, either central (e.g. dementia or myelopathy) or peripheral neuropathies.

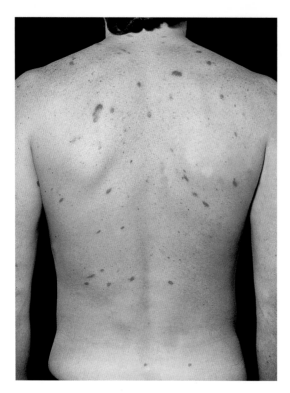

Fig. 10.14 Kaposi's sarcoma in acquired immune deficiency syndrome (AIDS): a vascular tumour of endothelial origin in a homosexual male (HIV-antigen positive).

Diagnosis

This is confirmed by the presence of antibodies to HIV or the direct detection of HIV RNA in the plasma. The blood count reveals a progressive lymphopenia and a fall of the CD4:CD8 ratio from the normal value of 1.5–2.5:1 to less than 1:1. A polyclonal rise in serum immunoglobulin is often found and a paraprotein occurs in the serum of about 10% of patients with AIDS.

Haematological aspects

The most frequent abnormalities are anaemia, thrombocytopenia and neutropenia either individually or combined, together with lymphopenia. Thrombocytopenia may be immune or secondary to marrow dysfunction. The bone marrow may be hypercellular (with an increase of plasma cells and lymphocytes), normocellular or hypocellular. The cells may be dysplastic and fibrosis may occur. Marrow examination is valuable for the diagnosis of some opportunistic infections, e.g. tuberculosis, atypical mycobacterial infection, *Cryptococcus*, leishmaniasis and histoplasmosis (Fig. 10.15). The drugs used in therapy, especially azidothymidine (AZT) but also ganciclovir, pentamidine and trimethoprim, may also cause cytopenias, especially if the patient is folate deficient. Thrombocytopenia may respond to corticosteroids and intravenous immunoglobulin (if autoimmune) or antiretroviral therapy. Lymphomas are treated in the usual way, although these tend to be high grade and, if the patient already has AIDS, the prognosis is poor.

Treatment

This is both supportive and specific. Supportive treatment is primarily aimed at preventing or treating infections, e.g. with prophylactic antibiotics such as co-trimoxazole, isoniazid or antifungals. Specific treatment is with agents that suppress viral replication. AZT was the first agent shown to have efficacy in reducing the viral load: this has been followed by the development of a range of other reverse transcriptase inhibitors such as lamivudine and nevirapine. The more recently introduced protease inhibitors, such as indinavir, ritonavir and saquinavir, are extremely potent at reducing virus load. Because of the high likelihood of viral resistance developing during monotherapy, combination therapy with at least three drugs is usually recommended. The optimal time to introduce therapy is still unclear, and the benefits have to be weighed against the likelihood of side-effects from combination antiretroviral therapy. Most clinicians would certainly start therapy when symptoms develop or the CD4+ count drops below $0.2 \times 10^9/l$, but treatment is increasingly being introduced earlier and particularly when primary HIV infection is recognized.

DIFFERENTIAL DIAGNOSIS OF LYMPHADENOPATHY

The principal causes of lymphadenopathy are listed in Fig. 10.16. The clinical history and examination give essential information. The age of the patient, length of history, associated

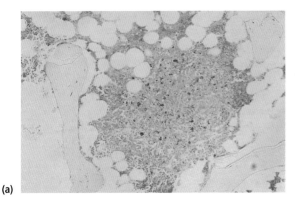

(a)

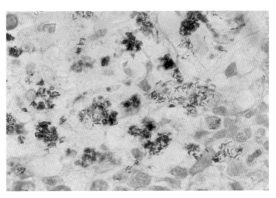

(b)

Fig. 10.15 Human immunodeficiency virus (HIV) infection: bone marrow trephine biopsy. (a) Granuloma showing positivity with Ziehl–Nielsen stain. (b) Higher power shows large numbers of acid-fast bacilli.

Localized

Local infection
- pyogenic infection,
  e.g. pharyngitis,
  dental abscess,
  otitis media,
  actinomyces
- viral infection
- cat scratch fever
- lymphogranuloma venereum
- tuberculosis

Lymphoma
- Hodgkin's disease
- non-Hodgkin's lymphoma

Carcinoma (secondary)

Generalized

Infection
- viral, e.g. infectious
  mononucleosis,
  measles, rubella,
  viral hepatitis, HIV
- bacterial, e.g. syphilis,
  brucellosis, tuberculosis,
  Salmonella, bacterial
  endocarditis
- fungal, e.g. histoplasmosis
- protozoal, e.g. toxoplasmosis

**Non-infectious inflammatory
diseases,** e.g. sarcoidosis,
rheumatoid arthritis, SLE,
other connective tissue diseases,
serum sickness

Malignant
- leukaemias, especially CLL, ALL
- lymphoma: non-Hodgkin's lymphoma,
  Hodgkin's disease
- Waldenström's macroglobulinaemia
- rarely secondary carcinoma
- angioimmunoblastic lymphadenopathy

Miscellaneous
- sinus histocytosis with massive lymphadenopathy
- reaction to drugs and chemicals, e.g. hydantoins
  and related chemicals, beryllium
- hyperthyroidism

Fig. 10.16 Causes of lymphadenopathy. ALL, acute lymphoblastic leukaemia; CLL, chronic lymphocytic leukaemia; SLE, systemic lupus erythematosus. Malignancies are listed in red.

symptoms of possible infectious or malignant disease, whether the nodes are painful or tender, consistency of the nodes and whether there is generalized or local lymphadenopathy, are all important. The size of the liver and spleen are assessed. In the case of local node enlargement, inflammatory or malignant disease in the associated lymphatic drainage area are particularly considered.

Further investigations will depend on the initial clinical diagnosis but it is usual to include a full blood count, blood film and erythrocyte sedimentation rate (ESR). Chest X-ray, monospot test, cytomegalovirus and *Toxoplasma* titres, and anti-HIV and Mantoux tests, are frequently needed. In many cases, it will be essential to make a histological diagnosis by node biopsy but a fine needle aspirate may sometimes avoid the need for this. Computed tomography (CT) scanning is valuable in determining the presence and extent of deep node enlargement. Subsequent investigations will depend on the diagnosis made and the patient's particular features. In some cases of deep node enlargement, where enlarged superficial nodes are not available for biopsy, bone marrow, liver biopsies, CT or ultrasound guided trucut node biopsy may be needed in an attempt to reach a histological diagnosis and avoid the need for a diagnostic laparotomy.

BIBLIOGRAPHY

Albert L.J. and Inman R.D. (2000) Molecular mimicry and autoimmunity. *N. Engl. J. Med.* **341**, 2068–74.

Bain B.J. (1997) The haematological features of HIV infection *Br. J. Haematol.* **99**, 1–8.

Buckley R.H. (2001) Primary immunodeficiency diseases due to defects in lymphocytes. *N. Engl. J. Med.* **343**, 1313–24.

Carpenter C.C. *et al.* (1998) Antiretroviral therapy for HIV infection in 1998: updated recommendations of the International AIDS Society—USA panel. *JAMA* **280**, 78.

Cohen J.J. (2000) Epstein–Barr virus infection. *N. Engl. J. Med.* **343**, 481–91.

Delves P.J. and Roitt I.M. (2000) The immune system. *N. Engl. J. Med.* **343**, 37–49, 108–17.

Klein U., Goosens T., Fischer M. *et al.* Somatic hypermutation in normal and transformed human B cells. *Immunol. Rev.* **162**, 261–80.

Roitt I.M. (2001) *Essential Immunology*, 10th edn. Blackwell Science, Oxford.

Walport M.J. (2001) Complement. *N. Eng. J. Med.* **344**, 1140–4.

CHAPTER 11

The genetics of haematological malignancies

The haemopoietic malignancies are clonal diseases which are thought to derive from a single cell in the marrow or peripheral lymphoid tissue which has undergone a genetic alteration (Fig. 11.1). Malignant transformation occurs as a result of the accumulation of genetic mutation in cellular genes. The genes that are involved in the development of cancer can be broadly divided into two groups—oncogenes and tumour-suppressor genes.

Oncogenes

Oncogenes arise because of gain-of-function mutations in normal cellular genes called proto-oncogenes Fig. 11.2. Proto-oncogenes are involved in a variety of important cellular processes, often in the pathway by which external signals are transduced to the cell nucleus to activate genes. Oncogenic versions are generated when the activity of proto-oncogenes is increased or they acquire a novel function. This can occur in a number of ways including translocation, mutation or duplication. One of the striking features of haematological malignancies (in contrast to most solid tumours) is their high frequency of chromosomal translocations. These have been of great value in characterizing the genes at the breakpoints, many of which are transcription factors (see Fig. 1.11). Translocation may lead to: (a) overexpression of an oncogene when it comes under the control of the promoter of another gene (usually an immunoglobulin or T-cell receptor gene, in lymphoid malignancies) or (b) fusion of segments of two genes creating a novel fusion gene and hence fusion protein, e.g. in chronic myeloid leukaemia (see Fig. 13.1) or acute myeloid leukaemia (AML M_3) (Fig. 11.12). A subset of proto-oncogenes are involved in control of apoptosis. The most important is BCL-2 which is overexpressed in follicular lymphoma (p. 209).

Tumour-suppressor genes

Tumour-suppressor genes may acquire loss-of-function mutations, usually by point mutation or deletion, which lead to malignant transformation (Fig. 11.2). Tumour-suppressor genes commonly act as components of control mechanisms which regulate entry of the cell from the G1 phase of the cell cycle into the S phase or passage through the S phase to G2 and mitosis. Examples of oncogenes and tumour-suppressor genes involved in haemopoietic malignances are shown in Tables 11.1 and 11.2.

Clonal progression

Malignant cells appear to arise as a multistep process with acquisition of mutations in different intracellular pathways (Fig. 11.3). Another feature of malignancy is clonal progression. In many cases the disease develops new characteristics during

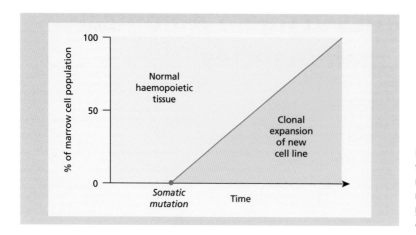

Fig. 11.1 Theoretical graph to show the replacement of normal bone marrow cells by a clonal population of malignant cells arising by successive mitotic divisions from a single cell with an acquired genetic alteration.

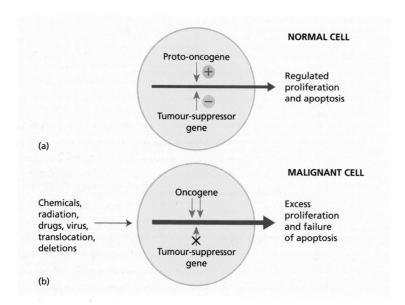

Fig. 11.2 Proliferation of normal cells depends on a balance between the action of proto-oncogenes (a) and tumour-suppressor genes (b). In a malignant cell this balance is disturbed leading to uncontrolled cell division.

its clinical course and this may be accompanied by new chromosome changes. Selection of subclones may occur during treatment or reflect disease acceleration. Drug resistance may arise through a variety of molecular mechanisms. In one example the cells express a protein which actively pumps a number of different drugs to the outside of the cells (multidrug resistance, MDR).

CHROMOSOME NOMENCLATURE

The normal somatic cell has 46 chromosomes and is called *diploid*; ova or sperm have 23 chromosomes and are called *haploid*. The chromosomes occur in pairs and are numbered 1–22 in decreasing size order; there are two sex chromosomes, XX in females, XY in males. *Karyotype* is the term used to describe the chromosomes derived from a mitotic cell which have been set out in numerical order (see Fig. 13.1d). A somatic cell with more or less than 46 chromosomes is termed *aneuploid*; more than 46 is *hyperdiploid*, less than 46 *hypodiploid*; 46 but with chromosome rearrangements, *pseudodiploid*.

Each chromosome has two arms, the shorter

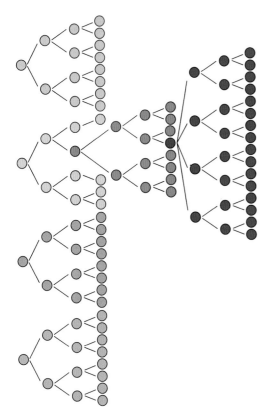

Fig. 11.3 Multistep origin of a malignant tumour. Successive mutations lead to a growth advantage of one subclone.

Table 11.1 Cellular oncogenes and tumour-suppressor genes implicated in human leukaemias and lymphomas

Membrane-associated tyrosine kinases (including growth factor receptors)	*FMS, KIT*
Intracellular signal transducers	
GTP-binding	*RAS*
Serine-threonine kinases	*RAF*
Nuclear	
Transcription factors	*CBFα* and *CBFβ, MYC, TAL-1, TAL-2, PBX*
Hormone receptor	Retinoic acid receptor α (*RARα*)
Tyrosine kinase	*ABL*, FGFR1*
Signalling of DNA damage and apoptosis	*p53, ATM*
Inhibitor of apoptosis	*BCL-2*
Control of cell cycle	*BCL-1* and *Rb***

*The BCR-ABL fusion protein in CML is cytoplasmic.
**Tumour suppressor gene.
GTP, guanosine triphosphate.

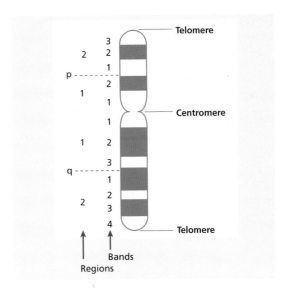

Fig. 11.4 A schematic representation of a chromosome. The bands may be divided into subbands according to staining pattern.

called 'p', the longer called 'q'. These meet at the *centromere* and the ends of the chromosomes are called *telomeres*. On staining each arm divides into regions numbered outwards from the centromere and each region divides into bands (Fig. 11.4).

When a whole chromosome is lost or gained, a – or + is put in front of the chromosome number. If part of the chromosome is lost it is prefixed with del for deletion. If there is extra material replacing part of a chromosome the prefix add for additional material is used. Chromosome translocations are denoted by t, the chromosomes involved placed in brackets with the lower numbered chromosome first. The prefix inv describes an inversion where part of the chromosome has been inverted to run in the opposite direction. An isochromosome, denoted by i, describes a chromosome with identical chromosome arms at each end, for example i(17q) would consist of two copies of 17q joined at the centromere.

Telomeres

Telomeres are repetitive sequences at the ends of chromosomes. They decrease by about 200 base

Table 11.2 Some of the more frequent genetic abnormalities in leukaemia and lymphoma

Disease	Genetic abnormality*	Oncogene(s) involved	Disease	Genetic abnormality*	Oncogene(s) involved
Myeloid			Burkitt's lymphoma, B-ALL	t(8; 14)†	*MYC* to *IgH* locus
AML M$_2$	t(8; 21) (q22; q22)	*ETO* and *CBFα* (*AML1*)		t(2; 8)	*MYC* to *IgK* locus
	t(6; 9)	*DEK, CAN*		t(8; 22)	*MYC* to *Igλ* locus
AML M$_3$	t(15; 17)	*RARα, PML*	T-ALL	t(1; 14)	*TAL-1* to TCRδ locus
				t(8; 14)†	*MYC*
AML M$_4$	inv(16) (p13q22), del(16q)	*CBFβ, MYH11*		t(11; 14)	*RBTN-1* or *RBTN-2*
				t(7; 9)	*TAL-2* to TCRβ locus
AML M$_5$	del(11q); t(9; 11); t(11; 19)	*MLL*	Follicular lymphoma	t(14; 18)	*BCL-2* to *IgH*
MDS	–5/del(5q)	Unclear	Anaplastic lymphoma	t(2; 5)	*ALK* to *NPM*
	–7/del(7q)				
	Point mutation	*N-RAS*	Mantle cell lymphoma	t(11; 14)†	*BCL-1* (cyclin D1) to *IgH*
Secondary myeloid leukaemia	11q23 translocations	*MLL* gene		Mutation	p53 and ATM
			B-CLL	Trisomy 12	Unknown
				13q14 deletion	Unknown
CML	t(9; 22)	*ABL, BCR*		11q22–23 mutation or deletion	*ATM*
Myeloproliferative disease	20q–			17p mutation or deletion	*p53*
	t(8; 13)	*DET* to *FGFR1*		6q21 deletion	Unknown
Lymphoid			MALT B-cell lymphoma	t(1; 14)	*BCL10* to *IgH* locus
Precursor B lineage	t(12; 21)	*TEL, AML1*			
	t(4; 11)	*AF4, MLL* (*ALL1, HRX*)	T-PLL	inv(14q) or t(14q) mutations	*ATM*
	t(9; 22)	*ABL, BCR*			
	t(1; 19)	*PBX-1, E2A*			
	Hyperdiploidy				
	Hypodiploidy				

* Other chromosomal abnormalities may occur in many of the conditions listed, e.g., Flt-3 mutation occurs in 30% of AML cases.
† The breakpoints on chromosome 14 are in different positions in T-ALL, B-ALL, mantle cell lymphoma and Burkitt's lymphoma.
ALL, acute lymphoblastic leukaemia; AML, acute myeloid leukaemia; CLL, chronic lymphocytic leukaemia; CML, chronic myeloid leukaemia; MALT, mucosa-associated lymphoid tissue; MDS, myelodysplasia.

pairs of DNA with every round of replication. When they decrease to a critical length, the cell exits from cell cycle. Germ cells and stem cells that need to self-renew and maintain a high proliferative potential contain an enzyme telomerase that can add extensions to the telomeric repeats and compensate for loss at replication and so enable the cells to continue proliferation. Telomerase is also often expressed in malignant cells but this is probably a consequence of the malignant transformation rather than an initiating factor.

METHODS USED TO STUDY GENETICS OF MALIGNANT CELLS

Karyotype analysis

Karyotype analysis involves direct morphological analysis of chromosomes from tumour cells under the microscope (Figs. 11.5 and see 13.1). This requires tumour cells to be in metaphase and so cells are cultured to encourage cell division prior to chromosomal preparation (see Fig. 13.1).

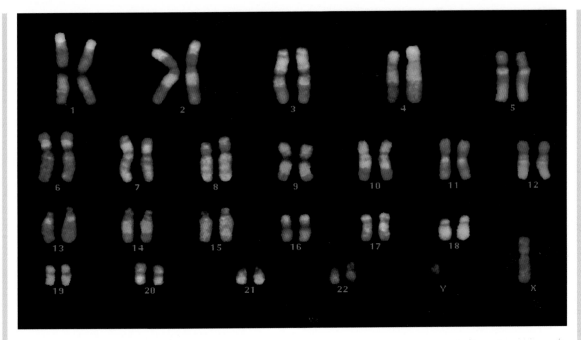

Fig. 11.5 A colour-banded karyotype from a normal male. Each chromosome pair shows an individual colour-banding pattern. This involves a cross-species multiple colour chromosome banding technique. Probe sets developed from the chromosomes of gibbons are combinatorially labelled and hybridized to human chromosomes. The success of cross-species colour banding depends on a close homology between host and human conserved DNA, divergence of repetitive DNA and a high degree of chromosomal rearrangement in the host relative to the human karyotype. (Courtesy Dr C.J. Harrison.)

Fluorescent *in situ* hybridization analysis

Fluorescent *in situ* hybridization (FISH) analysis involves the use of fluorescent-labelled genetic probes which hybridize to specific parts of the genome. It is possible to label each chromosome with a different combination of fluorescent labels (Fig. 11.5). This is a sensitive technique that can pick up extra copies of genetic material in both metaphase and interphase (non-dividing) cells (e.g. trisomy 12 in chronic lymphocytic leukaemia (CLL)) or, by using two different probes, reveal chromosomal translocations (Fig. 11.6).

Southern blot analysis

Southern blot analysis involves the extraction of cell DNA followed by restriction enzyme digestion, gel electrophoresis and transfer by 'blotting' to a suitable membrane. The DNA is then hybridized to a probe complementary to the gene of interest. When the probe recognizes a segment within the boundaries of a single restriction fragment one band is identified but if the gene has been translocated to a new area in the genome a novel band of different electrophoretic mobility is seen (see Fig. 6.24). Although time consuming and relatively insensitive this remains a powerful technique.

Polymerase chain reaction

Polymerase chain reaction (PCR) (see Fig. 6.22) can be performed on blood or bone marrow for a number of specific translocations such as

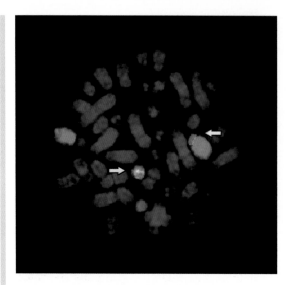

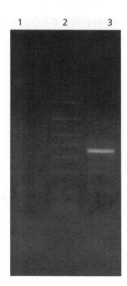

Fig. 11.6 An example of fluorescent *in situ* hybridization (FISH) analysis showing the t(12; 21) translocation. The green probe hybridizes to the region of the *TEL* gene on chromosome 12 and the red probe hybridizes to the region of the *AML1* gene on chromosome 21. The arrows point to the two derived chromosomes resulting from the reciprocal translocation. (Courtesy of Dr C.J. Harrison.)

Fig. 11.7 Reverse transcription PCR analysis of bone marrow from a patient with AML M₃ (acute promyelocytic leukaemia) at diagnosis. The PML-RARα fusion product (cDNA) formed by the t(15; 17) translocation has been amplified by PCR using oligonucleotide primers from the PML and RARα genes. Lane 1, water control; lane 2, low molecular weight DNA marker; lane 3, patient sample. A single 355 base pair fusion message has been amplified showing the presence of the fusion gene.

t(9; 22) and t(15; 17) (Fig. 11.7). It can also be used to detect 'clonal' cells of B- or T-cell lineage by immunoglobulin or T-cell receptor (TCR) gene rearrangement analysis. As it is relatively straightforward and extremely sensitive (detecting one abnormal cell in 10^5–10^6 normal cells) it has become of great value in the diagnosis and monitoring of minimal residual disease (see p. 160).

DNA microarray platforms

DNA microarray platforms allow a rapid and comprehensive analysis of cellular transcription by hybridizing labelled cellular mRNA to DNA probes which are immobilized on a solid support (Fig. 11.8). Oligonucleotides or complimentary (c)DNA arrays may be immobilized on the array and RNA from the tissue of interest is used to generate fluorescent cDNA or RNA which is

then annealed to this DNA matrix. This approach can rapidly determine mRNA expression from a large number of genes and may be used to determine the mRNA expression pattern of different leukaemia subtypes. It is likely to become an important methodology for the diagnosis and classification of haematological malignancies.

Immunofluorescence staining

Immunofluorescence staining can be performed for a few chromosomal abnormalities. An example is expression of the promyelocytic leukaemia (PML) protein which normally has a punctate distribution but is diffusely scattered in acute promyelocytic leukaemia with the t(15; 17) translocation (Fig. 11.9). In addition abnormal fusion proteins can sometimes be detected by specific monoclonal antibodies.

ESTABLISHMENT OF CLONALITY

Demonstration that a cellular expansion is clonal (derived by repeated mitosis from a single cell) rather than polyclonal is important both in haematology research and for diagnosing malignant disease. Various techniques have been used for this purpose (Table 11.3).

Glucose-6-phosphate dehydrogenase isoenzyme analysis

The glucose-6-phosphate dehydrogenase (*G6PD*) gene is on the X chromosome and in females two different alleles of the enzyme, G6PDA or G6PDB, may be present on each chromosome. Because of X-chromosome inactivation (Lyon hypothesis), a clonal proliferation will express only one type, G6PDA or G6PDB, but not a mixture of the two.

Cytogenetics

If an abnormal chromosome, e.g. Philadelphia (Ph), is present in all the tumour cells, the cells containing the abnormality are considered to derive from a common 'stem' cell in which the mutation occurred. The same chromosomal abnormality may be present in different types of leukaemia, e.g. the Ph chromosome in chronic myeloid leukaemia (CML) and in some cases of precursor B acute lymphoblastic leukaemia (c-ALL) (see Fig. 13.1). Moreover, different chromosome abnormalities may underlie apparently the same disease (Table 11.2).

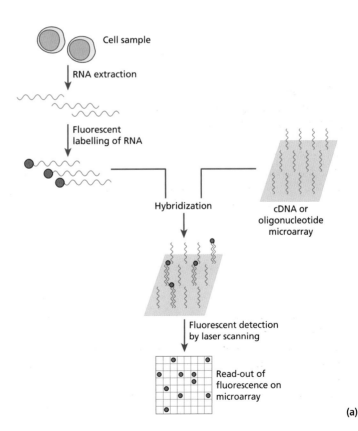

Fig. 11.8 (a) Principle of transcriptional profiling of RNA expression in leukaemia samples using DNA microarrays.

(a)

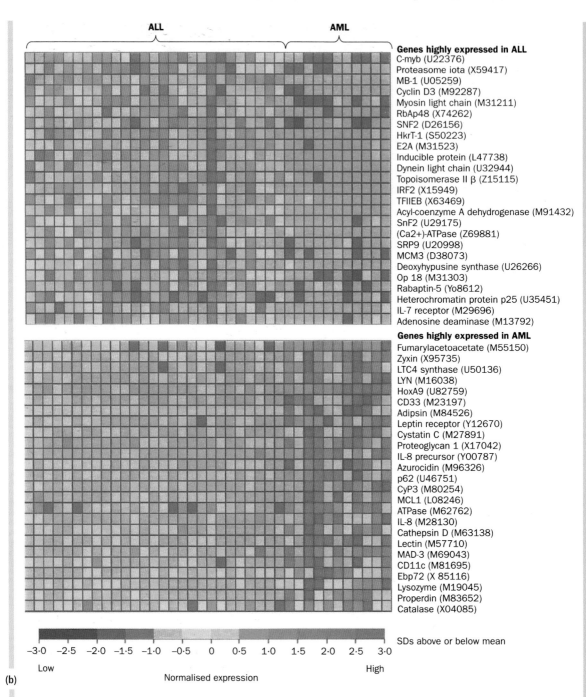

Fig. 11.8 *Continued.* (b) Microarray analysis of genes distinguishing acute lymphoblastic leukaemia (ALL) from acute myeloid leukaemia (AML). The 50 genes most highly correlated on gene-expression microarrays with each of these leukaemias are shown. Each row corresponds to a gene; each column corresponds to the expression value in a particular sample. Expression for each gene is normalized across the samples such that the mean is 0 and the SD is 1. Expression greater than the mean is shaded in red, and that below the mean is shaded in blue. Although the genes as a group appear correlated with the type of leukaemia under study, no single gene is uniformly expressed across the class, illustrating the value of a multigene prediction method. (Reproduced courtesy of Golub and colleagues.)

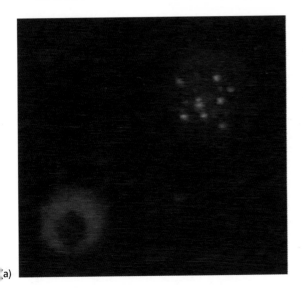

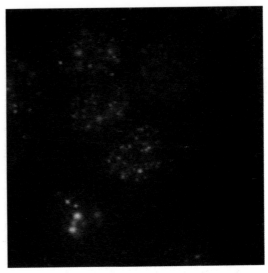

(a)

(b)

Fig. 11.9 Immunofluorescent staining of the promyelocytic leukaemia (PML) protein in acute promyelocytic leukaemia. In normal cells (a) the protein is expressed in a characteristic nuclear speckled pattern due to localization of the protein into discrete dots (5–20 per nucleus), named PML nuclear bodies. (b) In promyelocytic leukaemia cells the PML nuclear bodies are disrupted and the staining changes to a microgranular appearance. (Courtesy of Dr R. Johnson.)

Table 11.3 Establishment of clonality

G6PD isoenzyme analysis	Applicable to 'informative' females only
X-linked RFLP analysis	
Light chain restriction	Applicable to B-lymphoid tumours only
Immunoglobulin and TCR gene rearrangements	Applicable to lymphoid malignancies
Cytogenetics: chromosomal translocational analysis point mutations	

G6PD, glucose-6-phosphate dehydrogenase; RFLP, restriction fragment length polymorphism; TCR, T-cell receptor.

Restriction fragment length polymorphism analysis

Restriction fragment length polymorphism (RFLP) indicates the variation in the size of a DNA fragment, detectable with a given probe, after digestion with a restriction enzyme (p. 88). Differences in size of the RFLP detected can be caused by a point mutation in a restriction site, or by a shift in the position of the restriction site because of deletion or duplication of neighbouring DNA. In females, the two X chromosomes can be informative by having different RFLP haplotypes (see Fig. 6.25). In a clone of cells, only one of the X chromosomes will be active (see Lyon hypothesis above). DNA active in transcription is usually hypomethylated whereas resting DNA is methylated. Because the DNA of the active X chromosomes will be hypomethylated the use of a second restriction enzyme (e.g. Hpa I) sensitive to the methylation status of the DNA, followed by Southern blotting using a single X chromosome probe, will be informative of whether only one (as in a monoclonal tumour) or both (as in a polyclonal proliferation) X chromosomes are active in the tissue examined.

Light chain restriction

Mature B-lineage cells express surface immunoglobulin with κ or λ light chains. A polyclonal population usually shows a ratio of 2:1 of κ:λ expressing cells. In a clonal population, e.g. CLL or B-cell lymphoma, the cells will all express either κ or λ chains but not both (see Fig. 15.10).

Immunoglobulin or TCR rearrangement

The immunoglobulin or TCR genes each exist as separate segments in germline cells (see Fig. 10.4). Rearrangement of the immunoglobulin genes occurs in B-lineage cells and of the TCR genes in T-lineage cells. These rearrangements are all different in polyclonal cells but identical in a clonal population and these clonal rearrangements can be detected by Southern blotting or PCR technique.

INHERITED AND ACQUIRED PREDISPOSITION TO LEUKAEMIA AND LYMPHOMA

Exactly how genetic mutations accumulate in haemopoietic malignancies is largely unknown. As in most diseases it is the combination of genetic background and environmental influence that will determine the risk of developing a malignancy. However, in the majority of individual cases neither a genetic susceptibility nor an environmental agent are apparent.

Inherited factors

There is a greatly increased incidence of leukaemia in some genetic diseases, particularly Down's syndrome (where acute leukaemia occurs with a 20–30-fold increased frequency), Bloom's syndrome, Fanconi anaemia, ataxia-telangiectasia, Klinefelter's syndrome, osteogenesis imperfecta and Wiskott–Aldrich syndrome. As well as the increased incidence of leukaemia in these primary genetic diseases there is a weak familial tendency in diseases such as B-cell CLL (B-CLL), Hodgkin's disease and non-Hodgkin's lymphoma although the genes predisposing to this risk are unknown.

Interestingly it appears that a significant number of cases of childhood acute lymphoblastic leukaemia (ALL) may be initiated by genetic mutations that occur during development *in utero* (Fig. 11.10). Studies in identical twins have shown that both may be born with the same chromosomal abnormalities, e.g. t(12; 21) in their haemopoietic cells. This has presumably arisen spontaneously in a progenitor cell which has passed into both twins as a result of the sharing of blood as a consequence of a single placenta. One twin may develop ALL early, e.g. at age 5, presumably because of a second transforming event while the other remains well or develops ALL later. The nature of the second event is unclear but may be associated with proliferative stress put upon B-cell progenitors at the time of development of immunity to external antigens, e.g. infection.

Environmental influences

Chemicals
Chronic exposure to benzene may cause bone marrow hypoplasia, dysplasia and chromosome abnormalities and is an unusual cause of myelodysplasia or acute myeloid leukaemia (AML). Other industrial solvents and chemicals may less commonly cause leukaemia.

Drugs
The alkylating agents, e.g. chlorambucil, mustine, melphalan, procarbazine and nitrosoureas (e.g. BCNU, CCNU) predispose to AML especially if combined with radiotherapy or if used to treat patients with lymphocytic or plasmacytic disorders. Epipodophyllotoxins such as etoposide are powerful antileukaemic agents themselves but their use is associated with a risk of the development of secondary leukaemias associated with mutation of the *MLL* gene at 11q23.

Radiation
Radiation, especially to the marrow, is leukaemogenic. This is illustrated by an increased incidence of all types of leukaemia (except B-CLL) in survivors of the atom bomb explosions in Japan.

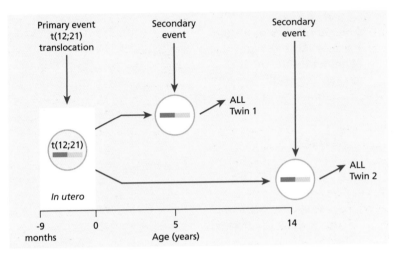

Fig. 11.10 Prenatal origin of acute lymphoblastic leukaemia (ALL) in a pair of identical twins. ALL was diagnosed in the first twin at age 5 years and in the second at age 14 years. Both tumours had an identical t(12;21) translocation indicating probable origin of the leukaemic clone in an haemopoietic cells *in utero* and dissemination to both twins via a shared placental blood supply. Because of the prolonged latency of the ALL it is presumed that a secondary event is required to initiate the development of frank leukaemia. At the time of the diagnosis of ALL in twin 1 the t(12;21) translocation could be detected in the bone marrow of twin 2. It is likely that such a 'fetal origin' of childhood ALL occurs in a significant number of sporadic ALL cases. (Based on J.L. Wiemels *et al*. 1999.)

Infection

Viruses (Table 11.4)

Human T-lymphotropic virus type 1 (HTLV-1) is implicated in the cause of adult T-cell leukaemia/lymphoma (ATLL) (p. 197) although most people infected with this virus do not develop the tumour. Epstein–Barr virus (EBV) DNA has been found integrated into the genome of endemic (African) Burkitt lymphoma cells but rarely in sporadic Burkitt lymphoma cells. The EBV genome is also present in the tumour cells of patients who develop post-transplant lymphoproliferative disease (PTLD) during immunosuppressive therapy after solid organ transplantation, in many patients with acquired immune deficiency syndrome (AIDS) developing lymphomas, and in a proportion of patients with Hodgkin's disease. Human herpes virus 8 (HHV-8) is associated with Kaposi's sarcoma and rare subtypes of lymphoma. Hepatitis C has been associated with B-cell non-Hodgkin's lymphoma.

Table 11.4 Infections associated with haemopoietic malignancies*

Infection	Tumour
Virus	
HTLV-1	Adult T-cell leukaemia/lymphoma
Epstein–Barr virus	Burkitt's and Hodgkin's lymphomas; PTLD
HHV-8	Primary effusion lymphoma
HIV-1	High-grade B-cell lymphoma
Bacteria	
Helicobacter pylori	Gastric lymphoma (MALT)
Protozoa	
Malaria	Burkitt's lymphoma

HHV-8, human herpes virus 8; HIV, human immunodeficiency virus; HTLV-1, human T-lymphotropic virus type 1; PTLD, post-transplant lymphoproliferative disease.

Bacteria

Helicobacter pylori infection has been implicated in the pathogenesis of gastric mucosa B-cell (MALT) lymphoma (see p. 211).

Protozoa

Endemic Burkitt's lymphoma occurs in the tropics particularly in malaria areas. It is thought that malaria may alter host immunity and predispose to tumour formation as a result of EBV infection.

GENETIC ABNORMALITIES ASSOCIATED WITH HAEMATOLOGICAL MALIGNANCIES

Some of the genetic abnormalities commonly associated with different types of leukaemia and lymphoma are listed in Table 11.2.

The mechanisms of gene abnormality include the following (Fig. 11.11).

Point mutations

These are best illustrated by activation of the *RAS* oncogenes which are seen in a wide variety of human tumours including AML (20–30%), ALL (15–20%), myelodysplasia (20–40%) and myeloma (20%). A point mutation in one of three codons (12, 13 or 61) accounts for virtually all of the activated *RAS* alleles in human malignancy. Activation of *N-RAS* is the usual mutation found in human haemopoietic malignancies.

Translocations

These are a characteristic feature of haematological malignancies and there are two main mechanisms whereby they may contribute to malignant change.

1 Fusion of parts of two genes to generate a chimeric gene that encodes a novel 'fusion protein', e.g. *BCR-ABL* in t(9; 22) in chronic myeloid leukaemia (CML) (see Fig. 13.1), *RARα-PML* in t(15; 17) in AML M$_3$ (Fig. 11.12) or *TEL-AML1* in t(12; 21) in pre-B-ALL (Fig. 11.6).

2 Overexpression of a normal cellular gene, for example overexpression of *BCL*-2 in the t(14; 18) translocation of follicular lymphoma or *MYC* in Burkitt's lymphoma (Fig. 11.13). Interestingly, this

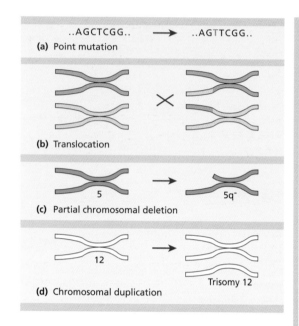

Fig. 11.11 Types of genetic abnormality which may lead to haemopoietic malignancy. (a) Point mutation; (b) chromosomal translocation; (c) chromosomal deletion or loss; (d) chromosomal duplication.

class of translocation nearly always involves a TCR or immunoglobulin gene locus presumably as a result of aberrant activity of the recombinase enzyme which is involved in immunoglobulin or *TCR* gene rearrangement in immature B or T cells.

Gene and chromosomal deletions

Gene and chromosomal deletions may involve a small part of a chromosome, the short or long arm (e.g. 5q–) or the entire chromosome (e.g. monosomy 7). Losses most commonly affect chromosomes 5, 6, 7, 11, 20 and Y. The critical event is probably loss of a tumour-suppressor gene.

Chromosomal duplication or gene amplification

In chromosomal duplication (e.g. trisomy 12 in B-CLL) or gene amplification, gains are common in chromosomes 8, 12, 19, 21 and Y. Gene amplification is not a common feature in haemopoietic malignancy but has been described involving the *MLL* gene.

SPECIFIC EXAMPLES OF TRANSLOCATIONS ASSOCIATED WITH HAEMATOLOGICAL MALIGNANCY

Retinoic acid receptor

In the t(15; 17) translocation associated with AML M_3 (p. 163), the promyelocytic leukaemia gene *PML* on chromosome 15 is fused to the retinoic acid receptor α gene, *RARα*, on chromosome 17 (Fig. 11.12). The resultant *PML-RARα* fusion protein functions as a transcriptional repressor whereas normal (wild-type) *RARα* is an activator. Normally the PML protein forms homodimers with itself whereas the RARα protein forms heterodimers with the retinoid X receptor protein, RXR. The PML-RARα fusion protein binds to PML and RXR, preventing them from linking with their natural partners. This results in the cellular phenotype of arrested differentiation. Cases of AML M_3 associated with the t(15; 17) translocation respond to treatment with high doses of all-transretinoic acid (ATRA) which causes differen-

tiation of the abnormal promyelocytes and results in improved prognosis (p. 174). Interestingly, in rare variants of AML M_3 *RARα* is fused to other genes. In these cases ATRA treatment is not successful. A common mechanism involved in all cases is the recruitment by the fusion proteins of a histone deacetylase that represses transcription. This interaction is overcome by ATRA in cases involving the t(15; 17) translocation but not those with t(5; 17) or t(11; 17).

This model may represent a unifying concept of how many of the different chromosomal translocations lead to the development of AML. Namely, that rearrangement of transcription factor genes leads to aberrant transcription as a result of recruitment of histone deacetylase and transcriptional corepressors rather than transcriptional activation. Chemical inhibitors of histone deacetylation are now being used in clinical trials.

Translocation of *MYC*

In Burkitt's lymphoma and B-ALL one of three translocations is normally found. All of these bring the *MYC* oncogene into close proximity with one of the immunoglobulin genes (Fig. 11.13); the most frequent is translocation to the heavy chain locus, t(8; 14). As a result, expression of the *MYC* gene is deregulated and the gene is expressed in parts of the cell cycle during which it should normally be switched off.

Translocation of the *BCL-2* gene

This oncogene is translocated from chromosome

Fig. 11.12 Generation of the t(15; 17) translocation. The *PML* gene at 15q22 may break at one of three different breakpoint cluster regions (BCR-1, -2 and -3) and joins with exons 3–9 of the *RARα* gene at 17q12. Three different fusion mRNAs are generated (termed long (L), variable (V) or short (S)) and these give rise to fusion proteins of different size. In this diagram only the long version resulting from a break at BCR-1 is shown.

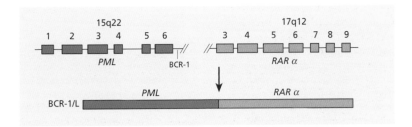

18 to chromosome 14 in the (14; 18) translocation found in about 85% of cases of follicular lymphoma and in some cases of diffuse lymphoma and B-CLL. The translocation leads to constitutive expression of the *BCL-2* gene with increased survival of cells because of reduced apoptosis.

Translocations involving the core binding factor genes

Core binding factor (CBF) is a heterodimeric transcription factor and is important in regulating expression of a number of genes such as *IL-3* and

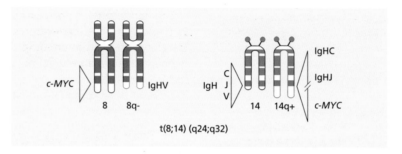

t(8;14) (q24;q32)

Fig. 11.13 The genetic events in one of the three translocations found in Burkitt's lymphoma and B-cell acute lymphoblastic leukaemia. The oncogene *c-MYC* is normally located on the long arm (q) of chromosome 8. In the (8; 14) translocation, *c-MYC* is translocated into close proximity to the immunoglobulin heavy chain gene on the long arm of chromosome 14. Part of the heavy chain gene (the V region) is reciprocally translocated to chromosome 8. C, constant region; IgH, immunoglobulin heavy chain gene; J, joining region; V, variable region.

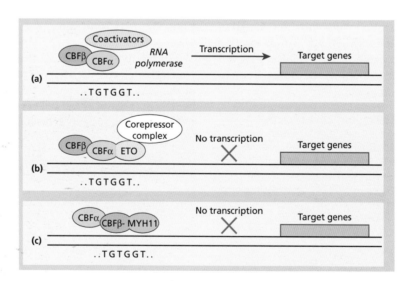

Fig. 11.14 Mechanism of action of the core binding factor (CBF) transcription factor and its disruption in acute myeloid leukaemia. CBF consists of two subunits, *CBFβ* and *CBFα* (or *AML1*) which together form a heterodimer (a). This complex binds to the DNA sequence TGTGGT in the regulatory region of certain target genes. This binding allows recruitment of coactivators which lead to transcription from these genes. (b) The t(8; 21) translocation leads to a fusion protein of CBFα with ETO. Although the CBF subunits can still form heterodimers their binding to DNA leads to recruitment of a corepressor complex which blocks transcription. (c) In the inv(16) mutation a CBFα-MYH11 fusion protein is generated which again can form CBF heterodimers but these do not gain access to DNA.

GM-CSF. Genes encoding the two components of CBF, *CBFα* and *CBFβ*, are involved in a number of chromosomal translocations associated with leukaemia (Fig. 11.14). These include t(8; 21) in which the *CBFα* gene, also known as *AML1*, is translocated to the *ETO* gene on chromosome 8. Another common rearrangement in AML is inv(16) in which the *CBFβ* gene is fused to the *SMMHC* (*MYH11*) gene. In the t(12; 21) translocation associated with pre-B-ALL the *TEL* gene is fused to the CBFα gene to generate a novel fusion protein. All three translocations appear to act as dominant inhibitors of normal wild-type CBF activity.

VALUE OF GENETIC MARKERS IN MANAGEMENT OF HAEMATOLOGICAL MALIGNANCY

The detection of genetic abnormalities may be important in several aspects of the management of patients with leukaemia or lymphoma.

For initial diagnosis

Many genetic abnormalities are so specific for a particular disease that their presence determines that diagnosis. An example is the t(15; 17) translocation which classifies an AML as promyelocytic leukaemia. Clonal immunoglobulin or TCR gene rearrangements are useful in establishing clonality and determining the lineage of a lymphoid malignancy.

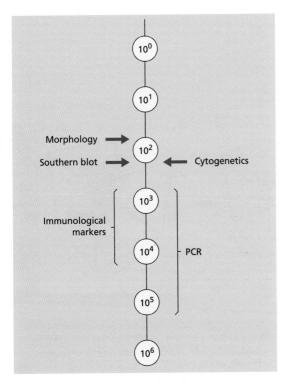

Fig. 11.15 Sensitivity of detection of leukaemic cells using five different techniques. 10^1–10^6 = 1 cell in 10 to 1 cell in 10^6 detected.

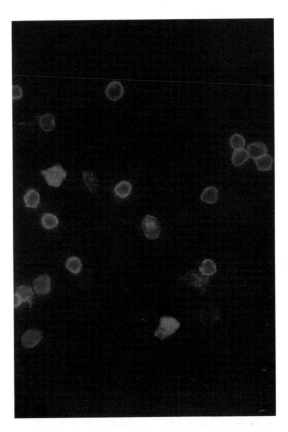

Fig. 11.16 Minimal residual disease in the bone marrow of a patient with T-ALL in remission detected by immunofluorescence microscopy. Three cells double stained by anti-CD3 (green) and TdT (red) are residual leukaemia cells. Normal bone marrow CD3+ T cells are TdT−. (Courtesy of D. Campana.)

For establishing a treatment protocol

There is a growing realization that haematological malignancies should not be grouped together as simply as has been the case until now. For instance, AML is a diverse group of genetic disorders and evidence suggests that individual subtypes respond differently to standard treatment. For instance, t(15; 17), inv(16) and t(8; 21) subgroups do well whereas monosomy 7 carries a poor prognosis. Treatment strategies are now tailored around the genetic disorder and in some instances knowledge of the genetic abnormality underlying the tumour can lead to rational treatment approaches. The best example is the use of retinoic acid in the treatment of promyelocytic leukaemia associated with the t(15; 17) translocation. Genetic information is also valuable for giving a prognosis. For instance, Ph+ ALL has a particularly poor prognosis, whereas hyperdiploidy in ALL is a favourable finding.

Monitoring the response to therapy
(Fig. 11.17)

The detection of minimal residual disease (MRD) (disease which cannot be seen by conventional staining and microscopy of the blood or bone marrow) in AML, ALL or CML after chemotherapy or bone marrow transplantation is possible using the following techniques (in increasing order of sensitivity, Fig. 11.15).

1 Cytogenetic analysis.

2 Southern blot analysis to look for a tumour-specific DNA rearrangement.

3 Immunoflorescence (Fig. 11.16) or fluorescence-activated cell sorting (FACS) to detect tumour cells using immunological markers which detect 'leukaemia-specific' combinations of antigens (Fig. 11.17).

4 PCR to amplify tumour-specific translocations or immunoglobulin/TCR sequences (see Fig. 11.7).

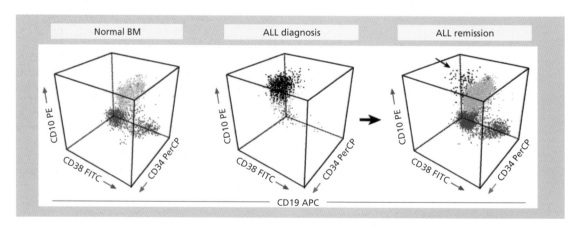

Fig. 11.17 Detection of minimal residual disease (MRD) by four-colour flow cytometry in: normal bone marrow mononuclear cells (BM), BM from a patient with B lineage ALL at diagnosis and in remission 6 weeks after diagnosis. The cells were detected with four different antibodies (anti-CD10, anti-CD19, anti-CD34, anti-CD38) attached to fluorescent labels abbreviated as PE, APC, PerCP and FITC, respectively. The tridimensional plot shows the immunophenotype of CD19 + lymphoid cells in the three samples. MRD of 0.03% of cells expressing the leukaemia-associated phenotype (CD10+, CD34+, CD38–) were detected at 6 weeks, confirmed by PCR analysis. (From D. Campana and E. Coustan-Smith 1999. Cytometry. *Commun Clin Cytometry* **38**, 139–52, with permission.)

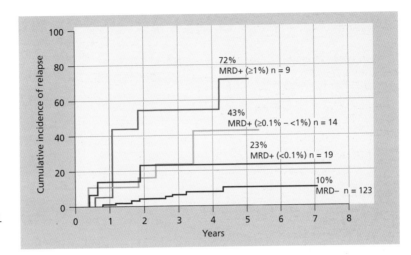

Fig. 11.18 Cumulative incidence of relapse according to minimal residual disease (MRD) levels at the end of remission induction in children with ALL treated at St Jude Children's Research Hospital. (Courtesy of Dr D. Campana.)

These approaches are being evaluated but they already play an important role in determining the treatment of individual patients, e.g. persistence of MRD in childhood ALL after the initial 1–3 months of therapy predicts probable relapse (Fig. 11.18) while persistence of the *BCR-ABL* fusion gene after allogeneic stem cell transplantation for CML suggests the need for treatment with donor leucocytes (see p. 110).

BIBLIOGRAPHY

Degos L., Linch D.C. and Lowenberg B. (eds) (1999) *A Textbook of Malignant Hematology*. Martin Dunitz, London.

Greaves M.F. (1999) Molecular genetics, natural history and the demise of childhood leukaemia. *Eur. J. Cancer* **35**, 173–85.

Kearney L. (1999) The impact of the new FISH technologies on the cytogenetics of haematological malignancies. *Br. J. Haematol.* **104**, 648–58.

Knuutila S. *et al.* (1997) Lineage specificity in haematological neoplasms. *Br. J. Haematol.* **96**, 2–11.

Kuzrock R. and Talpaz M. (eds) (1999) *Molecular Biology in Cancer Medicine*, 2nd edn. Martin Dunitz, London.

Preudhomme C. and Fenaux P. (1997) The clinical significance of mutations of the p53 tumour suppressor gene in haematological malignancies. *Br. J. Haematol.* **98**, 502–11.

Rabbitts T.H. (1991) Translocations, master genes, and differences between the origins of acute and chronic leukaemias. *Cell* **67**, 641–4.

Russell N.H. (1997) Biology of acute leukaemia. *Lancet* **349**, 118–22.

Stamatoyannopoulos G., Perlmutter R.M., Majerus P.W. and Varmus H. (eds) (2000) *The Molecular Basis of Blood Diseases*, 3rd edn. W.B. Saunders, Philadelphia.

Wickremasinghe R.G. and Hoffbrand A.V. (2000) Molecular basis of leukaemia and lymphoma. In: *Molecular Haematology*. Provan D. and Gribben J. (eds) Blackwell Science, Oxford. pp. 25–41.

Wiemels J.L., Ford A.M., Van Wering E.R., Postma A. and Greaves M. (1999) Protracted latency of acute lymphoblastic leukaemia after TEL-AML1 gene fusion *in utero. Blood* **94**, 1057–62.

Wiernick P.H., Canellos, G.P., Dutcher J.P. and Kyle R.A. (eds) (1996) *Neoplastic Diseases of the Blood*, 3rd edn. Churchill Livingstone, New York.

Willis T.G. and Dyer M.J.S. (2000) The role of immunoglobulin translocations in the pathogenesis of B-cell malignancies. *Blood* **96**, 808–22.

CHAPTER 12

Acute leukaemias

The leukaemias are a group of disorders characterized by the accumulation of malignant white cells in the bone marrow and blood. These abnormal cells cause symptoms because of: (a) bone marrow failure (i.e. anaemia, neutropenia, thrombocytopenia); and (b) infiltration of organs (e.g. liver, spleen, lymph nodes, meninges, brain, skin or testes).

CLASSIFICATION OF LEUKAEMIA

The main classification is into four types—acute and chronic leukaemias which are further subdivided into lymphoid or myeloid (Table 12.1).

Acute leukaemias are usually aggressive diseases in which the malignant transformation causes accumulation of early bone marrow haemopoietic progenitors, called blast cells. The dominant clinical feature of these diseases is usually bone marrow failure caused by accumulation of blast cells although tissue infiltration also occurs. If untreated these diseases are usually fairly rapidly fatal but, paradoxically, they are also easier to cure than chronic leukaemias.

CLASSIFICATION OF ACUTE LEUKAEMIA

Acute leukaemia is defined as the presence of over 30% of blast cells in the bone marrow at clinical presentation. It is further subdivided into acute myeloid leukaemia (AML) and acute lymphoblastic leukaemia (ALL) on the basis of whether the blasts are shown to be myeloblasts or lymphoblasts (Table 12.2).

Differentiation of ALL from AML

In most cases, the clinical features and morphology on routine staining distinguish ALL from AML. In ALL the blasts show no differentiation (with the exception of B-cell ALL (B-ALL)) whereas in AML some evidence of differentiation to granulocytes or monocytes is usually seen in the blasts or their progeny. Specialized tests are needed to confirm the diagnosis of AML or ALL and to subdivide cases of AML or ALL into their different subtypes (Tables 12.3 and 12.4).

In a minority of cases of acute leukaemia the blast cells show features of both AML and ALL. These features may be on the same cell (biphenotypic) or on separate populations (bilineal) and they include inappropriate expression of immunological markers or inappropriate gene rearrangements. This is termed hybrid acute leukaemia and treatment is usually given on the basis of the dominant pattern.

ACUTE LYMPHOBLASTIC LEUKAEMIA

This is caused by an accumulation of lymphoblasts and is the most common malignancy of childhood.

Classification

This may be on the basis of morphology or immunological markers. The French–American–British (FAB) group subclassifies ALL into three subtypes (Table 12.2 and Fig. 12.1):

1 the L_1 type show uniform, small blast cells with scanty cytoplasm;

2 the L_2 type comprise larger blast cells with more prominent nucleoli and cytoplasm and with more heterogeneity; and

3 the L_3 blasts are large with prominent nucleoli, strongly basophilic cytoplasm and cytoplasmic vacuoles.

Immunological markers in ALL are as follows (Table 12.4 and Fig. 12.2).

1 Precursor B-ALL: CD19+, cytoplasmic CD22+ and TdT+ three subtypes:

(a) early pre-B, CD10–
- also called pre-pre-B or pro-B-ALL
- often seen in infants;

(b) early pre-B, CD10+ is known as common ALL (cALL);

(c) pre-B
- intracytoplasmic μ+
- CD10– or CD10+.

2 T-ALL which shows T-cell antigens (e.g. CD7 and cytoplasmic CD3).

3 B-ALL which shows surface immunoglobulin and is TdT–.

Table 12.1 Classification of leukaemias

Acute (see Table 12.2)
Acute myeloid leukaemia: M_0–M_7
Acute lymphoblastic leukaemia: L_1–L_3

Chronic (see Tables 13.1 and 14.1)
Chronic myeloid leukaemias
Chronic lymphoid leukaemias

Table 12.2 Classification of acute myeloid (AML) and acute lymphoblastic (ALL) leukaemia according to the French–American–British (FAB) group

AML	ALL
M_0 undifferentiated	L_1 blast cells small, uniform high nuclear to cytoplasmic ratio
M_1 without maturation	
M_2 with granulocytic maturation	L_2 blast cells larger, heterogeneous, lower nuclear to cytoplasmic ratio
M_3 acute promyelocytic	L_3 vacuolated blasts, basophilic cytoplasm (usually B-ALL)
M_4 granulocytic and monocytic maturation	
M_5 monoblastic (M_{5a}) or monocytic (M_{5b})	
M_6 erythroleukaemia	
M_7 megakaryoblastic	

Table 12.3 Specialized tests for acute lymphoblastic leukaemia (ALL) and acute myeloid leukaemia (AML)

	ALL	AML
Cytochemistry		
Myeloperoxidase	—	+ (including Auer rods)
Sudan black	—	+ (including Auer rods)
Non-specific esterase	—	+ in M_4, M_5
Periodic acid–Schiff	+ (coarse block positivity in ALL)	+ (fine blocks in M_6)
Acid phosphatase	+ in T-ALL (Golgi staining)	+ in M_6 (diffuse)
Electron microscopy	—	+ (early granule formation)
Immunoglobulin and TCR genes	Precursor B-ALL: clonal rearrangement of immunoglobulin genes	Germline configuration of immunoglobulin and TCR genes
	T-ALL: clonal rearrangement of TCR genes	
Chromosomes (see Table 11.2)		
Immunological markers (see Table 12.4)		

TCR, T-cell receptor.

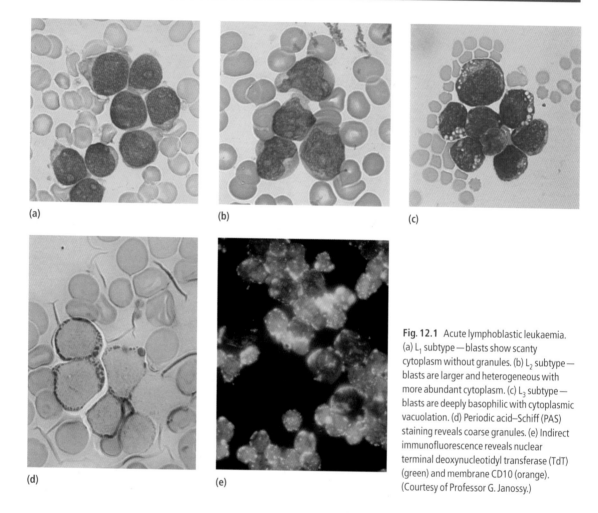

(a)

(b)

(c)

(d)

(e)

Fig. 12.1 Acute lymphoblastic leukaemia. (a) L_1 subtype — blasts show scanty cytoplasm without granules. (b) L_2 subtype — blasts are larger and heterogeneous with more abundant cytoplasm. (c) L_3 subtype — blasts are deeply basophilic with cytoplasmic vacuolation. (d) Periodic acid–Schiff (PAS) staining reveals coarse granules. (e) Indirect immunofluorescence reveals nuclear terminal deoxynucleotidyl transferase (TdT) (green) and membrane CD10 (orange). (Courtesy of Professor G. Janossy.)

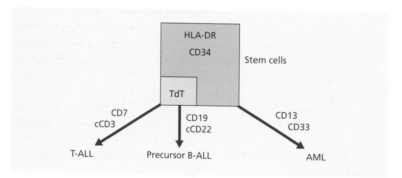

Fig. 12.2 Development of three cell lineages from pluripotential stem cells giving rise to the three main immunological subclasses of acute leukaemia. The immunological characterization using pairs of markers is shown, as well as the three markers characterizing the early 'stem' cells. ALL, acute lymphoblastic leukaemia; AML, acute myeloid leukaemia; c, cytoplasmic.

Table 12.4 Immunological markers for classification of acute myeloid (AML) and acute lymphoblastic (ALL) leukaemia

Marker	AML	ALL Precursor B*	T
Myeloid			
CD13	+	−	−
CD33	+	−	−
Glycophorin	+ (M$_6$)	−	−
Platelet antigens, e.g. CD41	+ (M$_7$)	−	−
Myeloperoxidase	+ (M$_0$)		
B lineage			
CD19	−	+	−
cCD22	−	+	−
CD10	−	+ or −	−
cIg	−	+ (pre-B)	−
T lineage			
CD7	−	−	+
cCD3	−	−	+
TdT	−	+	+

* B-ALL resembles precursor B-ALL immunologically but has surface immunoglobulin (Ig) and is terminal deoxynucleotidyl transferase negative (TdT−).
c, Cytoplasmic.

B-ALL usually corresponds to the morphological L$_3$ type whereas the precursor B or T types may be L$_1$ or L$_2$ and are morphologically indistinguishable.

Incidence and clinical features

ALL is the common form of leukaemia in children; its incidence is highest at 3–7 years, falling off by 10 years. The common (CD10+) precursor B type which is most usual in children has an equal sex incidence; there is a male predominance for T-ALL. There is a lower frequency of ALL after 10 years of age with a secondary rise after the age of 40.

Clinical features are secondary to the following.
1 Bone marrow failure—anaemia (pallor, lethargy and dyspnoea); neutropenia (fever, malaise, features of mouth, throat, skin, respiratory, perianal or other infections; Fig. 12.3); and

thrombocytopenia (spontaneous bruises, purpura, bleeding gums and menorrhagia; Fig. 12.4).
2 Organ infiltration—tender bones, lymphadenopathy (Fig. 12.5), moderate splenomegaly, hepatomegaly and meningeal syndrome (headache, nausea and vomiting, blurring of vision and diplopia). Fundal examination may reveal papilloedema and sometimes haemorrhage. Less common manifestations include testicular swelling (Fig. 12.5b) or signs of mediastinal compression in T-ALL (Fig. 12.6).

Investigations

Haematological investigations may reveal a normochromic, normocytic anaemia with thrombocytopenia in most cases. The total white cell count may be decreased, normal or increased up to $200 \times 10^9/l$ or more. Blood film examination typically shows variable numbers of blast cells. The bone marrow is hypercellular with >30% leukaemic blasts. The blast cells are characterized by morphology, immunological tests and cytogenetic analysis and, for follow-up, minimal residual disease analysis, by characterizing by PCR analysis, the V gene or TCR gene clonal rearrangement of the particular patient. Cytogenetic analysis shows differing patterns in infants, children and adults which partly explains the different prognoses of these groups (Fig. 12.7).

Lumbar puncture for cerebrospinal fluid examination should be performed and may show that the spinal fluid has an increased pressure and contains leukaemic cells. Biochemical tests may reveal a raised serum uric acid, serum lactate dehydrogenase and less commonly hypercalcaemia. Liver and renal function tests are performed as a baseline before treatment begins. X-rays may reveal lytic bone lesions and a mediastinal mass caused by enlargement of the thymus and/or mediastinal lymph nodes characteristic of T-ALL (Fig. 12.6).

The differential diagnosis includes AML, aplastic anaemia (with which ALL sometimes presents), marrow infiltration with other malignancies (e.g. rhabdomyosarcoma, neuroblastoma and Ewing's sarcoma), infections such as infec-

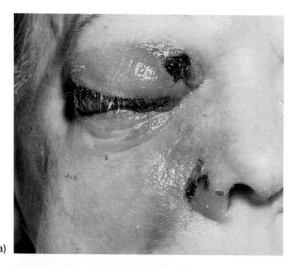

(a)

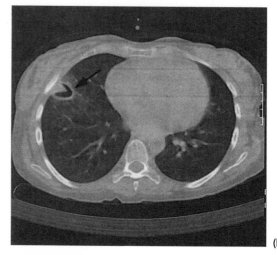

(b)

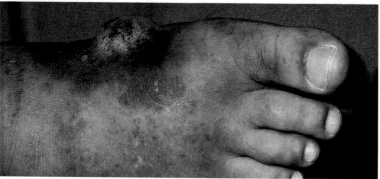

(c)

Fig. 12.3 (a) An orbital infection in a female patient (aged 68 years) with acute myeloid leukaemia and severe neutropenia (haemoglobin 8.3 g/dl, white cells 15.3×10⁹/l, blasts 96%, neutrophils 1%, platelets 30×10⁹/l). (b) CT scan of a chest showing cavitating mass (arrowed) in the periphery of the right upper lobe which at operation (lobectomy) proved to be an aspergilloma in a patient with acute leukaemia. (c) Skin infection (*Pseudomonas aeruginosa*) in a female patient (aged 33 years) with acute lymphoblastic leukaemia receiving chemotherapy and with severe neutropenia (haemoglobin 10.1 g/dl, white cells 0.7×10⁹/l, neutrophils <0.1×10⁹/l, lymphocytes 0.6×10⁹/l, platelets 20×10⁹/l).

tious mononucleosis and pertussis, juvenile rheumatoid arthritis and immune thrombocytopenic purpura.

Principles of cytotoxic drug therapy

Most of the cytotoxic drugs used in leukaemia therapy damage the capacity of cells for reproduction (Table 12.5). Combinations of at least three drugs are now usually used to increase the cytotoxic effect, improve remission rates and reduce the frequency of emergence of drug resistance. These multiple drug combinations have also been found to give longer remissions in acute leukaemias than single agents.

Initial therapy may be complicated by hyperkalaemia and hyperuricaemia with urate nephropathy (the 'tumour lysis syndrome'). Thus the patient should be given allopurinol before starting therapy, be well hydrated and if the white cell count is high and there is substantial organ infiltration, alkalization of the urine should be carried out with intravenous sodium bicarbonate.

Table 12.5 Drugs used in the treatment of leukaemia

	Mechanism of action	Particular side-effects*
Antimetabolites		
Methotrexate	Inhibit pyrimidine or purine synthesis or incorporation into DNA	Mouth ulcers, gut toxicity
6-Mercaptopurine†		Jaundice
6-Thioguanine†		Gut toxicity
Cytosine arabinoside		CNS especially cerebellar toxicity and conjunctivitis at high doses
Hydroxyurea		Pigmentation, nail dystrophy, skin ulceration
Alkylating agents		
Cyclophosphamide	Cross-link DNA, impede RNA formation	Haemorrhagic cystitis, cardiomyopathy, loss of hair
Chlorambucil		Marrow aplasia, hepatic toxicity, dermatitis
Busulphan (Myleran)		Marrow aplasia, pulmonary fibrosis, hyperpigmentation
Nitrosoureas BCNU, CCNU		Renal and pulmonary toxicity
DNA binding		
Anthracyclines, e.g.	Bind to DNA and interfere with mitosis	Cardiac toxicity, hair loss
Daunorubicin		
Hydroxodaunorubicin (Adriamycin)		
Mitoxantrone		
Idarubicin		
Bleomycin	DNA breaks	Pulmonary fibrosis, skin pigmentation
Mitotic inhibitors		
Vincristine (Oncovin)	Spindle damage, absent metaphase	Neuropathy (peripheral or bladder or gut), hair loss
Vinblastine		
Vindesine		
Purine analogues		
Fludarabine	Inhibit adenosine deaminase or other purine pathways	Immune suppression (low CD4 counts); autoimmune haemolytic anaemia; renal and neurotoxicity (at high doses)
2-Chlorodeoxyadenosine		
Deoxycoformycin		
Miscellaneous		
Corticosteroids	Lymphoblast lysis	Peptic ulcer, obesity, diabetes, osteoporosis, psychosis, hypertension
L-Asparaginase	Deprive cells of asparagine	Hypersensitivity, low albumin and coagulation factors, pancreatitis
Epipodophyllotoxin (etoposide, VP-16)	Mitotic inhibitor	Hair loss, oral ulceration
α-Interferon	Activation of RNAase and natural killer activity	Flu-like symptoms, thrombocytopenia, leucopenia, weight loss
Transretinoic acid	Induces differentiation	Liver dysfunction, skin hyperkeratosis, leucocytosis and hyperviscosity, pleural or pericardial effusion

* Most of the drugs cause nausea, vomiting, mucositis and bone marrow toxicity, and in large doses infertility. Tissue necrosis is a problem if the drugs are extravasated during infusion.

† Allopurinol potentiates the action and side-effects of 6-mercaptopurine and 6-thioguanine.

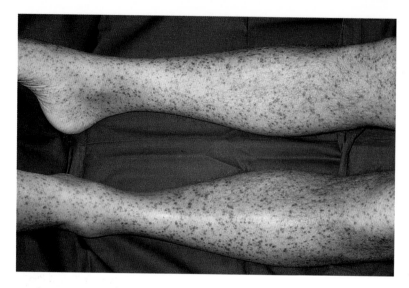

Fig. 12.4 Purpura over the lower limbs in a male patient (aged 53 years) with acute leukaemia.

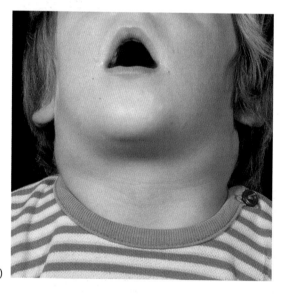

(a)

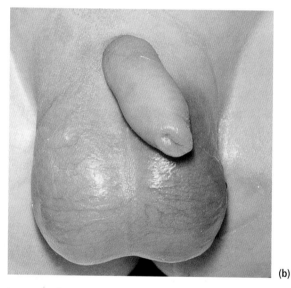

(b)

Fig. 12.5 Acute lymphoblastic leukaemia. (a) Marked cervical lymphadenopathy in a boy. (b) Testicular swelling and erythema on the left hand side of the scrotum caused by testicular infiltration. (Courtesy of Professor J.M. Chessels.)

The aim of cytotoxic therapy is first to induce a remission (absence of any clinical or conventional laboratory evidence of the disease) and then to eliminate the hidden leukaemic cell population by courses of consolidation therapy. Cyclical combinations of two, three or four drugs are given with treatment-free intervals to allow the bone marrow to recover. This recovery depends upon the differential regrowth pattern of normal haemopoietic and leukaemic cells. For ALL, long-term (2–3 years) maintenance therapy has been found to reduce the risk of relapse but this is not established in AML.

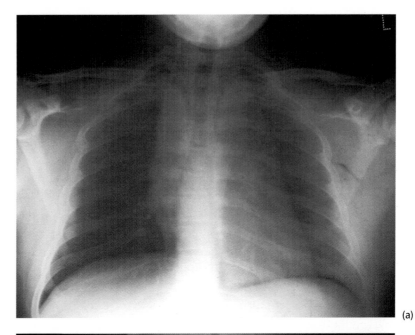

(a)

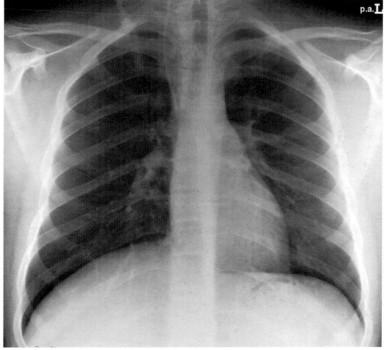

(b)

Fig. 12.6 Chest X-ray of a boy aged 16 years with acute lymphoblastic leukaemia (T-ALL). (a) There is a large mediastinal mass caused by thymic enlargement at presentation. (b) After 1 week of therapy with prednisolone, vincristine and daunorubicin, the mass has resolved.

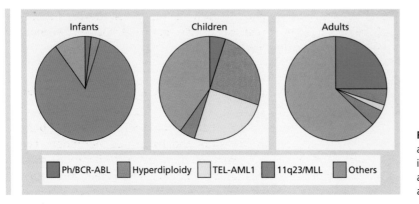

Fig. 12.7 Cytogenetic subsets of ALL: acute lymphoblastic leukaemia. The incidence of different cytogenic abnormalities in infants, children and adults.

Treatment

This may be conveniently divided into supportive and specific treatments.

General supportive therapy

General supportive therapy for bone marrow failure includes the following.

1 Insertion of a central venous catheter. It is usual to insert a central venous catheter (e.g. Hickman) via a skin tunnel from the chest into the superior vena cava to give ease of access for giving chemotherapy, blood products, antibiotics, intravenous feeding, etc., and for blood sampling for laboratory tests.

2 Prevention of vomiting. Drugs are used to prevent or treat drug-induced emesis and these include metoclopramide, phenothiazines (e.g. chlorpromazine or prochlorperazine), selective 5-hydroxytryptamine type 3 (5-HT$_3$) receptor antagonists (e.g. ondansetron, granisetron or tropisetron), steroids (e.g. dexamethasone), benzodiazepines (e.g. lorazepam) or cannabinoids (e.g. nabilone).

3 Blood product support with red cell and platelet transfusions. Fresh frozen plasma (FFP) may be needed to reverse coagulopathies.

4 Allopurinol and intravenous fluids, sometimes with alkalinization of the urine, to prevent tumour lysis syndrome.

5 Prophylaxis and treatment of infection. Infection is a great danger in the treatment of acute leukaemia. Neutropenia results from both the disease and the treatment and in many patients neutrophils are totally absent from the blood for 2 weeks or more. Infections are predominantly bacterial and usually arise from the patient's own commensal bacterial flora, most commonly Gram-positive skin organisms (e.g. *Staphylococcus* and *Streptococcus*) or Gram-negative gut bacteria (e.g. *Pseudomonas aeruginosa*, *Escherichia coli*, *Proteus*, *Klebsiella* and anaerobes). Organisms not normally considered pathogeneic, e.g. *Staphylococcus epidermidis*, may cause life-threatening infection. Moreover, in the absence of neutrophils, local superficial lesions may rapidly cause severe septicaemia. Viral (e.g. herpes simplex and zoster), fungal (e.g. *Candida*, *Aspergillus*) and protozoal (e.g. *Toxoplasma gondii*) infections also occur with increased frequency, particularly when neutropenia is prolonged, lymphopenia is present and multiple courses of antibiotics have been used to treat possible bacterial infection.

Prophylaxis of infection

The following measures may be taken to reduce the risk of infection but the various protocols in use vary from unit to unit. Isolation facilities may be used with patients nursed in separate rooms with reverse-barrier isolation and air filtration to prevent infection by airborne spores, e.g. *Aspergillus* species. Oral antimicrobial agents such as neomycin and colistin may be given to reduce gut and other commensal flora and antifungal agents such as amphotericin, fluconazole or itraconazole may be given prophylactically. Oral antibiotics such as ciprofloxacin may reduce Gram-negative infections and co-trimoxazole is used for prophylaxis of *Pneumocystis* infection. Regular surveillence cultures are taken to document the patient's bacterial flora and its sensitivity. Topical antiseptics are often used for bathing and mouthwashes.

Treatment of infection
Fever is the main indication that infection is present but because of neutropenia pus may not be formed and infections are often not localized. Cultures should be taken from any likely focus of infection and in addition blood cultures from central venous lines and peripheral blood, urine and mouth swabs should be taken. Direct examination of possibly infected material may help to identify the responsible organism. The mouth and throat, intravenous catheter site, and perineal and perianal areas are particularly likely foci. A chest X-ray is indicated.

Antibiotic therapy must be started immediately after blood and other cultures have been taken. In at least 50% of febrile episodes no organisms are isolated. There are many different antibiotic regimes in use. Typical are a penicillin active against *Pseudomonas* (tazocin); a single agent monobactam such as meropenem; a broad-spectrum cephalosporin such as ceftazidime with teicoplanin to deal with *Staphylococcus epidermidis* which is a common source of fever in patients with intravenous lines. Teicoplanin is often added after 24–48 h if the fever does not settle and it is not in the initial regime. As soon as the infective agent and its antibiotic sensitivities are known, appropriate changes in the regimen may be made. If no response occurs, the possibility of fungal or viral infection should be considered and appropriate therapy given, e.g. with amphotericin (liposomal if renal failure) or aciclovir.

Specific therapy
Specific therapy of ALL is with chemotherapy and sometimes radiotherapy (Fig. 12.8). These are used in various phases in a treatment course (Fig. 12.9) which usually has four components. The protocols differ in infants, children and adults and in cases, in the different age groups, considered to have different prognosis. The rare B-ALL is treated by a different protocol to the more common types.

Remission induction
When a patient presents with acute leukaemia they usually have a very high tumour burden and are at great risk from the complications of bone marrow failure and leukaemic infiltration. The aim of remission induction is to kill rapidly most of the tumour cells and get the patient into a state of remission. This is defined as less than 5% blasts in the bone marrow, normal peripheral blood counts and no other symptoms or signs of the disease. Prednisolone or dexamethasone, vincristine and asparaginase are the drugs usually used and they are very effective—achieving remission in over 90% of children and in 80–90% of adults (in whom daunorubicin is also usually added). However, it should be remembered that remission is not the same as cure. In remission a patient may still be harbouring large numbers of tumour cells and without further chemotherapy virtually all patients will relapse. Nevertheless, achievement of remission is a valuable first step in the treatment course and patients who fail to achieve remission have a poor prognosis.

Consolidation/intensification blocks
These courses use high doses of multidrug chemotherapy in order to reduce the tumour burden to very low levels. The doses of chemotherapy are near the limit of patient tolerability and during intensification blocks patients may need a great deal of support. Typical protocols involves the use of vincristine, cyclophosphamide, cytosine arabinoside, daunorubicin, etoposide, thioguanine or mercaptopurine given as blocks in different combinations. The optimal number of intensification blocks is under trial but two or three is typical in children, with more in adults.

Central nervous system (CNS) directed therapy
Few of the drugs given systemically reach the cerebrospinal fluid (CSF) and specific treatment is required. Options are high-dose methotrexate given intravenously, intrathecal methotrexate or cytosine arabinoside or cranial irradiation. Clini-

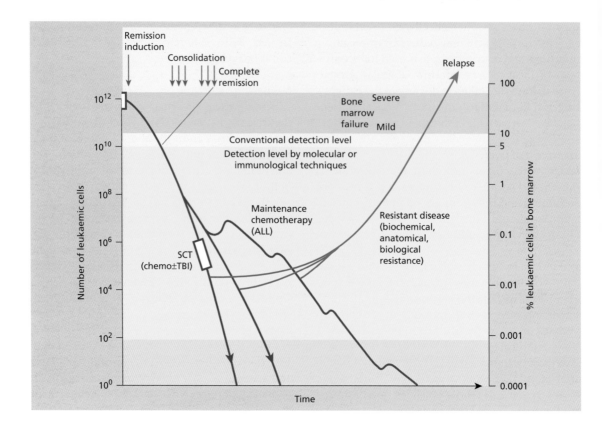

Fig. 12.8 Acute leukaemia: principles of therapy. ALL, acute lymphoblastic leukaemia; chemo ± TBI, chemotherapy ± total-body irradiation; SCT, stem cell transplantation.

cal trials are comparing these regimens. CNS relapses still occur and present with headache, vomiting, papilloedema and blast cells in the CSF. Treatment is with intrathecal methotrexate, cytosine arabinoside and hydrocortisone, with or without cranial irradiation and systemic reinduction because bone marrow disease is usually also present.

Maintenance

This is given for 2 years in girls and adults and for 3 years in boys, with daily oral mercaptopurine and once-weekly oral methotrexate. Intravenous vincristine with a short course (5 days) of oral corticosteroids is added at monthly or 3-monthly (in

adults) intervals. There is a high risk of varicella or measles during maintenance therapy in children who lack immunity to these viruses. If exposure to these infections occurs, prophylactic immunoglobulin should be given. In addition, oral co-trimoxazole is given to reduce the risk of *Pneumocystis carinii*.

Prognosis

There is a great variation in the chance of individual patients achieving a long-term cure based on a number of biological variables (Table 12.6). Age is important—around 70–90% of children can expect to be cured whereas in adults this drops significantly to less than 5% over the age of 65 years. Infants also do less well. Cytogenetics are important, particularly the presence of the Philadelphia chromosome, the incidence of which rises with

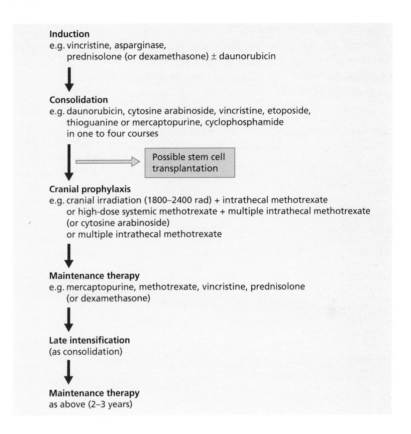

Induction
e.g. vincristine, asparginase,
  prednisolone (or dexamethasone) ± daunorubicin

Consolidation
e.g. daunorubicin, cytosine arabinoside, vincristine, etoposide,
  thioguanine or mercaptopurine, cyclophosphamide
  in one to four courses

Possible stem cell
transplantation

Cranial prophylaxis
e.g. cranial irradiation (1800–2400 rad) + intrathecal methotrexate
  or high-dose systemic methotrexate + multiple intrathecal methotrexate
  (or cytosine arabinoside)
  or multiple intrathecal methotrexate

Maintenance therapy
e.g. mercaptopurine, methotrexate, vincristine, prednisolone
  (or dexamethasone)

Late intensification
(as consolidation)

Maintenance therapy
as above (2–3 years)

Fig. 12.9 Acute lymphoblastic leukaemia: flow chart illustrating typical treatment regimen.

age (Fig. 12.7). Hyperdiploidy and *TEL* rearrangement are associated with good outcome. B-ALL (L₃ or Burkitt's type) has a poor prognosis with conventional precursor B-ALL treatment protocols; regimes similar to those in use for high-grade non-Hodgkin's lymphoma are generally used. When treatment fails, death usually occurs because of resistant disease or from infections or other complications during treatment.

Treatment of relapse

The treatment of this is unsatisfactory at present. If it occurs during or soon after initial chemotherapy the outlook is very poor. It is usual to give further chemotherapy and then stem cell transplantation using either a human leucocyte antigen (HLA) matching sibling donor or HLA-matched volunteer donor. The role of autologous stem cell transplantation in first or second remission.

ACUTE MYELOID LEUKAEMIA

Incidence and clinical features

AML occurs in all age groups. It is the common form of acute leukaemia in adults and is increasingly common with age. AML forms only a minor fraction (10–15%) of the leukaemias in childhood. An important distinction is between primary AML which appears to arise *de novo* and secondary AML which can develop from myelodysplasia and other haematological diseases or follow previous treatment with chemotherapy. Both types are associated with distinct genetic markers and have different prognoses. In addition, cytogenetic abnormalities and response to initial treatment have a major influence on prognosis (Table 12.7).

Clinical features resemble those of ALL. Anaemia and thrombocytopenia are often profound. A bleeding tendency caused by thrombocytopenia and disseminated intravascular coagulation (DIC) is characteristic of the M_3

Table 12.6 Prognosis in acute lymphoblastic leukaemia (ALL)

	Favourable	Unfavourable
WBC	Low	High (e.g. $> 50 \times 10^9$/l)
Sex	Girls	Boys
Immunophenotype	c-ALL (CD10+)	B-ALL
Age	Child	Adult (or infant < 2 years)
Cytogenetics	Normal or hyperdiploidy (> 50)	Ph+, 11q23 rearrangements
	TEL rearrangement	
Time to clear blasts from blood	< 1 week	> 1 week
Time to remission	< 4 weeks	> 4 weeks
CNS disease at presentation	Absent	Present
Minimal residual disease	Negative at 1–3 months	Still positive at 3–6 months

CNS, central nervous system; Ph+, Philadelphia chromosome positive; WBC, white blood cell count.

variant of AML. Tumour cells can infiltrate a variety of tissues. Gum hypertrophy and infiltration (Fig. 12.10), skin involvement and CNS disease are characteristic of the myelomonocytic (M_4) and monocytic (M_5) types. An isolated mass of leukaemic blasts is usually referred to as a granulocytic sarcoma.

Classification is usually based on the morphological criteria of the FAB scheme. This divides AML into eight variants (Table 12.2 and Fig. 12.11) and the FAB subtypes are associated with characteristic patterns of cytochemical stains

Table 12.7 Prognosis in acute myeloid leukaemia (AML)

	Favourable	Unfavourable*
Cytogenetics	t(15; 17) t(8; 21) inv(16)	Deletions of chromosome 5 or 7 Flt-3 mutation 11q23 t(6; 9) abn(3q) Complex rearrangements
Bone marrow response to remission induction	< 5% blasts after first course	> 20% blasts after first course
Age	< 60 years	> 60 years

*High expression of multidrug resistance protein (see p. 146) is also a poor prognostic feature.

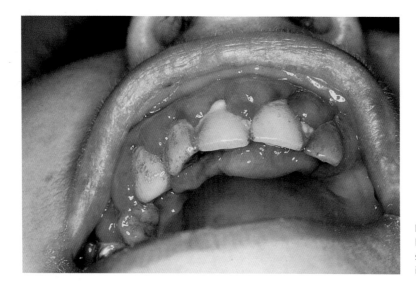

Fig. 12.10 Acute myeloid leukaemia FAB type M_5 (monocytic): the gums are swollen and haemorrhagic because of infiltration by leukaemic cells.

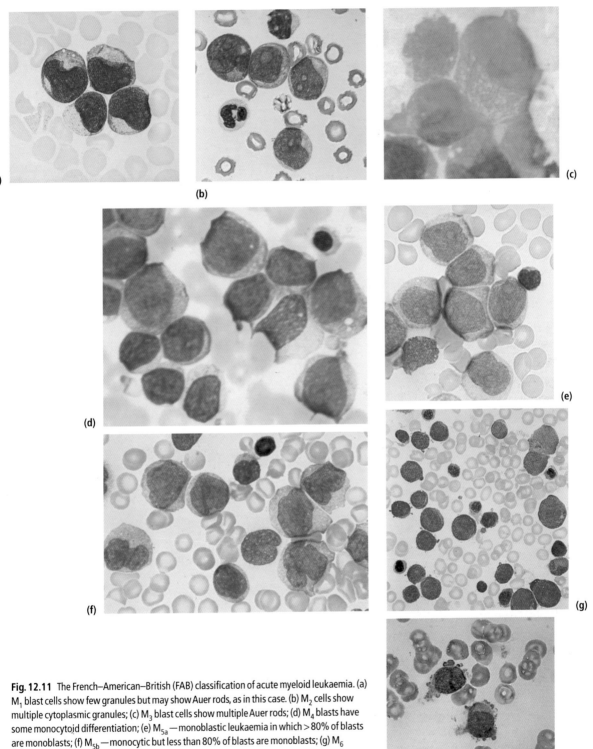

Fig. 12.11 The French–American–British (FAB) classification of acute myeloid leukaemia. (a) M_1 blast cells show few granules but may show Auer rods, as in this case. (b) M_2 cells show multiple cytoplasmic granules; (c) M_3 blast cells show multiple Auer rods; (d) M_4 blasts have some monocytoid differentiation; (e) M_{5a}—monoblastic leukaemia in which >80% of blasts are monoblasts; (f) M_{5b}—monocytic but less than 80% of blasts are monoblasts; (g) M_6 showing preponderance of erythroblasts; (h) M_7—megakaryoblastic leukaemia showing cytoplasmic blebs on blasts.

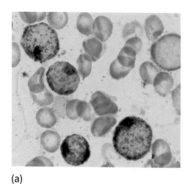
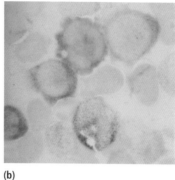

(a)

(b)

Fig. 12.12 Cytochemical staining in acute myeloid leukaemia. (a) Sudan black B shows black staining in the cytoplasm. (b) M_4 (myelomonocytic): non-specific esterase/chloracetate staining shows orange-staining monoblast cytoplasm and blue-staining (myeloblast) cytoplasm.

(Fig. 12.12), immunophenotype and chromosomal changes (see also Chapter 11). The typical 'myeloid immunophenotype' is CD13+, CD33+ and TdT– (Table 12.4 and Fig. 12.8) and special antibodies are helpful in the diagnosis of AML M_0, M_6 or M_7 (Table 12.4).

Although the distinct AML subtypes are in fact different genetic diseases their grouping together is valid as generally their treatment and prognosis is similar. However, differences in treatment according to subtype have been introduced.

Cytogenetic abnormalities have a major influence on prognosis (Table 12.7).

Investigation and management

The general haematological and biochemical findings are similar to those seen in ALL. Tests for DIC are positive in patients with the promyelocytic (M_3) variant of AML. Blood and urinary lysozyme may be raised in monocytic leukamias.

Management is both supportive and specific.
1 Supportive treatment is based on the same principles as that for ALL. Problems unique to AML include the haemorrhagic syndrome associated with the AML M_3 variant. The disease may present with catastrophic haemorrhage or this may develop in the first few days of treatment. It is treated as for DIC with replacement of clotting factors with FFP and multiple platelet transfusions. In addition all-transretinoic acid (ATRA) therapy is given in conjunction with chemotherapy.

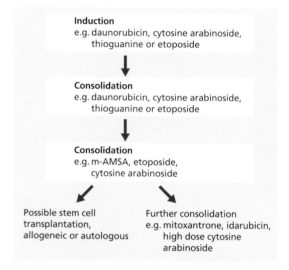

Induction
e.g. daunorubicin, cytosine arabinoside, thioguanine or etoposide

↓

Consolidation
e.g. daunorubicin, cytosine arabinoside, thioguanine or etoposide

↓

Consolidation
e.g. m-AMSA, etoposide, cytosine arabinoside

Possible stem cell transplantation, allogeneic or autologous

Further consolidation e.g. mitoxantrone, idarubicin, high dose cytosine arabinoside

Fig. 12.13 Acute myeloid leukaemia: flow chart illustrating typical treatment regimen.

2 Specific therapy of AML is primarily with the use of intensive chemotherapy. This is usually given in four or five blocks each of approximately 1 week and the most commonly used drugs include cytosine arabinoside, daunorubicin, idarubicin, 6-thioguanine, mitoxantrone or etoposide (Fig. 12.13). All the AML subtypes (FAB M_0–M_7) are treated similarly except for the promyelocytic (M_3) variant associated with the t(15; 17) translocation in which ATRA is added to the initial chemotherapy. A typical good response in AML to cytotoxics is shown in Fig. 12.14. The drugs

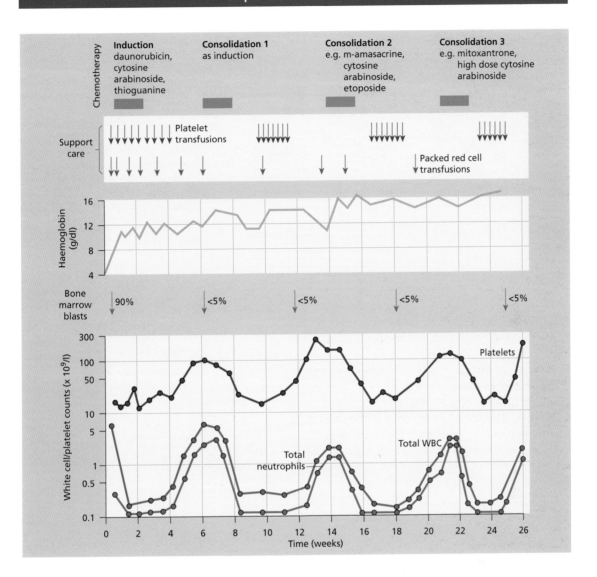

Fig. 12.14 Typical flow chart for the management with chemotherapy of acute myeloid leukaemia.

are myelotoxic with limited selectivity between leukaemic and normal marrow cells and so marrow failure is severe, and prolonged and intensive supportive care is required. Maintenance therapy is not needed and CNS prophylaxis is not usually given in AML.

An important concept developing in AML therapy is that of basing the treatment schedule of individual patients on their risk group. Remission after one course of chemotherapy is also favourable. In contrast, monosomy 5 or 7 abnormalities, blast cells with Flt-3 mutations or poorly responsive disease places patients into poor risk groups which may need more intensive treatments. Radiolabelled monoclonal antibodies targeted against CD33 or CD45 are being developed as a possible addition to AML therapy.

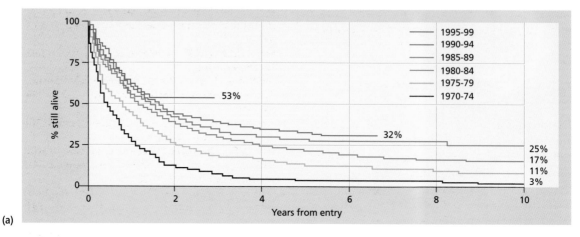

(a)

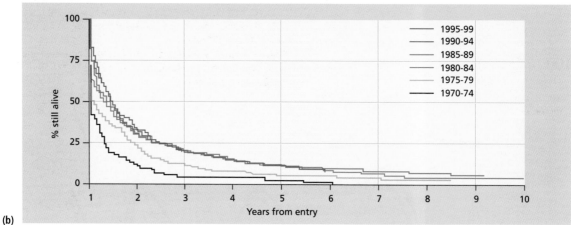

(b)

Fig. 12.15 Survival in children and adults with acute myeloid leukaemia (Medical Reseach Council trials). (a) Patients under 60 years old; (b) patients 60 years or greater.

Stem cell transplantation

Autologous transplantation reduces the rate of relapse but adds further toxicity to the treatment regime. Its role in treatment is the subject of continuing debate but it tends to be reserved until relapse for good risk groups and children. Allogeneic SCT is used in some centres in patients under 45 years old with an HLA matching sibling donor with standard or poor risk AML in first remission although some groups save it as an option for relapsed disease. Patients with t(8; 21), t(15; 17) and inv16 who go into remision after the first course do not have SCT unless they subsequently relapse.

Patients over 60 years of age

Results of AML therapy in the elderly are poor because of primary disease resistance and poor tolerability of intensive treatment protocols. Death from haemorrhage, infection or failure of the heart, kidneys or other organs is more frequent than in younger patients. In elderly patients with serious disease of other organs, the decision may be made to use supportive care with or without gentle, single drug chemotherapy. However, in those otherwise well, combination chemotherapy similar to that used in younger patients may produce long-term remissions.

Prognosis

The prognosis for patients with AML has been improving steadily, particularly for younger patients. Perhaps 50% of children and young adults may expect a long-term 'cure' (Fig. 12.15). Cytogenetic abnormalities and initial response to treatment are major predictors of prognosis. For the elderly the situation is poor and only 5% of those over 65 years of age can expect long-term remission.

BIBLIOGRAPHY

Burnett A. (ed) Acute myeloid leukaemia. *Clin. Haematol.* **14**, 1–23.

Fenaux P. and Degos L. (1997) Differentiation therapy for acute promyelocytic leukaemia. *N. Engl. J. Med.* **337**, 1076–7.

Greaves M.F. (1997) Aetiology of acute leukaemia. *Lancet* **349**, 344–9.

Hann I.M. *et al.* (1997) Results of the Medical Research Council's 10th AML trial (MRC AML10) *Blood* **89**, 2311–18.

Harousseau J.L. (1998) Acute myeloid leukaemia in the elderly. *Blood Rev.* **12**, 145–53.

Harrison C.J. (2000) The management of patients with leukaemia: the role of cytogenetics in this moleuclar era. *Br. J. Haematol.* **108**, 19–30.

Lowenberg B., Downing J.R. and Burnett A. (1999) Acute myeloid leukameia. *N. Engl. J. Med.* **341**, 1051–62.

Reilly J.T. *et al.* (1996) The role of cytology, cytochemistry, immunophenotyping and cytogenetic analysis in the diagnosis of haematological neoplasms. *Clin. Lab. Haem.* **18**, 231–6.

Vora A. and Lilleyman J.S. (1999) Management of childhood lymphoblastic leukaemia. *CME Bull. Haematol.* **2**, 85–9.

CHAPTER 13

Chronic myeloid leukaemia and myelodysplasia

The chronic leukaemias are distinguished from acute leukaemias by their slower progression. Paradoxically, they are also more difficult to cure. Chronic leukaemias can be broadly subdivided into myeloid and lymphoid groups (see Chapter 14).

The chronic myeloid leukaemias constitute six different types of leukaemia (Table 13.1) but by far the most common type is chronic myeloid leukaemia associated with the Philadelphia (Ph) chromosome.

PHILADELPHIA-POSITIVE CHRONIC MYELOID LEUKAEMIA

Chronic myeloid leukaemia (CML) is a clonal disorder of a pluripotent stem cell and is classified as one of the myeloproliferative disorders.

The disease accounts for around 15% of leukaemias and may occur at any age. The diagnosis of CML is rarely difficult and is assisted by the characteristic presence of the Ph chromosome (Fig. 13.1). This results from the t(9; 22)(q34; q11) translocation between chromosomes 9 and 22 as a result of which part of the Abelson proto-oncogene *ABL* is moved to the *BCR* gene on chromosome 22 (Fig. 13.1a) and part of chromosome 22 moves to chromosome 9. The abnormal chromosome 22 is the Ph chromosome. In the Ph translocation 5' exons of *BCR* are fused to the 3' exons of *ABL* (Fig. 13.1b, c). The resulting chimeric *BCR-ABL* gene codes for a fusion protein of size 210 kDa (p210). This has tyrosine kinase activity in excess of the normal 145-kDa ABL product. The Ph translocation is also seen in a minority of cases of acute lymphoblastic leukaemia (ALL) and in some of these the breakpoint in *BCR* occurs in the same region as in CML. However, in other cases the breakpoint in *BCR* is further upstream, in the intron between the first and second exons, leaving only the first *BCR* exon intact. This chimeric *BCR-ABL* gene is expressed as a p190 protein which like p210 has enhanced tyrosine kinase activity. In a minority of patients the Ph abnormality cannot be seen by microscopic karyotypic analysis but the same molecular rearrangement is detectable by more sensitive techniques. This Ph-negative BCR-ABL-positive CML behaves clinically like Ph-positive CML. As the Ph chromosome is an acquired abnormality of haemopoietic stem cells it is found in cells of both the myeloid (granulocytic, erythroid and megakaryocytic) and lymphoid (B and T cell) lineages.

A great increase in total body myeloid cell mass is responsible for most of the clinical feaures. In at least 70% of patients there is a terminal metamorphosis to acute leukaemia, often preceded by an accelerated phase.

Clinical features

This disease occurs in either sex (male:female ratio of 1.4:1), most frequently between the ages of 40 and 60 years. However, it may occur in children and neonates, and in the very old. In most cases there are no predisposing factors but the

Table 13.1 Classification of chronic myeloid leukaemias (CML)

Chronic myeloid leukaemia, Ph positive (CML, Ph+) (chronic granulocytic leukaemia, CGL)
Chronic myeloid leukaemia, Ph negative (CML, Ph–)
Juvenile chronic myeloid leukaemia
Chronic neutrophilic leukaemia
Eosinophilic leukaemia
Chronic myelomonocytic leukaemia (CMML) (see myelodysplasia, p. 186)

incidence was increased in survivors of the atom bomb exposures in Japan. Its clinical features include the following:

1 Symptoms related to hypermetabolism, e.g. weight loss, lassitude, anorexia or night sweats.
2 Splenomegaly is nearly always present and is frequently massive. In some patients splenic enlargement is associated with considerable discomfort, pain or indigestion.
3 Features of anaemia may include pallor, dyspnoea and tachycardia.
4 Bruising, epistaxis, menorrhagia or haemorrhage from other sites because of abnormal platelet function.
5 Gout or renal impairment caused by hyperuricaemia from excessive purine breakdown may be a problem.
6 Rare symptoms include visual disturbances and priapism.
7 In up to 50% of cases the diagnosis is made incidentally from a routine blood count.

Laboratory findings

1 Leucocytosis is usually $>50 \times 10^9/l$ and sometimes $>500 \times 10^9/l$ (Fig. 13.2). A complete spectrum of myeloid cells is seen in the peripheral blood. The levels of neutrophils and myelocytes exceed those of blast cells and promyelocytes (Fig. 13.3).
2 Increased circulating basophils.
3 Normochromic, normocytic anaemia is usual.
4 Platelet count may be increased (most frequently), normal or decreased.
5 Neutrophil alkaline phosphatase score is invariably low (Table 13.2).
6 Bone marrow is hypercellular with granulopoietic predominance.

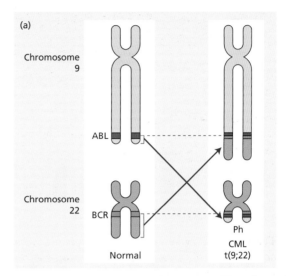

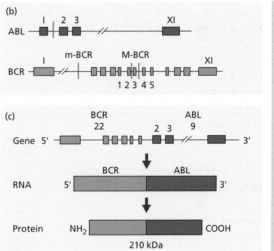

Fig. 13.1 The Philadelphia chromosome. (a) There is translocation of part of the long arm of chromosome 22 to the long arm of chromosome 9 and reciprocal translocation of part of the long arms of chromosome 9 to chromosome 22 (the Philadelphia chromosome). This reciprocal translocation brings most of the *ABL* gene into the *BCR* region on chromosome 22 (and part of the *BCR* gene into juxtaposition with the remaining portion of *ABL* on chromosome 9). (b) The breakpoint in *ABL* is between exons 1 and 2. The breakpoint in *BCR* is at one of the two points in the major breakpoint cluster region (M-BCR) in CML or in some cases of Ph+ ALL. (c) This results in a 210-kDa fusion protein product derived from the *BCR-ABL* fusion gene. In other cases of Ph+ ALL, the breakpoint in *BCR* is at a minor breakpoint cluster region (m-BCR) resulting in a smaller *BCR-ABL* fusion gene and a 190-kDa protein.

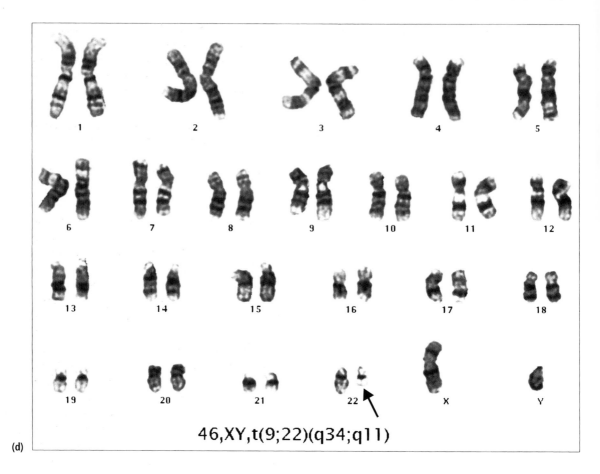

$$46,XY,t(9;22)(q34;q11)$$

(d)

Fig. 13.1 (*Continued*) (d) Karyotype showing the t(9; 22) (q34; q11) translocation. The Ph chromosome is arrowed.

7 Ph chromosome on cytogenetic analysis of blood or bone marrow (Fig. 13.1).
8 Serum vitamin B_{12} and vitamin B_{12}-binding capacity are increased.
9 Serum uric acid is usually raised.

Treatment

Treatment of chronic phase

Chemotherapy Hydroxyurea is effective at bringing the disease under control and maintaining a normal white count in the chronic phase but usually needs to be given indefinitely (Fig. 13.4). A

Table 13.2 Neutrophil alkaline phosphatase score (p. 121); the normal score is 20–100

Raised in	Low in
Infections	Chronic myeloid leukaemia
Pregnancy	
Polycythaemia (rubra) vera	
Myelofibrosis	
Leukaemoid reactions	

typical regimen would be to start with 1.0–2.0 g/day and then to reduce this in weekly increments to a maintenence dosage of 0.5–1.5 g/day. The alkylating agent busulphan is also effective in controlling the disease but has considerable long-term side-effects and is now reserved for patients who are intolerant of hydroxyurea. Allopurinol is often used in the initial phase of treatment to prevent attacks of gout.

Tyrosine kinase inhibitors These are now being assessed in clinical trials and are showing great promise. The agent STI 571 is a specific inhibitor of the ABL protein tyrosine kinase (Fig. 13.5) and is able to produce a complete haematological response in virtually all patients in the chronic phase with a high rate of conversion of the bone marrow from Ph positive to Ph negative. It is likely to become the first-line treatment for CML either alone or with interferon or other drugs.

Interferon-α This is usually used when the white cell count has been controlled by hydroxyurea, and is currently the drug of choice in the chronic phase although it may be superceded by tyrosine kinase inhibitors (see above). A typical regimen would be from 3 to 9 megaunits between three to seven times each week given as a subcutaneous injection. The aim is to keep the white cell count low (around 4×10^9/l). Almost all patients suffer symptoms of a 'flu-like' illness in the first few days of treatment which responds to paracetamol and gradually wears off. More serious complications include anorexia, depression and cytopenias (see Table 12.5). A minority (approximately 15%) of patients may achieve long-term remission with loss of the Ph chromosome on cytogenetic analysis although the *BCR-ABL* fusion gene can still be detected by PCR. Interferon produces an overall prolongation of the chronic phase with increased life expectancy. Combinations of interferon with

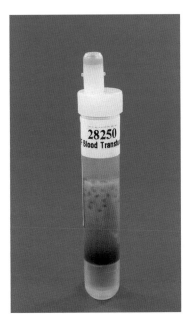

Fig. 13.2 Chronic myeloid leukaemia: peripheral blood showing a vast increase in buffy coat. The white cell count was 532×10^9/l.

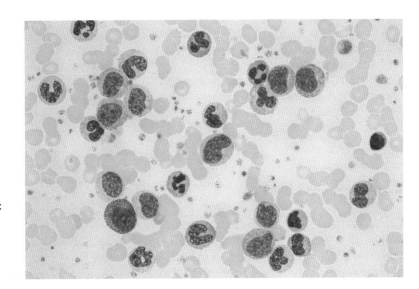

Fig. 13.3 Chronic myeloid leukaemia: peripheral blood film showing various stages of granulopoiesis including promyelocytes, myelocytes, metamyelocytes and band and segmented neutrophils.

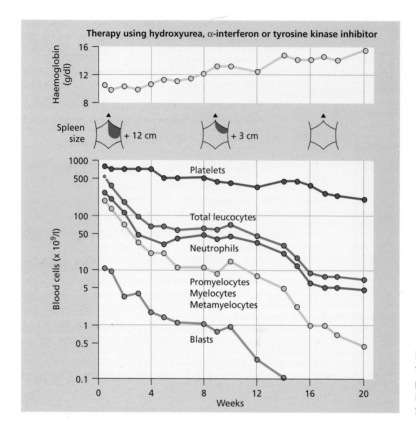

Fig. 13.4 Chronic myeloid leukaemia: typical haematological course of a patient treated with hydroxyurea, α-interferon or tyrosine kinase inhibitor STI-571.

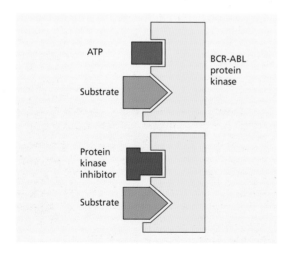

Fig. 13.5 Mode of action of the tyrosine kinase inhibitor STI-571. It blocks the adenosine triphosphate (ATP)-binding site.

pulses of cytosine arabinoside may be more effective than α-interferon alone.

Stem cell transplantation (SCT) This may be either allogeneic or autologous. Allogeneic bone marrow transplantation (BMT) is the only established curative treatment for CML. The results are better when it is performed in chronic rather than acute or accelerated phases. Only patients below approximately 60 years of age can tolerate the procedure and only 30% of these will have a matched sibling. The 5-year survival is around 50–70%. Although international bone marrow donor panels are playing an increasingly important part in providing human leucocyte antigen (HLA) matching unrelated donors, allogeneic SCT can only be offered to a minority of patients. Leukaemia relapse post-transplant is a significant problem but donor leucocyte infusions are highly effective in CML (p. 110) particularly if relapse is diagnosed early by molecular detection of the

BCR-ABL transcript. Autologous BMT is an experimental approach and trials are in progress to assess its role.

Course and prognosis

CML usually shows an excellent response to chemotherapy in the chronic phase (Fig. 13.4). The median survival is 5–6 years. Death usually occurs from terminal acute transformation or from intercurrent haemorrhage or infection. Twenty per cent of patients survive 10 years or more. The patients may be divided into prognostic groups according to age, spleen size, platelet count, blast cells on presentation and ease of response to therapy; these are only rough guides to outcome.

Accelerated phase and metamorphosis (blast cell or acute transformation)

Acute transformation (30% blasts in the marrow) may occur rapidly over days or weeks (Fig. 13.6). More commonly the patient has an accelerated phase with anaemia, thrombocytopenia and an increase in basophils, eosinophils or blast cells in the blood and marrow. The spleen may be enlarged despite control of the blood count and the marrow may become fibrotic. The patient may be in this phase for several months during which the disease is less easy to control than in the chronic phase. In either the accelerated or acute phase,

new chromosome abnormalities (e.g. double Ph chromosome) are often present. In about one-fifth of cases acute transformation is lymphoblastic and patients may be treated in a similar way to acute lymphoblastic leukaemia with a number of patients returning to the chronic phase for months or even a year or two. In the majority, transformation is into acute myeloid leukaemia (AML) or mixed types. These are more difficult to treat. Marrow or peripheral blood stem cells stored during the chronic phase may be used to restore haemopoiesis after intensive chemotherapy with or without total-body radiotherapy (autologous BMT). Survival following AML transformation is brief, however, and rarely more than 12 months. The role of STI–571 in the acute phase is being assessed.

PHILADELPHIA-NEGATIVE CHRONIC MYELOID LEUKAEMIA

Less than 5% of patients with features suggestive of CML are negative for the Philadelphia chromosome and *BCR-ABL* translocation. These patients usually have haematological features typical of myelodysplasia and the prognosis appears to be worse than for Ph-positive CML.

JUVENILE CHRONIC MYELOID LEUKAEMIA

This rare condition affects young children and has characteristic clinical features including skin rashes, lymphadenopathy, hepatosplenomegaly and recurrent infections. The blood film shows monocytosis. A high haemoglobin F (Hb F) level is a useful diagnostic feature, the neutrophil alkaline phosphatase score is normal and the Philadelphia chromosome test is negative. The prognosis is poor and SCT is the treatment of choice.

CHRONIC MYELOMONOCYTIC LEUKAEMIA

Chronic myelomonocytic leukaemia (CMML)

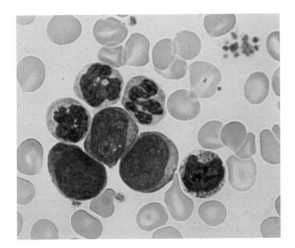

Fig. 13.6 Chronic myeloid leukemia: acute myeloblastic transformation peripheral blood showing frequent myeloblasts.

represents an area of overlap between myeloproliferative disorders and myelodysplasia but is classified in the latter group (see below).

EOSINOPHILIC LEUKAEMIA AND CHRONIC NEUTROPHILIC LEUKAEMIA

These are very rare conditions in which there is a relatively pure proliferation of mature cells. Splenomegaly may be present and, in general, the prognosis is good.

MYELODYSPLASTIC SYNDROMES (MYELODYSPLASIA)

This is a group of acquired neoplastic disorders of multipotent haemopoietic stem cells characterized by increasing bone marrow failure with quantitative and qualitative abnormalities of all three myeloid cell lines. A hallmark of the disease is ineffective haemopoiesis so that cytopenias often accompany a marrow of normal or increased cellularity. Increased apoptosis within the mar-

row is a common feature. There is a tendency to progress to AML, although death often occurs before this develops. In most cases, the disease arises *de novo*, but in a significant proportion of patients chemotherapy and/or radiotherapy has previously been given for another haematological disease, lymphoma or other solid tumour.

Classification of myelodysplastic syndromes

The myelodysplastic syndromes (MDS) are classified into five subgroups (Table 13.3). These are separated according to:
1 the proportion of blasts in the blood and marrow;
2 whether or not ring sideroblasts are frequent (>15%) in the marrow; and
3 the proportion of monocytes in the peripheral blood.

The prognosis is substantially better in patients with a normal proportion of marrow blasts (<5%) than in those with increased marrow blasts (5% or more).

Table 13.3 Classification of the myelodysplastic syndromes. The changes in the provisional new World Health Organization (WHO) classification are also given

	Peripheral blood	Bone marrow	Approximate median survival (months)
Refractory anaemia (RA)*	Blasts <1%	Blasts <5%	50
RA with ring sideroblasts (RARS)	Blasts <1%	Blasts <5% Ring sideroblasts >15% of total erythroblasts	50
RA with excess blasts (RAEB)	Blasts <5%	Blasts 5–20%	11
RAEB in transformation (RAEB-t)†	Blasts >5%	Blasts 20–30% or Auer rods present	5
Chronic myelomonocytic leukaemia (CMML)	As any of the above with >1.0 × 10^9/l monocytes	As any of the above with promonocytes	11

* In some cases neutropenia or thrombocytopenia is present without anaemia. These cases are classified as refractory cytopenia (WHO). Patients, usually elderly females with deletion of part of the long arm of chromosome 5 have a relatively good prognosis and are separately classified as 5q⁻, syndrome (WHO).

† Now classified as acute myeloid leukaemia (WHO).

Chromosomal abnormalities

Cytogenetic abnormalities are more frequent in secondary than primary MDS and most commonly constitute partial or total loss of chromosomes 5, 7 or Y, or trisomy 8. The loss of chromosome 5 bands q13 to q33 in elderly females with macrocytic anaemia, normal or raised platelet counts and micromegakaryocytes has been termed the 5q-syndrome and has a good prognosis. *RAS* oncogene (usually *N-RAS*) mutations occur in about 20% of cases and mutations of *FMS* in about 15%.

Clinical features

About half the patients are over 70 and fewer than 25% are less than 50 years old. Males are more commonly affected. The evolution is often slow and the disease may be found by chance when a patient has a blood count for some unrelated reason. The symptoms, if present, are those of anaemia, infections or of easy bruising or bleeding (Fig. 13.7). In some patients transfusion-dependent anaemia dominates the course, while in others recurring infections or spontaneous bruising and bleeding is the major clinical problem. Because the neutrophils, monocytes and platelets are often functionally impaired, spontaneous infections in some cases, or bruising or bleeding in others, may occur out of proportion to the severity of the cytopenia. The spleen is not usually enlarged except in CMML in which gum hypertrophy and lymphadenopathy may also occur.

Laboratory findings

Peripheral blood Pancytopenia is a frequent finding. The red cells are usually macrocytic or dimorphic but occasionally hypochromic; normoblasts may be present. The reticulocyte count is low. Granulocytes are often reduced and may show lack of granulation (Fig. 13.8). Their chemotactic,

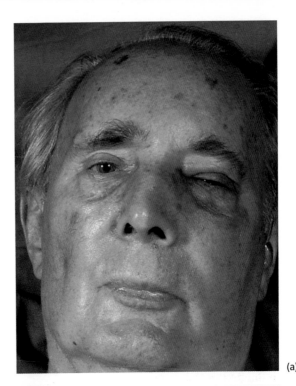

(a)

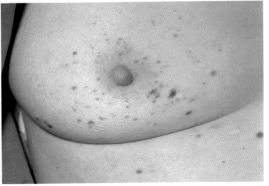

(b)

Fig. 13.7 Myelodysplasia. (a) A 78-year-old male patient with refractory anaemia had recurring infections of the face and maxillary sinuses associated with neutropenia (haemoglobin 9.8 g/dl; white cells 1.3×10^9/l; neutrophils 0.3×10^9/l; platelets 38×10^9/l). (b) Purpura in a 58-year-old female with refractory anaemia (haemoglobin 10.5 g/dl; white cells 2.3×10^9/l; platelets 8×10^9/l).

phagocytic and adhesive functions are impaired. The Pelger abnormality (single or bilobed nucleus) is often present. In CMML monocytes are $>1.0 \times 10^9$/l in the blood and the total white blood count may be $>100 \times 10^9$/l. The platelets

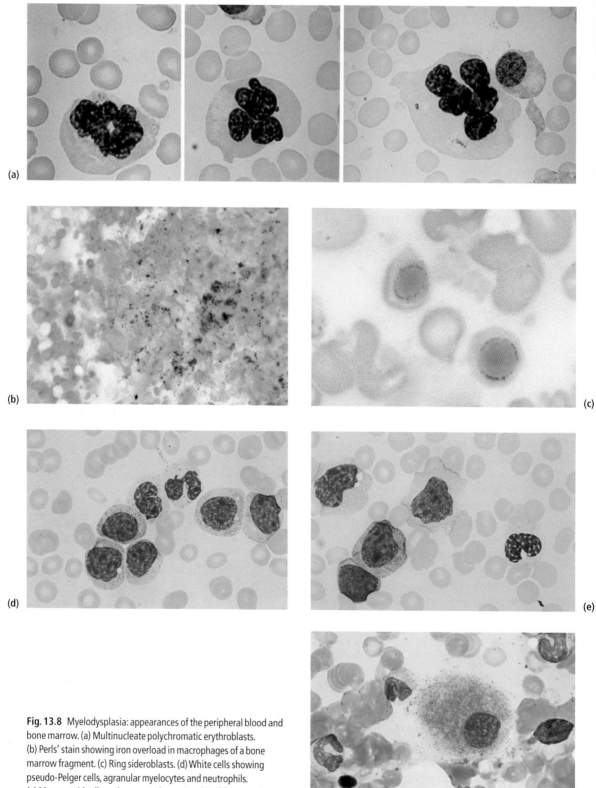

Fig. 13.8 Myelodysplasia: appearances of the peripheral blood and bone marrow. (a) Multinucleate polychromatic erythroblasts. (b) Perls' stain showing iron overload in macrophages of a bone marrow fragment. (c) Ring sideroblasts. (d) White cells showing pseudo-Pelger cells, agranular myelocytes and neutrophils. (e) Monocytoid cells and an agranular neutrophil. (f) Mononuclear megakaryocyte.

may be unduly large or small and are usually decreased in number but in 10% of cases are elevated. In poor prognosis cases variable numbers of myeloblasts are present in the blood.

Bone marrow The cellularity is usually increased. Ring sideroblasts may occur in all five of the French–American–British (FAB) types but by definition constitute >15% of the normoblasts in refractory anaemia with ring sideroblasts. Multinucleate normoblasts and other dyserythropoietic features are seen (Fig. 13.8). The granulocyte precursors show defective primary and secondary granulation, and cells which are difficult to identify as either agranular myelocytes, monocytes or promonocytes are frequent. Megakaryocytes are abnormal with micronuclear, small binuclear or polynuclear forms. Bone marrow biopsy shows fibrosis in 10% of cases.

Treatment

This is often extremely difficult because no therapy has been found regularly to revert haemopoiesis to normal and intensive or even low-dose chemotherapy may, in some cases, make the situation worse rather than better.

Low-risk myelodysplastic syndromes

Patients with less than 5% blasts in the marrow are defined as having low-grade myelodysplastic syndromes. They are usually managed conservatively with red cell transfusions, platelet transfusions or antibiotics as required. Attempts are being made to improve marrow function with haemopoietic growth factors, either singly or in combination. Erythropoietin in high doses may raise the haemoglobin concentration and obviate the need for blood transfusions. Cyclosporin or antilymphocyte globulin (ALG) occasionally improve patients, particularly those with a hypocellular bone marrow. In the long term, iron overload may be a problem after multiple transfusions; iron chelation therapy (p. 80) should be started after 30–50 units have been transfused and if the anaemia and the need for transfusion continues to be the dominant problem. In selected young patients, allogeneic transplantation may offer a permanent cure.

High-risk myelodysplastic syndromes

In these patients with 5% or more blasts in the marrow, a variety of treatments have been attempted to improve the overall prognosis with varying degrees of success. These treatments extend from general support only to intensive chemotherapy.

General support care only This is most suitable in elderly patients with other major medical problems. Transfusions of red cells and platelets, and therapy with antibiotics and antifungals, are given as needed.

Single agent chemotherapy Hydroxyurea, etoposide, mercaptopurine, azacytidine or low-dose cytosine arabinoside may be given with some benefit to patients with CMML or with refractory anaemia with excess blasts (RAEB) or RAEB in transformation (RAEB-t) with high circulating white cell counts.

Intensive chemotherapy Chemotherapy as given in AML (p. 176) may be tried in high-risk patients. The combination of fludarabine with high-dose cytosine arabinoside (ara-C) with granulocyte colony-stimulating factor (G-CSF) (FLAG) may be particularly valuable for obtaining remission in MDS. Topetecan, ara-C and G-CSF (TAG) may also help. Full remission is less frequent than in *de novo* AML and the risks of intensive chemotherapy as for AML, are greater because prolonged pancytopenia may occur in some cases without normal haemopoietic regeneration, presumably because normal stem cells are not present.

Stem cell transplantation In younger patients (less than 50–55 years) with an HLA matching brother or sister or an unrelated but HLA matching donor, SCT offers a prospect of complete cure. SCT is usually carried out in MDS without a complete remission being first obtained with chemotherapy, although in high-risk cases initial chemotherapy may be tried to reduce the blast proportion and the risk of recurrence of the MDS. Because of the usual old age of the MDS patient, SCT is only feasible in a small minority of the patients.

BIBLIOGRAPHY

Dansey R. (2000) Myelodysplasia. *Curr. Opin. Oncol.* **12**, 13–21.

Deininger M.W.N. and Goldman J.M. (1998) Chronic myeloid leukaemia. *Curr. Opin. Hematol.* **5**, 302–8.

Druker B.J., Sawyers C.L., Kantarjian H. *et al.* (2001) Activity of a specific inhibitor of the BCR-ABL tyrosine kinase in the blast crisis of the chronic myeloid leukemia and acute lymphoblastic leukemia with the Philadelphia Chromosome. *N. Engl. J. Med.* **344**, 1038–42.

Druker B.J., Talpaz M., Resta R.N. *et al.* (2001) Efficacy and safety of a specific inhibitor of the BCR-ABL tyrosine kinase in chronic myeloid leukemia. *N. Engl. J. Med.* **344**, 1031–7.

Greenberg P. (2001) Implications of pathogenic and prognostic features for management of myelodysplastic syndromes. *Lancet* **357**, 1059–60.

Goldman J.M. (ed.) (1997) Treatment of chronic myeloid leukaemia. *Clin. Haematol.* **10**, 187–228.

Hansen J.A., Gooley T.A., Martin P.J. *et al.* (1998) Bone marrow transplants from unrelated donors for patients with chronic myeloid leukemia. *N. Engl. J. Med.* **338**, 962–8.

Heaney M.L. and Golde D.W. (1999) Myelodysplasia. *N. Engl. J. Med.* **340**, 1649–60.

Heinrich M.C., Griffith D.J., Druker B.J. *et al.* (2000) Inhibition of c-kit receptor tyrosine kinase activity by STI 571, a selective tyrosine kinase inhibitor. *Blood* **96**, 925–32.

Koeffler H.D. (ed.) (1996) Myelodysplastic syndromes I and II. *Semin. Hematol.* **33**, Nos 2 and 3.

O'Dwyer M.E.O. and Druker B.J. (2000) STI/571: an inhibitor of the BCR-ABL tyrosine kinase for the treatment of chronic myelogenous leukaemia. *Lancet Oncol.* **1**, 207–11.

Sole F., Espinet B., Sanz G.F. *et al.* (2000) Incidence, characterization and prognostic significance of chromosomal abnormalities in 640 patients with primary myelodysplastic syndromes. *Br. J. Haematol.* **180**, 346–56.

The chronic lymphoid leukaemias

Several disorders are included in this group characterized by proliferation of mature looking lymphocytes of either B- or T-cell type (Table 14.1). There is considerable overlap with the lymphomas. In many cases of non-Hodgkin's lymphoma, lymphoma cells are found in the blood and in some cases the distinction between chronic leukaemia and lymphoma is arbitrary, depending on the relative proportion of the disease in soft tissue masses compared to blood and bone marrow. In general the diseases are incurable but tend to run a chronic and fluctuating course.

Diagnosis

This group is characterized by a chronic persistent lymphocytosis and subtypes can be distinguished by morphology, immunophenotype and cytogenetics. DNA may be useful in showing a monoclonal rearrangement of either immunoglobulin or T-cell receptor genes.

CHRONIC LYMPHOCYTIC LEUKAEMIA

Chronic lymphocytic leukaemia (CLL) is by far the most common of the chronic lymphoid leukaemias and has a peak incidence between 60 and 80 years of age. The aetiology is unknown but there are geographical variations in incidence. It is the most common of the leukaemias in the West but rare in the Far East. There is no higher incidence with previous radiotherapy or chemotherapy. The tumour cell appears to be a relatively mature B cell with weak surface expression of im-

munoglobulin M (IgM) or IgD. The cells accumulate in the blood, bone marrow, liver, spleen and lymph nodes as a result of a prolonged lifespan with impairment of normal apoptosis.

Clinical features

1 The disease occurs in older subjects and is rare before 40 years of age. The male to female ratio is 2:1.
2 Many cases (usually stage 0) are diagnosed when a routine blood test is performed. With increasing routine medical check-ups, this proportion is rising.
3 Symmetrical enlargement of superficial lymph nodes is the most frequent clinical sign (Fig. 14.1). The nodes are usually discrete and non-tender. Tonsillar enlargement may be a feature.
4 Features of anaemia may be present.
5 Splenomegaly and hepatomegaly are usual in later stages.
6 Bacterial or fungal infections are common in later stages because of immune deficiency and neutropenia (caused by marrow infiltration, chemotherapy or hypersplenism). There is also an association with herpes zoster (Fig. 14.2).
7 Patients with thrombocytopenia may show bruising or purpura.

Laboratory findings

1 Lymphocytosis. The absolute lymphocyte count is $>5\times10^9/l$ and may be up to $300\times10^9/l$ or more. Between 70 and 99% of white cells in

Table 14.1 Classification of the chronic lymphoid leukaemias and leukaemia/lymphoma syndromes

B-cell	T-cell
Chronic lymphoid leukaemias	
B-cell chronic lymphocytic leukaemia (B-CLL, CLL)	Large granular lymphocytic leukaemia
B-cell prolymphocytic leukaemia (B-PLL)	T-cell prolymphocytic leukaemia (T-PLL)
Hairy cell leukaemia (HCL)	
Plasma cell leukaemia	
Leukaemia/lymphoma syndromes	
Splenic lymphoma with villous lymphocytes	Sézary syndrome
Follicular lymphoma	Adult T-cell leukaemia/lymphoma
Mantle cell lymphoma	Large cell lymphoma
Lymphoplasmacytic lymphoma	
Large cell lymphoma	

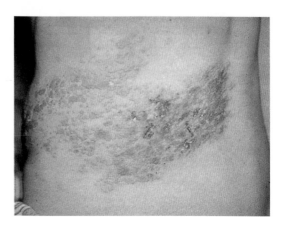

Fig. 14.2 Chronic lymphocytic leukaemia: herpes zoster infection in a 68-year-old female.

Table 14.2 Immunophenotype of the chronic B-cell leukaemias/lymphomas (all cases CD19+)

	CLL	PLL	HCL	FL	MCL
SIg	weak	++	++	++	+
CD5	+	–	–	–	+
CD22/FMC7	–	+	+	+	+
CD79b	–	++	–/+	++	++

CLL, chronic lymphocytic leukaemia; FL, follicular lymphoma; HCL, hairy cell leukaemia; MCL, mantle cell lymphoma; PLL, prolymphocytic leukaemia.
NB. CD103 is positive only in HCL.

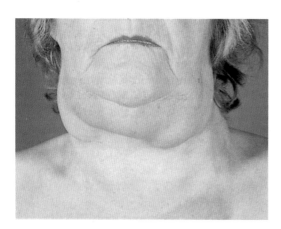

Fig. 14.1 Chronic lymphocytic leukaemia: bilateral cervical lymphadenopathy in a 67-year-old woman. Haemoglobin 12.5 g/dl; white blood count 150×10^9/l (lymphocytes 146×10^9/l); platelets 120×10^9/l.

the blood film appear as small lymphocytes. Smudge or smear cells are also present (Fig. 14.3).

2 Immunophenotyping of the lymphocytes shows them to be B cells (surface CD19 positive), weakly expressing surface immunoglobulin (IgM or IgD). This is shown to be monoclonal because of expression of one form of light chain (κ or λ only, p. 153). Characteristically the cells are also surface CD5 and CD23 positive but CD79b and FMC7 negative (Table 14.2).

3 Normocytic, normochromic anaemia is present in later stages as a result of marrow infiltration or hypersplenism. Autoimmune haemolysis may also occur (see below).

4 Thrombocytopenia occurs in many patients.

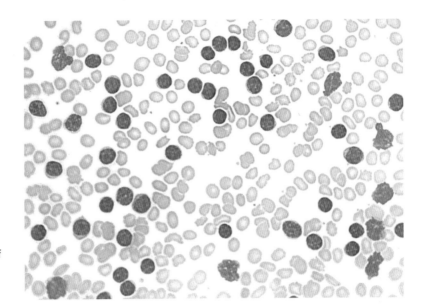

Fig. 14.3 Chronic lymphocytic leukaemia: peripheral blood film showing lymphocytes with thin rims of cytoplasm, coarse condensed nuclear chromatin and rare nucleoli. Typical smudge cells are present.

5 Bone marrow aspiration shows lymphocytic replacement of normal marrow elements. Lymphocytes comprise 25–95% of all the cells. Trephine biopsy reveals nodular, diffuse or interstitial involvement by lymphocytes.

6 Reduced concentrations of serum immunoglobulins are found and this becomes more marked with advanced disease. Rarely a paraprotein is present.

7 The four most common chromosome abnormalities are deletion of 13q14, trisomy 12, deletions at 11q23 and structural abnormalities of 17p involving the p53 gene. These abnormalities carry prognostic significance (Table 14.3).

8 The B cells VH genes undergo somatic hypermutation in germinal centres (p. 137). In CLL the VH genes are hypermutated in about 50% of cases suggesting origin from postgerminal follicle centre cells; in the other 50% the VH genes are non-mutated suggesting origin from pre-germinal centre cells. This latter group have a poorer prognosis (Table 14.3).

Table 14.3 Prognostic factors in chronic lymphocytic leukaemia

	Favourable	Unfavourable
Stage	Binet A (Rai 0–I)	Binet B, C (Rai II–IV)
Sex	Female	Male
Lymphocyte doubling time	Slow	Rapid
Bone marrow biopsy appearance	Nodular	Diffuse
Chromosomes	Deletion 13q14	Trisomy 12 p53 mutations (17p13.3) deletion 11q23
VH immunoglobulin genes	Hypermutated	Unmutated
LDH	Normal	Raised
CD38 expression	Negative	Positive

LDH, lactate dehydrogenase.

Staging

It is useful to stage patients at presentation as the information is useful both for prognosis and for deciding on therapy. The Rai and Binet staging systems are shown in Table 14.4. Typical survival ranges from 12 years for Rai stage 0 to less than 3 years for stage IV.

Table 14.4 Staging of chronic lymphocytic leukaemia (CLL)

(a) Rai classification

Stage	
0	Absolute lymphocytosis $> 15 \times 10^9/l$*
I	As stage 0 + enlarged lymph nodes (adenopathy)
II	As stage 0 + enlarged liver and/or spleen ± adenopathy
III	As stage 0 + anaemia (Hb < 10.0 g/dl)* ± adenopathy ± organomegaly
IV	As stage 0 + thrombocytopenia (platelets $< 100 \times 10^9/l$)* ± adenopathy ± organomegaly

(b) International Working Party classification (from J.L. Binet et al. 1981)

Stage	Organ enlargement*	Haemoglobin† (g/dl)		Platelets† ($\times 10^9/l$)
A (50–60%)	0, 1 or 2 areas			
B (30%)	3, 4 or 5 areas	≥10		≥100
C (<20%)	Not considered	<10	and/or	<100

* One area = lymph nodes > 1 cm in neck, axillae, groins or spleen, or liver enlargement.

† Secondary causes of anaemia (e.g. iron deficiency) or autoimmune haemolytic anaemia or autoimmune thrombocytopenia must be treated before staging.

Treatment

Cures are rare in CLL and so the approach to therapy is conservative, aiming for symptom control rather than a normal blood count. Indeed, chemotherapy given too early in the disease can shorten rather than prolong life expectancy. Treatment is given for troublesome organomegaly, haemolytic episodes and bone marrow suppression. The lymphocyte count alone is not a good guide to treatment. Usually patients in Binet stage C will need treatment as will some in stage B.

Chemotherapy

Chlorambucil The traditional treatment for CLL has been with the oral alkylating agent chlorambucil. Used as a daily treatment (e.g. 4–6 mg/day) or 6 mg/m² daily for 10 days the drug is effective

in reducing disease bulk in the majority of cases. Typically the drug will need to be given for 2–4 months after which a remission of variable duration will be obtained. Chlorambucil can be reintroduced when required although resistance may develop.

Purine analogues These drugs are effective in the treatment of chronic lymphoid leukaemias and lymphomas. The most effective agent in CLL appears to be fludarabine and initial evidence suggests that this drug is more effective as a single agent than chlorambucil. The place of fludarabine in the overall management of CLL is currently under trial. It may have a place as the drug of first choice as well as having value in patients resistant to chlorambucil. Both intravenous and oral formulations of the drug can be used in monthly courses. Myelosuppression and prolonged reduction of CD4 (helper) T lymphocytes leads to an increased infection risk and prophylaxis against *Pneumocystis carinii* infection with co-trimoxazole is given until CD4 counts recover. If patients are resistant to one of the purine analogues it may be worth trying another drug from the group, e.g. 2-chlorodeoxyadenosine. Combinations of fludarabine with for example cyclophosphamide (FC) or methotrexate and dexamethasone (FMD) may be more effective than fludarabine alone.

Corticosteroids Patients in bone marrow failure should be treated initially with prednisolone alone until there is significant recovery of the platelet, neutrophil and haemoglobin levels. The peripheral lymphocyte count initially rises as infiltrated organs shrink, but later the count falls. Corticosteroids are also indicated in autoimmune haemolytic anaemia or thrombocytopenia.

Other forms of treatment

Radiotherapy This is valuable in reducing the size of bulky lymph node groups which are unresponsive to chemotherapy.

Combination chemotherapy For example with cyclophosphamide, hydroxodaunorubicin. Oncovin (vincristine) and prednisone (CHOP, p. 213), is sometimes effective in late-stage cases and in patients refractory to chlorambucil.

Cyclosporin Red cell aplasia may respond to cyclosporin.

Monoclonal antibodies Both Campath IH (anti-CD52) and Rituximab (anti-CD20) produce responses in a proportion of patients. Campath-1H particularly effective against bone marrow disease.

Splenectomy This is generally reserved for those patients with immune-mediated cytopenias which do not respond to short courses of steroids or with painful bulky enlargement of the spleen.

Immunoglobulin replacement Immunoglobulin replacement (e.g. 250 mg/kg/month by intravenous infusion) is useful for patients with hypogammaglobulinaemia and recurrent infections.

Stem cell transplantation (SCT) This is currently an experimental approach in younger patients. Allogeneic SCT may be curative but has a high mortality rate. Autologous SCT after prior therapy with fludarabine and other drugs is undergoing clinical trials.

Course of disease

Many patients in Binet stage A or Rai stage 0 or I never need therapy. Indeed females aged 60 or more in Rai stage 0 have a life expectancy similar to a control population. For those that do need therapy, a typical pattern is that of a disease which is responsive to several courses of chemotherapy before the gradual onset of extensive bone marrow infiltration, bulky disease and recurrent infection. The disease may transform into a localized high-grade lymphoma (Richter's transformation) or there may be the appearance of an increasing number of prolymphocytes which are resistant to treatment.

PROLYMPHOCYTIC LEUKAEMIA

Although prolymphocytic leukaemia (PLL) may initially appear similar to B-cell CLL (B-CLL), the diagnosis is made by the appearance of a majority of prolymphocytes in the blood. The prolymphocyte is around twice the size of a CLL lymphocyte and has a large, central nucleolus (Fig. 14.4). B-cell PLL (B-PLL) is three times more common than T-cell PLL (T-PLL).

PLL and CLL also differ in their clinical features.

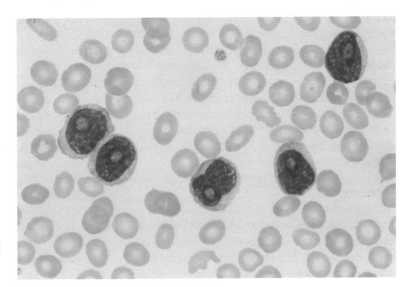

Fig. 14.4 Prolymphocytic leukaemia: blood film showing prolymphocytes that have prominent central nucleoli and an abundance of pale cytoplasm.

PLL typically presents with splenomegaly without lymphadenopathy and with a high and rapidly rising lymphocyte count. Anaemia is a poor prognostic feature.

Treatment is difficult in PLL. Splenectomy is usually of benefit and purine nucleoside analogues may help.

HAIRY CELL LEUKAEMIA

Hairy cell leukaemia (HCL) is an uncommon B-cell lymphoproliferative disease with a male to female ratio of 4 : 1 and a peak of incidence at 40–60 years. Patients typically present with infections, anaemia or splenomegaly. Lymphadenopathy is very uncommon. Pancytopenia is usual at presentation and the lymphocyte count is rarely over $20 \times 10^9/l$. Monocytopenia is a distinctive feature. The blood film reveals a variable number of unusual large lymphocytes with villous cytoplasmic projections (Fig. 14.5). Immunophenotyping is characteristic with CD22, FMC7 and CD103 positive in most cases (Table 14.2). The hairy cells stain for tartrate-resistant acid phosphatase (TRAP). The bone marrow trephine shows a characteristic appearance of mild fibrosis and a diffuse cellular infiltrate.

There are several effective treatments for HCL and a patient can expect a long-term remission. The treatment of choice is now probably 2-chlorodeoxyadenosine or deoxycoformycin and both agents achieve responses in over 90% of cases. HCL was one of the first diseases in which α-interferon was shown to be effective and it remains an excellent treatment. Typically 1 year of interferon is given after which a prolonged remission may be obtained. These treatments have largely replaced the need for splenectomy.

Hairy cell leukaemia variant

Some cases of HCL have clear differences from the typical disease and warrant a separate classification. The white cell count is typically higher, the hairy cells have a prominent nucleolus and

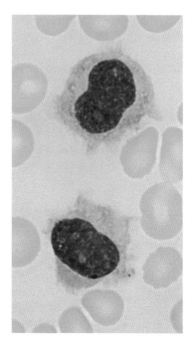

Fig. 14.5 Hairy cell leukaemia: peripheral blood film showing typical 'hairy' cells with oval nuclei and finely mottled pale grey/blue cytoplasm with an irregular edge.

response to interferon and purine analogues is less satisfactory.

SPLENIC LYMPHOMA WITH VILLOUS LYMPHOCYTES

Splenic lymphoma with villous lymphocytes (SLVL) (splenic marginal zone lymphoma) is characterized by massive splenomegaly and circulating populations of monoclonal B cells with a villous appearance. It is a disease of the elderly with a benign clinical course. Although many patients will not need treatment, splenectomy is valuable and purine nucleoside analogues are also effective.

PLASMA CELL LEUKAEMIA

This rare disease is characterized by a high

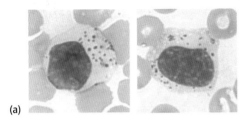

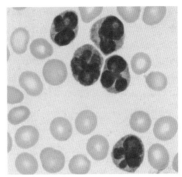

Fig. 14.6 (a) Large granular lymphocytes in the peripheral blood. (b) Adult T-cell leukaemia/lymphoma. Typical convoluted lymphoid cells in peripheral blood.

number of circulating plasma cells. The clinical features tend to be a combination of those found in acute leukaemia (pancytopenia and organomegaly) with features of myeloma (hypercalcaemia, renal involvement and bone disease) (Chapter 16). Treatment is with supportive care and systemic chemotherapy, e.g. with CHOP, cyclophosphamide-VAMP (vincristine, Adriamycin and methylprednisolone) or ABCM as for multiple myeloma (Chapter 16).

LARGE GRANULAR LYMPHOCYTIC LEUKAEMIA

Large granular lymphocytic leukaemia (LGL-L) is characterized by the presence of circulating lymphocytes with abundant cytoplasm and large azurophilic granules (Fig. 14.6a). Such cells may be either T cells or natural killer (NK) cells and show variable expression of CD16, CD56 and CD57. Cytopenia, especially neutropenia, is the main clinical problem although anaemia, splenomegaly and arthropathy with positive serology for rheumatoid arthritis are also common. The mean age is 50 years. Treatment may not be needed but, if required, steroids, cyclophosphamide, cyclosporin or methotrexate may relieve the cytopenia. G-CSF and GM-CSF (granulocyte–macrophage colony-stimulating factor) have been used in cases associated with neutropenia.

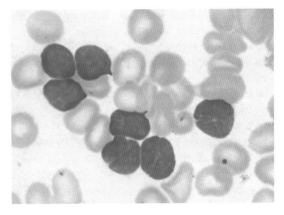

Fig. 14.7 Follicle centre lymphoma: small cleaved lymphoid cells in peripheral blood.

ADULT T-CELL LEUKAEMIA/LYMPHOMA

Adult T-cell leukaemia/lymphoma (ATLL) was the first malignancy to be associated with a human retrovirus, human T-cell leukaemia/lymphoma virus type 1 (HTLV-1). The virus is endemic in parts of Japan and the Caribbean and the disease is very rare in people who have not lived in these areas. ATLL lymphocytes have a bizarre morphology with a convoluted, 'clover-leaf' nucleus and a consistent CD4+ phenotype (Fig. 14.6b).

Many subjects infected with the virus and serologically positive do not develop the disease. The clinical presentation is often acute and dominated by hypercalcaemia, skin lesions, hepatospleno-megaly and lymphadenopathy. Diagnosis is by morphology and serology and although combination chemotherapy may be tried the prognosis is poor. Antiretroviral drugs may prove to have a valuable role.

SÉZARY SYNDROME

Patients with Sézary syndrome present with skin disease, usually a pruritic, exfoliative erythroderma affecting the palms, soles and face ('red man syndrome'). Biopsy of the skin reveals lymphocytic infiltration and Sézary cells in peripheral blood have a characteristic morphology with deep nuclear clefting, similar to ATLL cells. A variety of treatments are available including chemotherapy, radiotherapy and a photoactivable drug (psoralens) combined with ultraviolet A light (PUVA).

LYMPHOMA/LEUKAEMIA SYNDROMES

Circulating malignant lymphoid cells occur in a variety of syndromes in association with otherwise typical cases of non-Hodgkin's lymphoma such as mantle cell lymphoma (Table 14.1). This syndrome is most frequently seen in B-cell tumours of the follicle centre cell type (with circulating indented or cleaved nuclei) (Fig. 14.7) and the course is that of the non-Hodgkin's lymphoma (p. 209). Other types of lymphoma may also show tumour cells in the peripheral blood and bone marrow and in some cases it is difficult to define the disease as either lymphoma (with mainly soft tissue masses) or leukaemia.

BIBLIOGRAPHY

Binet J.L., Auquier A., Dighiero G. *et al.* (1981) A new prognostic classification of chronic lymphocytic leukemia derived from a multivariate survival analysis. *Cancer* **48**, 198–206.

Caligaris-Cappio F. (2000) Biology of chronic lymphocytic leukemia. *Rev. Clin. Exp. Hematol.* **4**, 5–21.

Esteve J. and Montserrat E. (2000) Hematopoietic stem-cell transplantation for B-cell chronic lymphocytic leukemia: current status. *Rev. Clin. Exp. Hematol.* **4**, 167–78.

Hallek M. (2000) New concepts in the pathogenesis, diagnosis, prognostic factors and clinical presentation of chronic lymphocytic leukemia. *Rev. Clin. Exp. Hematol.* **4**, 103–17.

Keating M.J. (1999) Chronic lymphocytic leukemia. *Semin. Oncol.* **26**, 107–14.

Keating M.J. and O'Brien S. (2000) Conventional management of chronic lymphocytic leukemia. *Rev. Clin. Exp. Hematol.* **4**, 118–33.

Kipps T.J. (2000) Chronic lymphocytic leukaemia. *Curr. Opin. Hematol.* **7**, 223–34.

Matutes E. and Polliack A (2000) Morphological and immunophenotypic features of chronic lymphocytic leukemia. *Rev. Clin. Exp. Hematol.* **4**, 22–47.

Rai K.R., Sawitsky A., Cronkite E.P., Chanana A.D., Levy R.N. and Pasternack B.S. (1975) Clinical staging of chronic lymphocytic leukemia. *Blood* **46**, 219–34.

Wierda W.G. and Kipps T.J. (1999) Chronic lymphocytic leukemia. *Curr. Opin. Hematol.* **6**, 253–61.

Malignant lymphomas

Lymphomas are a heterogeneous group of diseases caused by malignant lymphocytes which usually accumulate in lymph nodes and cause the characteristic clinical feature of lymphadenopathy. Occasionally they may spill over into blood ('leukaemic phase') or infiltrate organs outside the lymphoid tissue. Lymphomas are divided into Hodgkin's disease (lymphoma) and non-Hodgkin's lymphoma based on the histological presence of Reed–Sternberg (RS) cells in Hodgkin's lymphoma.

HODGKIN'S LYMPHOMA

Pathogenesis

Hodgkin's disease is a malignant lymphoma in which RS cells are found. It appears that the characteristic RS cells and the associated abnormal mononuclear cells are neoplastic whereas the associated inflammatory cells are reactive. Immunoglobulin gene rearrangement studies suggest that the RS cell is of B-lymphoid lineage and that it is often derived from a B cell with a 'crippled' immunoglobulin gene caused by the acquisition of mutations that prevent synthesis of full length immunoglobulin. The Epstein–Barr virus (EBV) genome has been detected in 50% or more of cases in Hodgkin tissue but its role in the pathogenesis is unclear.

Clinical features

The disease can present at any age but is rare in children and has peak incidences in the third decade and the elderly. In developed countries the ratio of young adult to child cases and of nodular sclerosing disease to other types is increased. There is an almost 2:1 male predominance. The following symptoms are common.

1 Most patients present with painless, non-tender, asymmetrical, firm, discrete and rubbery enlargement of superficial lymph nodes (Fig. 15.1). The cervical nodes are involved in 60–70% of patients, axillary nodes in about 10–15% and inguinal nodes in 6–12%. In some cases the size of the nodes decreases and increases spontaneously. They may become matted. Typically the disease is localized initially to a single peripheral lymph node region and its subsequent progression is by contiguity within the lymphatic system. Retroperitoneal nodes are also often involved but usually only diagnosed by computed tomography (CT) scan.

2 Clinical splenomegaly occurs during the course of the disease in 50% of patients. The splenic enlargement is seldom massive. The liver may also be enlarged because of liver involvement.

3 Mediastinal involvement is found in 6–11% of patients at presentation. This is a feature of the nodular sclerosing type, particularly in young women. There may be associated pleural effusions or superior vena cava obstruction.

4 Cutaneous Hodgkin's disease occurs as a late complication in about 10% of patients. Other organs (e.g. bone marrow, gastrointestinal tract, bone, lung, spinal cord or brain) may also be involved even at presentation but this is unusual.

5 Constitutional symptoms are prominent in patients with widespread disease. The following may be seen:

   (a) fever occurs in about 30% of patients and is continuous or cyclic;

   (b) pruritus, which is often severe, occurs in around 25% of cases;

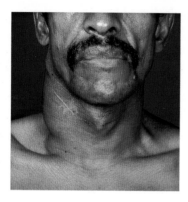

Fig. 15.1 Cervical lymphadenopathy in a patient with Hodgkin's disease.

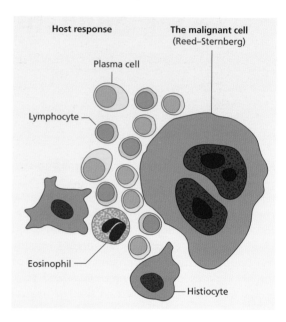

Fig. 15.2 Diagrammatic representation of the different cells seen histologically in Hodgkin's disease.

(c) alcohol-induced pain in the areas where disease is present occurs in some patients;
(d) other constitutional symptoms include weight loss, profuse sweating (especially at night), weakness, fatigue, anorexia and cachexia. Haematological and infectious complications are discussed below.

Haematological and biochemical findings

1 Normochromic, normocytic anaemia is most common. With marrow infiltration, bone marrow failure may occur with a leucoerythroblastic anaemia.
2 One-third of patients have a leucocytosis caused by a neutrophil increase.
3 Eosinophilia is frequent.
4 Advanced disease is associated with lymphopenia and loss of cell-mediated immunity.
5 The platelet count is normal or increased during early disease, and reduced in later stages.
6 The erythrocyte sedimentation rate (ESR) and C-reactive protein are usually raised and are useful in monitoring disease progress.
7 Bone marrow involvement is unusual in early disease. It may be demonstrated by trephine biopsy, usually in patients with disease at many sites. Bilateral trephine biopsy is performed in some units.
8 Serum lactate dehydrogenase (LDH) is raised initially in 30–40% of cases, and elevated levels

of serum transaminases may indicate liver involvement.

Diagnosis and histological classification

The diagnosis is made by histological examination of an excised lymph node. The distinctive multinucleate, polyploid RS cell is central to the diagnosis (Figs 15.2 and 15.3). Inflammatory components consist of lymphocytes, histiocytes, polymorphs, eosinophils, plasma cells and variable fibrosis. Histological classification is into five types (Table 15.1), each of which implies a different prognosis. Nodular sclerosis and mixed cellularity are more frequent. Patients with lymphocyte predominant histology have the most favourable prognosis. The nodular sclerosis type predominates in young adults; the other types have a bimodal age distribution with a second peak in old age.

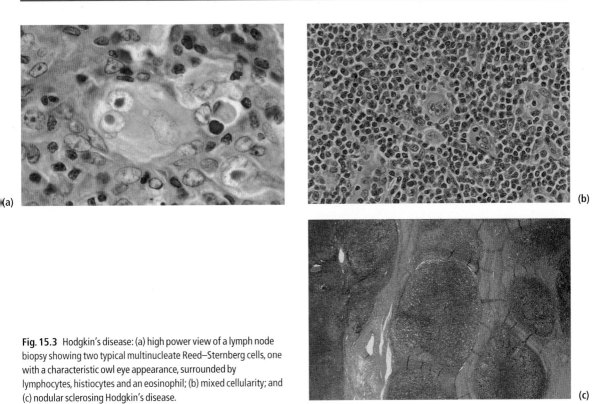

Fig. 15.3 Hodgkin's disease: (a) high power view of a lymph node biopsy showing two typical multinucleate Reed–Sternberg cells, one with a characteristic owl eye appearance, surrounded by lymphocytes, histiocytes and an eosinophil; (b) mixed cellularity; and (c) nodular sclerosing Hodgkin's disease.

Table 15.1 Histology of Hodgkin's disease (REAL/WHO classification)

Lymphocyte predominant/ nodular ± diffuse areas	Reed–Sternberg cells are absent; abnormal polymorphic B cells (lymphocytic and histiocytic) present
Classical Hodgkin's disease	
Nodular sclerosis	Collagen bands extend from the node capsule to encircle nodules of abnormal tissue. A characteristic lacunar cell variant of the Reed–Sternberg cell is often found. The cellular infiltrate may be of the lymphocyte-predominant, mixed cellularity or lymphocyte-depleted type; eosinophilia is frequent
Mixed cellularity	The Reed–Sternberg cells are numerous and lymphocyte numbers are intermediate
Lymphocyte depleted	There is either a reticular pattern with dominance of Reed–Sternberg cells and sparse numbers of lymphocytes or a diffuse fibrosis pattern where the lymph node is replaced by disordered connective tissue containing few lymphocytes. Reed–Sternberg cells may also be infrequent in this latter subtype
Lymphocyte rich	Scanty Reed–Sternberg cells; multiple small lymphocytes with few eosinophils and plasma cells; nodular and diffuse types

REAL, Revised American European Lymphoma; WHO, World Health Organization.

Clinical staging

The selection of appropriate treatment depends on accurate staging of the extent of disease (Table 15.2). Figure 15.4 shows the scheme (Ann Arbor) now recommended. Staging is performed by thorough clinical examination together with chest X-ray to detect mediastinal, hilar node or lung involvement (Fig. 15.5) and CT scan to detect intrathoracic, intra-abdominal or pelvic disease (Fig. 15.6). It is also used to monitor response to therapy. Magnetic resonance imaging (MRI) scanning may be needed for particular sites (Table 15.2). Bone marrow trephine is carried out; liver biopsy may also be needed in difficult cases. Gallium scanning or positron emission tomography (PET) scanning may also be useful in

Table 15.2 Techniques for staging of lymphoma

Laboratory	Full blood count
	ESR
	Bone marrow aspirate and trephine
	Liver function
	LDH
	C-reactive protein
Radiology	Chest radiograph
	CT of thorax, abdomen, chest and pelvis
	Ultrasound
Special tests	Magnetic resonance imaging
	Lymphangiography
	Bone scan
	Gallium scan
	Positron emission tomography

CT, computed tomography; ESR, erythrocyte sedimentation rate; LDH, lactate dehydrogenase.

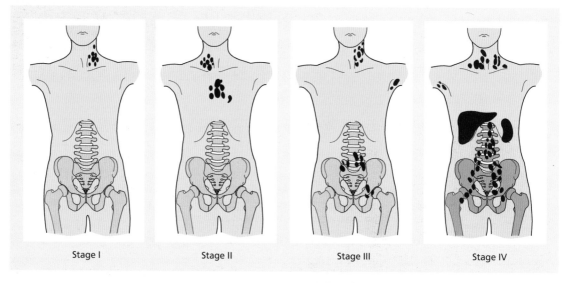

Stage I   Stage II   Stage III   Stage IV

Fig. 15.4 Staging of Hodgkin's disease. Stage I indicates node involvement in one lymph node area. Stage II indicates disease involving two or more lymph nodal areas confined to one side of the diaphragm. Stage III indicates disease involving lymph nodes above and below the diaphragm. Splenic disease is included in stage III but this has special significance (see below). Stage IV indicates involvement outside the lymph node areas and refers to diffuse or disseminated disease in the bone marrow, liver and other extranodal sites. NB. The stage number in all cases is followed by the letter A or B indicating the absence (A) or presence (B) of one or more of the following: unexplained fever above 38°C; night sweats; or loss of more than 10% of body weight within 6 months. Localized extranodal extension from a mass of nodes does not advance the stage but is indicated by the subscript E. Thus mediastinal disease with contiguous spread to the lung or spinal theca would be classified as I_E. As involvement of the spleen is often a prelude to widespread haematogenous spread of the disease, patients with lymph node and splenic involvement are staged as III_S. Bulky disease (widening of the mediastinum by more than one-third, or the presence of a nodal mass > 10 cm in diameter) is relevant to therapy at any stage.

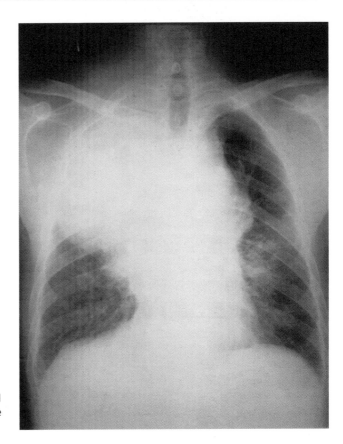

Fig. 15.5 Chest X-ray in Hodgkin's disease showing widespread enlargement of hilar and mediastinal lymph nodes with associated collapse of the right upper lobe and infiltration or possibly pneumonic changes in the mid zone of the left lung.

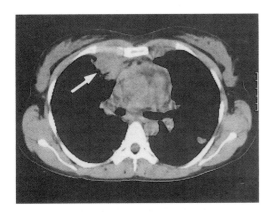

Fig. 15.6 Hodgkin's disease (nodular sclerosing type): CT scan of chest showing anterior mediastinal mass of enlarged lymph nodes (arrowed).

staging and detecting small foci of residual disease following treatment.

The patients are also classified as A or B according to whether or not constitutional features (fever or weight loss) are present (Fig. 15.4).

Treatment

This is with radiotherapy, chemotherapy or a combination of both. The choice depends primarily on the stage although histological grading is an additional factor.

Radiotherapy

Patients with stage I and IIA Hodgkin's disease may be cured by radiotherapy alone. A dose of 4000 rad (40 Gy) is able to destroy lymph node Hodgkin's tissue in about 80% of these patients. Improved high voltage radiotherapy techniques allow the treatment of all lymph node areas above or below the diaphragm by single 'upper mantle' or 'inverted Y' blocks. Radiotherapy also has a role in the treatment of bulky tumour masses, e.g. mediastinal tumour in nodular sclerosing disease or painful skeletal, nodal or soft tissue deposits. Short courses of chemotherapy are sometimes combined with radiotherapy in an attempt to reduce the relapse rate.

Chemotherapy

Cyclical chemotherapy is used for stage III and IV disease and also in stage I and II patients who have bulky disease, type B symptoms or have relapsed following initial radiotherapy. The combination of Adriamycin, bleomycin, vinblastine and dacarbazine (ABVD) is now most widely used. Quadruple therapy with mustine, vincristine (Oncovin), procarbazine and prednisolone (MOPP) is more likely to cause sterility or secondary leukaemia. Variants replace mustine with chlorambucil or cyclophosphamide. It is usual to give six cycles (or four after full remission). More intensive chemotherapy, e.g. Stanford V, which also uses radiotherapy to sites of bulky disease, is being investigated for patients with advanced or relapsed disease.

Relapsed cases

The patient is treated with an alternative combination chemotherapy to the initial regimen and, if necessary, with radiotherapy to sites of bulky disease. If the disease remains chemosensitive autologous stem cell transplantation improves the probability of cure. Allogeneic transplantation may also be used.

Prognosis

Approximate 5-year survival rates range from 50% to over 90% depending on age, stage and histology.

There is an increased incidence of myelodysplasia or acute myeloid leukaemia (AML) with a peak at 4 years after treatment for Hodgkin's disease with alkylating agents, especially if radiotherapy has also been given. Non-Hodgkin's lymphomas

and other cancers also occur with greater frequency than in controls. Non-malignant complications include sterility (semen storage should be carried out before therapy is commenced), intestinal complications, myocardial infarction and other cardiac or pulmonary complications of the mediastinal radiation and chemotherapy.

NON-HODGKIN'S LYMPHOMAS

The clinical presentation and natural history of these malignant lymphomas are more variable than in Hodgkin's disease, the pattern of spread is not as regular, and a greater proportion of patients present with extranodal disease or leukaemic manifestations.

Classification and histopathology

No area of diagnostic histopathology has been associated with greater confusion than the classification of non-Hodgkin's lymphomas. A number of classifications have been used over the years with no one scheme receiving unanimous support. In 1994 the Revised American European Lymphoma (REAL) classification was released and has gained widespread application (Table 15.3). The REAL/WHO classification includes all lymphoid malignancies as well as lymphomas and is more clinically based than previous classification schemes. In general terms there is a move away from subdividing lymphomas simply on the basis of subtle histological appearance and more in terms of syndromes with characteristic morphological, immunophenotypic, genetic and clinical features. It is also useful to think of the likely origin of individual lymphoid malignancies based on their phenotype and immunoglobulin gene rearrangement status (Fig. 15.7). In this chapter we consider each of the common lymphoma subtypes within this classification.

Predisposing diseases

HTLV-1 is the causative agent in adult T-

Table 15.3 The Revised American European Lymphoma (REAL) classification of lymphoid neoplasms. NB. Hodgkin's disease is also included in the full REAL classification. (The full WHO classification is included in Appendix 3)

B cell (85%)	T cell and NK cell (15%)
Precursor B-cell neoplasm	**Precursor T-cell neoplasms**
Precursor B-lymphoblastic leukaemia / lymphoma (B-ALL/LBL)	*Precursor T-lymphoblastic lymphoma / leukaemia (T-ALL/LBL)*
Mature (peripheral) B-cell neoplasms	**Mature (peripheral) T-cell neoplasms**
B-cell chronic lymphocytic leukaemia / small lymphocytic lymphoma	T-cell prolymphocytic leukaemia
B-cell prolymphocytic leukaemia	T-cell granular lymphocytic leukaemia
Lymphoplasmacytic lymphoma	Aggressive NK-cell leukaemia
Splenic marginal zone B-cell lymphoma (± villous lymphocytes)	Adult T-cell lymphoma / leukaemia (HTLV-1+)
Hairy cell leukaemia	
Plasma cell myeloma / plasmacytoma	Extranodal NK/T-cell lymphoma, nasal type
	Enteropathy-type T-cell lymphoma
Extranodal marginal zone B-cell lymphoma of MALT type	*Mycosis fungoides / Sézary syndrome*
	Anaplastic large cell lymphoma, primary cutaneous type
Mantle cell lymphoma	
Follicular lymphoma	*Peripheral T-cell lymphoma, unspecified*
Nodal marginal zone B-cell lymphoma	*Angioimmunoblastic T-cell lymphoma*
Diffuse large B-cell lymphoma	*Anaplastic large cell lymphoma, primary systemic type*
Burkitt's lymphoma	

ALL, acute lymphoblastic leukaemia; HTLV, human T-cell leukaemia / lymphoma virus; MALT, mucosa-associated lymphoid tissue; NK, natural killer.

cell leukaemia/lymphoma. Immunodeficiency, either inherited or acquired, predisposes to B-cell lymphomas. In acquired immune deficiency syndrome (AIDS) there is an increased incidence of lymphomas at unusual sites, e.g. in the central nervous system. The lymphomas are usually of B-cell origin and of high-grade or intermediate histology. EBV is usually present in the posttransplant lymphoproliferative disease (PTLD) which may begin with a polyclonal B-cell proliferation. EBV underlies the endemic form of Burkitt's lymphoma which is restricted to areas of holoendemic malaria. It also underlies nasal type (angiocentric) lymphoma in South-East Asia and South America. Gluten-induced enteropathy and angioimmunoblastic; lymphadenopathy predispose to T-cell lymphomas, and in some mucosa-associated lymphoid tissue (MALT) lymphomas of the stomach, *Helicobacter* infection has been implicated as a predisposing factor. Hepatitis C infection has also been suggested as a risk factor for the development of non-Hodgkin's lymphomas.

Low-grade and high-grade non-Hodgkin's lymphomas

The non-Hodgkin's lymphomas are a diverse group of diseases varying from highly proliferative and rapidly fatal diseases, to some of the most indolent and well-tolerated malignancies found in humans. For many years clinicians have subdivided lymphomas into low-grade and high-grade disease with some falling into an intermediate grade. This approach has been extremely valuable as, in general terms, the low-grade disorders are relatively indolent, respond well to chemotherapy and are very difficult to cure whereas high-grade lymphomas are aggressive and need urgent treatment but are often curable.

CLINICAL FEATURES OF NON-HODGKIN'S LYMPHOMAS

1 Superficial lymphadenopathy. The majority of patients present with asymmetric painless

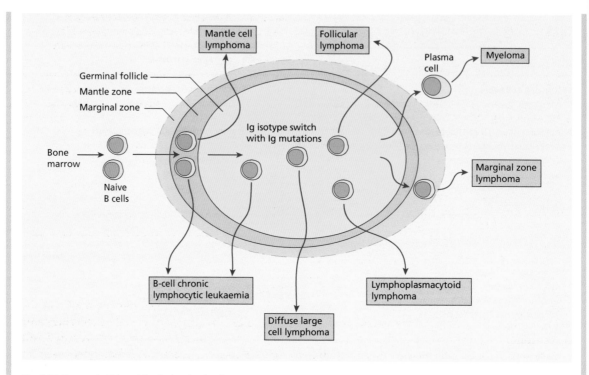

Fig. 15.7 Proposed cellular origin of B-lymphoid malignancies. Normal B cells migrate from the bone marrow and enter secondary lymphoid tissue. When they encounter antigen a germinal centre is formed and B cells undergo somatic hypermutation of the immunoglobulin genes. Finally B cells exit the lymph node as memory B cells or plasma cells. The cellular origin of the different lymphoid malignancies can be inferred from immunoglobulin gene rearrangement status and membrane phenotype. Mantle cell lymphoma and a proportion of B-CLL cases have unmutated immunoglobulin genes whereas marginal zone lymphoma, diffuse large cell lymphoma, follicle cell lymphoma, lymphoplasmacytoid lymphoma and some B-CLL cases have mutated immunoglobulin genes.

enlargement of lymph nodes in one or more peripheral lymph node regions.

2 Constitutional symptoms. Fever, night sweats and weight loss occur less frequently than in Hodgkin's disease and their presence is usually associated with disseminated disease. Anaemia and infections of the type seen in Hodgkin's disease may occur.

3 Oropharyngeal involvement. In 5–10% of patients there is disease of the oropharyngeal lymphoid structures (Waldeyer's ring) which may cause complaints of a 'sore throat' or noisy or obstructed breathing.

4 Anaemia, neutropenia with infections or thrombocytopenia with purpura may be present-

ing features in patients with diffuse bone marrow disease. Cytopenias may also be autoimmune in origin.

5 Abdominal disease. The liver and spleen are often enlarged and involvement of retroperitoneal or mesenteric nodes is frequent (Fig. 15.11). The gastrointestinal tract is the most commonly involved extranodal site after the bone marrow, and patients may present with acute abdominal symptoms.

6 Other organs. Skin, brain, testis or thyroid involvement is not infrequent. The skin is also primarily involved in two unusual, closely related T-cell lymphomas: mycosis fungoides and Sézary syndrome.

Haematological findings

1 A normochromic, normocytic anaemia is usual but autoimmune haemolytic anaemia may also be occur.

2 In advanced disease with marrow involvement there may be neutropenia, thrombocytopenia (especially if the spleen is enlarged) or leucoerythroblastic features.

3 Lymphoma cells (e.g. mantle zone cells, 'cleaved follicular lymphoma' or 'blast' cells) with variable nuclear abnormalities may be found in the peripheral blood in some patients (see Fig. 14.7).

4 Trephine biopsy of marrow is valuable (Fig. 15.12). Paradoxically, bone marrow involvement is found more frequently in low-grade malignant lymphomas. Immunological marker studies using fluorescence or peroxidase techniques may detect minimal involvement (e.g. with a clonal population of B cells shown by restricted immunoglobulin light chain (κ or λ) usage) not easily recognized by conventional microscopy.

Immunological markers

Monoclonal antibodies to antigens expressed on cells at sequential stages of lymphoid development and in different lineages or states of activation are used in the classification of malignant lymphoma (Table 15.4).

Chromosome findings

The various subtypes of non-Hodgkin's lymphoma are associated with characteristic chromosomal translocations which are of diagnostic and prognostic value (Chapter 11). These are described in Table 11.2. Particularly characteristic are: t(8; 14) (Burkitt's lymphoma), t(14; 18) (follicular lymphoma), t(11; 14) (mantle cell lymphoma) and t(2; 5) (anaplastic large cell lymphoma).

Table 15.4 Cluster differentiation (CD) antigens useful in lymphoma diagnosis. Other antigens which may be useful in lymphoma diagnosis include CD10, terminal deoxynucleotidyl transferase (TdT) and adhesion molecules

T cell	B cell	Activation markers	Leucocyte common antigen
CD2	CD19	CD23	CD45
CD3	CD20	CD25	
CD5	CD22	CD30	
CD7	CD24		
T-cell subsets	*Rare B cell*		
CD4	CD5		
CD8			

Gene rearrangements

In B-cell lymphomas the immunoglobulin genes are clonally rearranged, usually involving both heavy and light chain genes; whereas in T-cell lymphomas, the immunoglobin genes are in germline configuration but there is clonal rearrangement of the T-cell receptor genes (see Chapter 10).

Blood chemistry

Elevation of serum uric acid may occur. Abnormal liver function tests suggest disseminated disease. The serum LDH level is raised in more rapidly proliferating and extensive disease and may be used as a prognostic marker (Table 15.5).

Investigation and staging

Lymph node biopsy is the definitive investigation (Figs 15.8 and 15.9) and morphological examination may be assisted by immunophenotypic and genetic analysis.

Trephine biopsy of marrow, gene rearrangement studies and immunophenotyping may all be valuable (Fig. 15.10). Serum LDH is frequently raised and is useful as a prognostic indicator and for monitoring response to treatment.

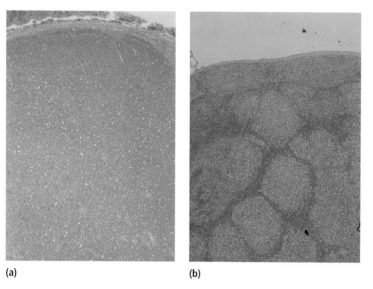

(a)   (b)

Fig. 15.8 Non-Hodgkin's lymphoma: histological sections of lymph nodes showing (a) a diffuse pattern of involvement in lymphocytic lymphoma with the normal architecture totally replaced by neoplastic lymphocytic cells; (b) a follicular or nodular pattern in follicular lymphoma — the 'follicles' or 'nodules' of neoplastic cells compress surrounding tissue and lack a mantle of small lymphocytes.

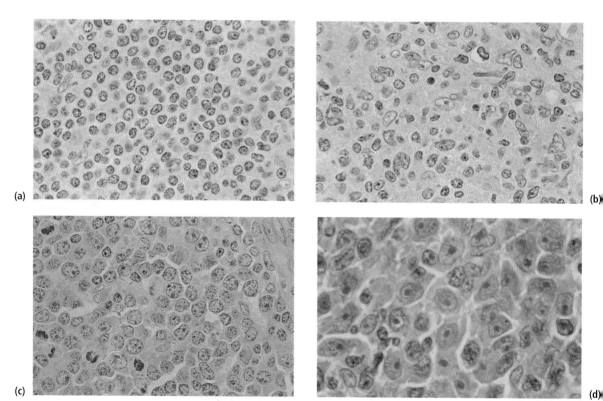

(a)   (b)

(c)   (d)

Fig. 15.9 Non-Hodgkin's lymphoma: high power view of lymph node biopsies showing (a) lymphocytic lymphoma showing predominantly small lymphocytes with round nuclei containing densely clumped heterochromatin. (b) Mantle cell lymphoma: showing characteristic deformed pattern of small lymphocytes with angular nuclei ('centrocytes'). (c) Diffuse large B-cell lymphoma: the neoplastic cells are much larger than normal lymphocytes and have a round nucleus with prominent nucleoli, many of which are adjacent to the nuclear membrane ('centroblasts'). A number of mitotic figures are seen. (d) Diffuse large B-cell lymphoma showing large neoplastic cells with a single prominent nucleolus and abundant dark staining cytoplasm (previously termed immunoblasts).

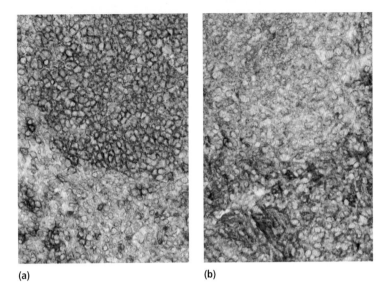

(a)   (b)

Fig. 15.10 Non-Hodgkin's lymphoma: lymph node stained by immunoperoxidase shows (a) brown ring staining for κ in the malignant lymphoid nodule, and (b) no labelling for λ confirming the monoclonal origin of the lymphoma.

Immunoglobulin electrophoresis may reveal a paraprotein.

The staging system is the same as that described for Hodgkin's disease but is less clearly related than histological type to prognosis. Staging procedures usually include chest X-ray, CT scanning or MRI (Fig. 15.11), and bone marrow aspiration and trephine (Fig. 15.12). Gallium or positron-emission tomography may detect disease not seen on CT scan and is useful for following treatment response (Fig. 15.11).

SPECIFIC SUBTYPES OF NON-HODGKIN'S LYMPHOMA

Lymphocytic lymphomas

Lymphocytic lymphomas are closely related to chronic lymphocytic leukaemia (CLL) and many regard this lymphoma as a tissue phase of CLL (Figs. 15.8 and 15.9). Many patients with this condition are elderly with slowly progressive disease and may not require treatment for extended periods. Treatment is along the lines of that for B-cell CLL (p. 194).

Lymphoplasmacytoid lymphomas

Lymphoplasmacytoid lymphomas are often associated with the production of monoclonal immunoglobulin M (IgM), in which case they tend to be termed Waldenström's macroglobulinaemia (p. 221). Complications are anaemia and hyperviscosity syndrome. Treatment is with oral chlorambucil or fludarabine.

Mantle cell lymphoma

Mantle cell lymphoma is derived from naïve pregerminal centre cells localized in the primary follicles or in the mantle region of secondary follicles. It has a characteristic phenotype of CD19+ and CD5+ (like CLL) but in contrast is CD22+, CD23–. A specific t(11; 14)(q13; q32) translocation is seen in most cases and leads to deregulation of the cyclin D1 (*BCL-1*) gene. Clinical presentation is typically with lymphadenopathy and often there is bone marrow infiltration and tumour cells in the blood. The cells have characteristically angular nuclei in histological sections (Fig. 15.9b). Current treatment regimes are not very effective and new protocols are being investigated. The prognosis is poor and the median survival is around 3 years.

Follicular lymphoma

This is the most common form of non-Hodgkin's lymphoma and is associated with the t(14; 18) translocation and constitutive BCL-2 expression in the great majority of cases (Fig. 15.13). Patients are likely to be middle-aged or elderly and their

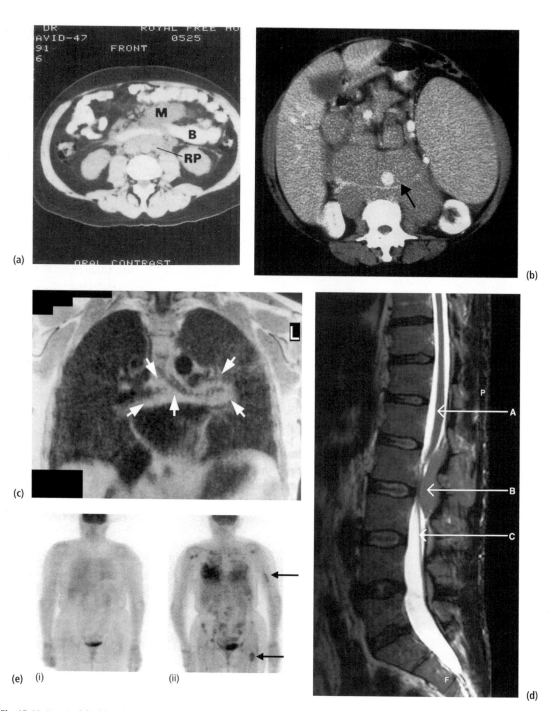

Fig. 15.11 Non-Hodgkin's lymphoma. (a) CT scan of the abdomen showing enlarged mesenteric (M) and retroperitoneal (RP; para-aortic) lymph nodes. B, bowel (courtesy of Dr L. Berger). (b) CT scan of the abdomen: enlarged retroperitoneal and mesenteric nodes from a man causing the 'floating aorta' (arrowed) appearance (courtesy of Professor A. Dixon and Dr R.E. Marcus). (c) MRI scan of the chest showing large mediastinal lymph nodes (white and arrowed) adjacent to the great vessels (black). (d) MRI T$_2$ weighted midline saggital image of a lumbosacral spine showing compression of the dual sac by an extradural mass. A, spinal cord; B, extradural mass; C, roots of corda equina. (Courtesy of Dr A. Valentine.) (e) PET body scan of a 59-year-old-lady with high-grade non-Hodgkin's lymphoma. The first scan (i) showed no evidence of disease prior to allogeneic transplant. Normal physiological uptake is seen in the brain and bladder. Two months post-transplant the patient relapsed clinically with a mass on the anterior chest wall. The PET scan (ii) showed evidence of widespread relapse in nodal (para-aortic and iliac nodes) and extranodal sites including the lung and bone. The uptake in bone is clearly demonstated in the left humerus and femur (arrowed). This scan illustrates how well PET can detect both nodal and extranodal disease and allows whole body assessment at a single scanning session. (Courtesy of Dr S.F. Barrington.)

disease is often characterized by a benign course for many years. The median survival from diagnosis is around 9 years.

Presentation is usually with painless lymphadenopathy, often widespread, and the majority of patients will have stage III or stage IV

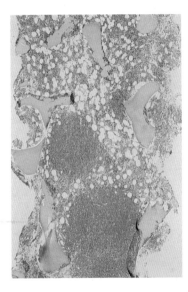

Fig. 15.12 Iliac crest trephine biopsy in lymphocytic lymphoma. Prominent nodules of lymphoid tissue are seen in the intertrabecular space and paratrabecular areas.

disease. However, sudden transformation may occur to aggressive diffuse tumours which are sometimes associated with a leukaemic phase.

Treatment options range from simple observation through oral chemotherapy to experimental high-dose treatment with stem cell support. When used as initial treatment chlorambucil or COP (cyclophosphamide, vincristine and prednisolone) achieve a response in up to 90% of patients with a median duration of around 2 years. However, with successive relapses the response rates and duration fall. Localized disease may respond very well to radiotherapy. CHOP (see below) is useful in relapsed cases. Fludarabine alone or in combination with cyclophosphamide or mitozantrone and dexamethasone (FMD) may produce remission and α-interferon (α-IFN) may help to extend remission time. In addition, humanized monoclonal antibody to CD20 is finding a place in management.

Marginal zone lymphomas

Marginal zone lymphomas are typically extranodal and are usually localized. MALT lymphomas come into this category and usually arise as a consequence of a pre-existing inflammatory or autoimmune disorder at sites such as the stomach or thyroid. Gastric MALT lymphoma is the

Fig. 15.13 Follicular lymphoma: immunohistological detection of BCL-2 protein. (a) Follicular lymphoma positive because the BCL-2 is activated by the (14; 18) translocation; (b) reactive node with unstained for BCL-2 germinal centres surrounded by positive mantle zone B and T cells. Immunoalkaline phosphatase (APAPP) stain. (Courtesy of Professors K.C. Gatter and D.Y. Mason.)

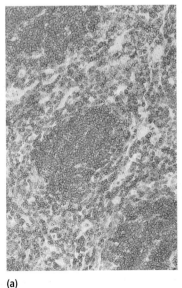

(a)

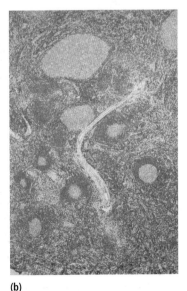

(b)

most common form and is preceded by *Helicobacter pylori* infection. In the early stages it may respond to antibiotic therapy aimed at eliminating *H. pylori*. Splenic marginal zone B-cell lymphoma usually is associated with circulating 'villous' lymphocytes (p. 196).

Burkitt's lymphoma

Burkitt's lymphoma is the lymphomatous correlate of L_3 acute lymphoblastic leukaemia (p. 164) and occurs in endemic or sporadic forms.

Endemic (African) Burkitt's lymphoma is seen in areas with chronic malaria exposure and is associated with EBV infection. In addition, in virtually all cases the *C-MYC* oncogene is translocated to an immunoglobulin gene, usually the heavy chain locus t(8;14). Typically the patient, usually a child, presents with massive lymphadenopathy of the jaw (Fig. 15.14) which is initially very responsive to chemotherapy although long-term cure is uncommon.

Sporadic Burkitt's lymphoma may occur anywhere in the world and is not associated with EBV infection. The histological picture of Burkitt's lymphoma is distinctive (Fig. 15.15). The prognosis for such patients had always been poor until recently when the introduction of chemotherapy regimes which include high-dose methotrexate and cyclophosphamide has transformed the outlook. Now the majority of patients may expect cure.

Diffuse large B-cell lymphomas

Diffuse large cell lymphomas (DLCL) are a heterogeneous group of disorders representing the classical 'high-grade' lymphomas. As such they typically present with rapidly progressive lymphadenopathy associated with a fast rate of cellular proliferation. Progressive infiltration may affect the gastrointestinal tract, the spinal cord, the kidneys or other organs.

A variety of clinical and laboratory findings are relevant to the outcome of therapy. According to the international prognostic index these include age, performance status, stage, number of extranodal sites and serum LDH (Table 15.5). Bulky disease (major mass > 5cm in diameter) and prior history of low-grade disease or AIDS are also associated with a poorer prognosis. The cell of origin of DLCL has recently been suggested to be of prog-

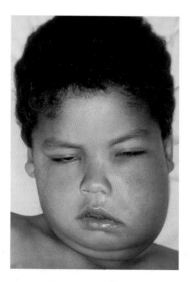

Fig. 15.14 Burkitt's lymphoma: characteristic facial swelling caused by extensive tumour involvement of the mandible and surrounding soft tissues.

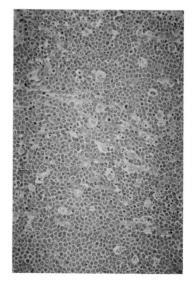

Fig. 15.15 Burkitt's lymphoma: histological section of lymph node showing sheets of lymphoblasts and 'starry sky' tingible body macrophages.

Table 15.5 International prognostic index for high-grade lymphoma

	Good	Bad
Age	< 60 years	> 60 years
Performance status	0 or 1	> 2
Stage (see p. 202)	I or II	III or IV
Number of extranodal sites	0 or 1	> 2
Serum LDH	Normal	Raised

LDH, lactate dehydrogenase.

nostic significance. If this is germinal centre the outlook has been found to be more favourable than if the origin is from an activated peripheral B cell. Cases associated with 3q27 translocation also have a relatively good prognosis.

Treatment

The mainstay of treatment of DLCL is the CHOP regimen (see p. 194). This is given in 3- or 4-weekly cycles, typically for six to eight courses. More aggressive chemotherapy regimes have not been proven to be more effective. Recent data, however, suggest that addition of anti-CD20 (Rituximab) to CHOP therapy improves remission rate in DLCL and trials of anti-CD20 radioactively linked to yttrium-90 or iodine-131 are promising. For localized disease, combined radiotherapy and chemotherapy (e.g. three courses of CHOP) may be optimal. For patients who relapse and have chemotherapy-sensitive disease, high-dose chemotherapy, e.g. with ifosfamide, epirubicin and etoposide (IVE), followed by autologous stem cell transplantation can be effective. For those with primary refractory or chemoresistant disease the outlook is poor. Overall long-term survival is around 45%.

Lymphoblastic lymphomas

Lymphoblastic lymphomas occur mainly in children and young adults and these conditions merge clinically and morphologically with acute lymphoblastic leukaemia (ALL).

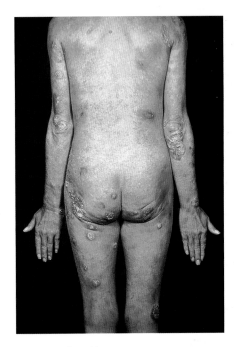

Fig. 15.16 Mycosis fungoides.

T-CELL LYMPHOMAS

Peripheral T-cell lymphomas which present with lymphadenopathy rather than extranodal disease are a heterogeneous group of rare tumours, usually of CD4+ phenotype. Several variants of T-cell lymphomas are recognized.

Angioimmunoblastic lymphadenopathy usually occurs in elderly patients with lymphadenopathy, hepatosplenomegaly, skin rashes and a polyclonal increase in serum IgG.

Mycosis fungoides is a chronic cutaneous T-cell lymphoma which presents with severe pruritus and psoriasis-like lesions (Fig. 15.16). Ultimately deeper organs are affected, particularly lymph nodes, spleen, liver and bone marrow.

In Sézary syndrome there is dermatitis, erythroderma, generalized lymphadenopathy and circulating T-lymphoma cells. The cells are usually CD4+ and have a folded or cerebriform nuclear chromatin. Initial treatment of these conditions is by local irradiation, topical chemotherapy or photochemotherapy with psoralen and ultraviolet light (PUVA). Chemotherapy may be needed.

Adult T-cell leukaemia/lymphoma is associated with human T-cell leukaemia/lymphoma virus type 1 (HTLV-1) infection and presents with lymphadenopathy, hepatic and splenic enlargement, cutaneous infiltrations and hypercalcaemia (p. 197).

Angiocentric lymphomas typically involve the nasal sinuses whereas T-cell intestinal lymphoma is associated with gluten-induced enteropathy in many cases.

Anaplastic large cell lymphoma is particularly common in children and is of T-cell or null cell phenotype. The disease is CD30+ and associated with the t(2; 5)(p23; q35) translocation. It has an aggressive course characterized by systemic symptoms and extranodal involvement.

BIBLIOGRAPHY

Aisenberg A.C. (1999) Problems in Hodgkin's disease management. *Blood* **93**, 761–79.

Alizadeh A.A., Elsen M.B., Davis R.E. *et al.* (2000) Distinct types of diffuse large B-cell lymphoma identified by gene expression profiling. *Nature* **403**, 503–11.

Armitage J.O., Cavalli F. and Longo D.L. (1999) *Text Atlas of Lymphomas*. Martin Dunitz, London.

Cheson B.D. (ed.) (2001) *Chronic Lymphoid Leukemias*, 2nd edn. Marcel Dekker Inc. New York.

Child J.A., Jack A.S. and Morgan G.J. (1998) *The Lymphoproliferative Disorders*. Chapman & Hall, London.

Fisher R.I. (2000) Diffuse large-cell lymphoma. *Ann. Oncol.* **11**, Suppl. 1, 529–33.

Gregory Bociek R. and Armitage J.O. (1999) Hodgkin's disease and non-Hodgkin's lymphoma. *Curr. Opin. Hematol.* **6**, 205–15.

Harris N.L. *et al.* (1994) A revised European–American classification of lymphoid neoplasms: a proposal from the International Lymphoma Study Group. *Blood* **84**, 1361–92.

Harris N.L., Jaffe E.S., Diebold J. *et al.* (2000) The WHO classification of neoplasms of the hematopoietic and lymphoid tissues. *Hematol. J.* **1**, 53–66.

Horning S.J. (2000) Follicular lymphoma: have we made progress? *Ann. Oncol.* **11**, Suppl. 1, 523–27.

Krackhardt A. and Gribben J.G. (1999) Stem cell transplantation for indolent lymphoma. *Curr. Opin. Hematol.* **6**, 388–93.

Kuppers R., Klein U., Hansmann M.-L. *et al.* (1999) Cellular origin of human B-cell lymphomas. *N. Engl. J. Med.* **341**, 1520–9.

Mauch P.M., Armitage J.O., Diehl V. *et al.* (1999) *Hodgkin's Disease*. Lippincott, Williams & Wilkins, Hagerstown.

Pinkerton C.R. (1999) The continuing challenge of treatment for non-Hodgkin's lymphoma in children. *Br. J. Haematol.* **107**, 220–34.

Yuen A.R. and Horning S.J. (1997) Recent advances in the treatment of Hodgkin's disease. *Curr. Opin. Haematol.* **4**, 286–90.

Multiple myeloma and related disorders

PARAPROTEINAEMIA

This term refers to the presence of a monoclonal immunoglobulin band in the serum. Normally serum immunoglobulins are polyclonal and represent the combined output from millions of different plasma cells. A monoclonal band, or paraprotein, reflects the synthesis of immunoglobulin from a single plasma cell clone. There are several situations in which this may occur (Table 16.1) and not all require treatment.

MULTIPLE MYELOMA

Multiple myeloma (myelomatosis) is a neoplastic proliferation of bone marrow plasma cells, characterized by lytic bone lesions, plasma cell accumulation in the bone marrow, and the presence of monoclonal protein in the serum and urine. Ninety-eight per cent of cases occur over the age of 40 with a peak incidence in the seventh decade.

The malignant plasma cells have clonally rearranged immunoglobulin genes and secrete the same paraprotein that is present in serum. The aetiology of the disease is unknown but cytokines have an important role. Interleukin (IL)-6 is a potent growth factor for myeloma, possibly by an autocrine mechanism. In addition, the osteolytic lesions in this disease are probably the result of osteoclast-activating factor (OAF) mainly tumour necrosis factor (TNF) and IL-1, secreted by the myeloma cells. Gains, losses and structural alterations to different chromosomes are frequent with clonal evolution. The most frequent monosomy is of chromosome 13 which carries a poor prognosis. A variety of other clonal chromosomal changes have been found.

Clinical features

1 Bone pain (especially backache) and pathological fractures.
2 Features of anaemia: lethargy, weakness, dyspnoea, pallor, tachycardia, etc.
3 Recurrent infections; related to deficient antibody production, abnormal cell-mediated immunity and, in advanced disease, neutropenia.
4 Features of renal failure and/or hypercalcaemia: polydipsia, polyuria, anorexia, vomiting, constipation and mental disturbance.
5 Abnormal bleeding tendency: myeloma protein may interfere with platelet function and coagulation factors; thrombocytopenia occurs in advanced disease.
6 Other features include macroglossia, carpal tunnel syndrome and diarrhoea caused by amyloid disease. In about 2% of cases there is a hyperviscosity syndrome with purpura, haemorrhages, visual failure, central nervous system (CNS) symptoms and neuropathies, and heart failure. This results from polymerization of the abnormal immunoglobulin and is particularly likely when this is immunoglobulin A (IgA), IgM or IgD.

Diagnosis

This depends on three principal findings.

1 Monoclonal protein in serum or urine (or both) (Fig. 16.1). The serum paraprotein is IgG in two-thirds, IgA in one-third, with rare IgM or IgD or mixed cases. Normal serum immunoglobulin levels (IgG, IgA and IgM) are reduced, a feature known as immuneparesis. The urine contains Bence Jones protein in two-thirds of cases. This consists of free light chains, either κ or λ, of the same type as the serum paraprotein. In 15% of cases, Bence Jones proteinuria is present without a serum paraprotein. Rare cases of myeloma are non-secretory and therefore not associated with a paraprotein.

2 Increased plasma cells in the bone marrow (usually >20%), often with abnormal forms (Fig. 16.2).

Table 16.1 Diseases associated with M proteins

Malignant or uncontrolled production
  Multiple myeloma
  Waldenström's macroglobulinaemia
  Malignant lymphoma
  Chronic lymphocytic leukaemia
  Primary amyloidosis
  Plasma cell leukaemia
  Heavy chain disease

Benign or stable production
  Benign monoclonal gammopathy
  Solitary plasmacytoma
  Chronic cold haemagglutinin disease
  Transient, e.g. with infections
  Acquired immune deficiency syndrome (AIDS)
  Gaucher's disease
  Rarely with carcinoma and other conditions

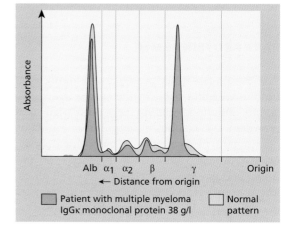

Fig. 16.1 Serum protein electrophoresis in multiple myeloma showing an abnormal paraprotein in the γ-globulin region with reduced levels of background β and γ globulins.

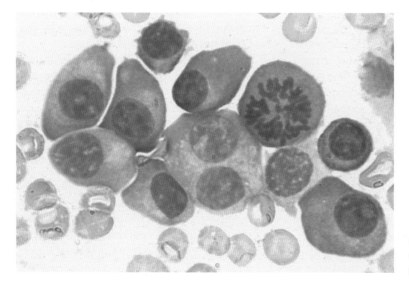

Fig. 16.2 The bone marrow in multiple myeloma showing large numbers of plasma cells, with many abnormal forms.

3 Bone lesions. Skeletal surveys show: osteolytic areas without evidence of surrounding osteoblastic reaction or sclerosis (60%) (Fig. 16.3); generalized osteoporosis (20%) (Fig. 16.4); or no bone lesions (20%). In addition, pathological fractures or vertebral colapse (Fig. 16.4b) are common.

Two of these three diagnostic features should be present to make the diagnosis.

Other laboratory findings include the following:

1 There is usually a normochromic, normocytic or macrocytic anaemia. Rouleaux formations are marked in most cases (Fig. 16.5). Neutropenia and thrombocytopenia occur in advanced disease. Abnormal plasma cells appear in the blood film in 15% of patients.

2 High erythrocyte sedimentation rate (ESR).

3 Serum calcium elevation occurs in 45% of patients. Typically the serum alkaline phosphatase is normal (except following pathological fractures).

4 The serum urea and creatinine are raised in 20% of cases. Proteinaceous deposits from heavy Bence Jones proteinuria, hypercalcaemia, uric acid, amyloid and pyelonephritis may all contribute to renal failure (Fig. 16.6).

5 A low serum albumin occurs with advanced disease.

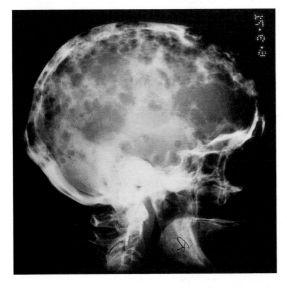

Fig. 16.3 Skull X-ray in multiple myeloma showing many 'punched-out' lesions.

6 Serum β_2-microglobulin is a useful indicator of prognosis. It partly reflects renal function. Levels less than 4 mg/l imply a relatively good prognosis.

Treatment

This may be divided into specific and supportive.

Specific

Chemotherapy The first major advance in the treatment of myeloma was the introduction of the oral alkylating agent melphalan. In elderly patients this may be used on its own or in combination with prednisolone and is effective in bringing the disease under control in the majority of patients. Typically, paraprotein levels gradually fall, bone lesions show improvement and blood counts may improve. Cyclophosphamide is also effective and simple to use as a single agent. However, after a variable number of courses a 'plateau phase' is reached in which the paraprotein level stops falling. At this point treatment is stopped and the patient seen at regular intervals in the outpatient clinic. After a variable period of time, often around 1 year, the disease 'escapes' from plateau with rising paraprotein and worsening symptoms. At this point treatment becomes difficult. Weekly oral or intravenous cyclophosphamide is one option.

In patients of less than 60 years of age more intensive chemotherapy is used initially such as the C-VAMP protocol (cyclophosphamide, vincristine, Adriamycin and methylprednisolone). Following several cycles of treatment most patients proceed to autologous stem cell transplantation (SCT) (see below). Other combinations may be used, e.g. ABCM (Adriamycin, BCNU, cyclophosphamide and melphalane).

Stem cell transplantation SCT using high-dose melphalan and autologous stem cells has a role in younger patients and prolongs life. Unfortunately it does not seem to cure the disease. Allogeneic transplantation may achieve this, but carries a greater procedure-related mortality.

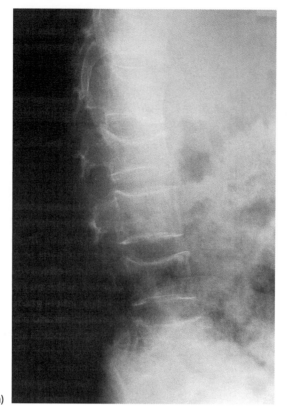

(a)

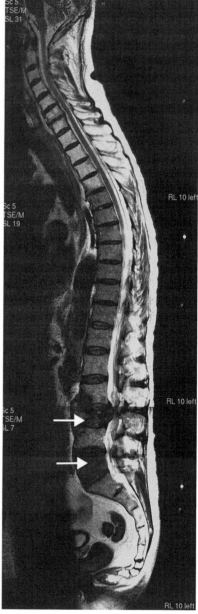

(b)

Fig. 16.4 (a) Multiple myeloma: X-ray of lumbar spine showing severe demineralization with partial collapse of L_3. (b) MRI of spine: T_2 weighted study. There is infiltration and destruction of L_3 and L_5 with bulging of the posterior part of the body of L_3 into the spinal canal compressing the corda equina (arrowed). Radiotherapy has caused a marrow signal change in vertebrae C_2–D_4 due to replacement of normal red marrow by fat (bright white signal). (Courtesy of Dr A. Platts.)

Interferon alpha This may prolong the plateau phase following chemotherapy or transplantation but has little, if any, effect on overall survival.

Radiotherapy This is highly effective in treating the symptoms of myeloma. It may be used for areas of bone pain or spinal cord compression.

Thalidomide This is showing promise in relapsed disease and is now being evaluated in trials in both early and late disease. Its precise mechanism of action is unknown.

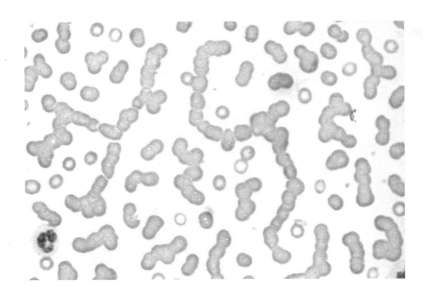

Fig. 16.5 The peripheral blood film in multiple myeloma showing rouleaux formations.

Supportive

Renal failure Rehydrate and treat the underlying cause (e.g. hypercalcaemia, hyperuricaemia). Dialysis is generally well tolerated. It is important that all patients with myeloma drink at least 3 litres of fluid each day throughout the course of their disease.

Bone disease and hypercalcaemia Bisphosphonates such as pamidronate and clodronate are effective in reducing the progression of bone disease. They may also improve overall survival. In acute hypercalcaemia bisphosphonates are given following rehydration with isotonic saline.

Compression paraplegia Use decompression laminectomy or irradiation; corticosteroid therapy may help.

Anaemia Transfusion or erythropoietin are used.

Bleeding Bleeding caused by paraprotein interference with coagulation and hyperviscosity syndrome may be treated by repeated plasmapheresis.

Infections Rapid treatment of any infection is essential. Prophylactic infusions of immunoglobulin concentrates together with oral broad-spectrum antibiotics and antifungal agents may be needed for recurrent infections.

Prognosis

The median survival with chemotherapy is 3–4 years with a 20% 5-year survival. However, this may be improved with autologous transplantation. An increased β_2-microglobulin level is a bad prognostic feature.

OTHER PLASMA CELL TUMOURS

Solitary plasmacytoma

These are isolated plasma cell tumours, usually of bone or soft tissue, e.g. the mucosa of the upper respiratory and gastrointestinal tracts or the skin. The associated M protein may disappear following radiotherapy to the primary lesion.

Plasma cell leukaemia

This occurs either as a late complication of

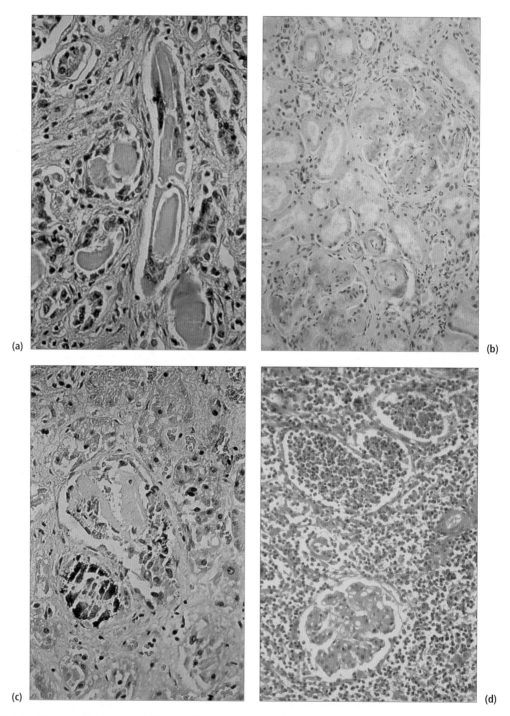

Fig. 16.6 The kidney in multiple myeloma. (a) Myeloma kidney — the renal tubules are distended with hyaline protein (precipitated light chains or Bence Jones protein). Giant cells are prominent in the surrounding cellular reaction. (b) Amyloid deposition — both glomeruli and several of the small blood vessels contain an amorphous pink-staining deposit characteristic of amyloid (Congo red stain). (c) Nephrocalcinosis — calcium deposition (dark 'fractured' material) in the renal parenchyma. (d) Pyelonephritis — destruction of renal parenchyma and infiltration by acute inflammatory cells.

myeloma or, often in younger patients, as a primary disease characterized by the presence of 20% or more plasma cells in the blood, with an absolute count of $>2.0\times10^9/l$ (Chapter 14). The outlook is poor.

Heavy chain disease

In these rare disorders the neoplastic cells secrete only incomplete immunoglobulin heavy chains (γ, α or μ). The most common form is α-heavy chain disease which occurs mainly in the Mediterranean area and starts as a malabsorption syndrome which may progress to lymphoma.

WALDENSTRÖM'S MACROGLOBULINAEMIA

This is an uncommon condition, seen most frequently in men over 50 years of age, in which there is a lymphoplasmacytoid lymphoma which produces a monoclonal IgM paraprotein (Fig. 16.7). The cell of origin appears to be a postgerminal centre B cell with the characteristics of an IgM-bearing memory B cell.

Clinical features

These are usually of insidious onset, with fatigue and weight loss. Hyperviscosity syndrome (p. 226) is common. IgM paraprotein increases blood viscosity more than equivalent concentrations of IgG or IgA, and small increases above 30 g/l in concentration lead to large increases in viscosity. Visual upset is frequent and the retina may show a variety of changes: engorged veins, haemorrhages, exudates and a blurred disc (Fig. 16.8). If the macroglobulin is a cryoglobulin features of cryoprecipitation, such as Raynaud's phenomenon, may be present. Anaemia, at least partly caused by an increased plasma volume, is usually a significant problem and a bleeding tendency may result from macroglobulin interference with coagulation factors and platelet function. Neurological symptoms, dyspnoea and heart failure may be presenting symptoms. Moderate lymphadenopathy and enlargement of the liver and spleen are frequently seen.

Diagnosis

This is made by the finding of a serum monoclonal IgM (usually > 15 g/l) together with bone marrow

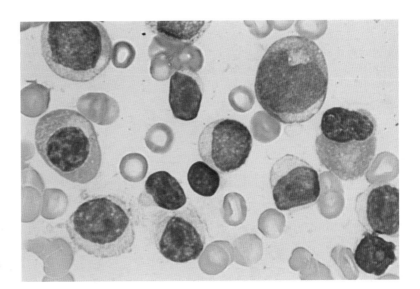

Fig. 16.7 Lymphoplasmacytoid lymphoma associated with Waldenström's macroglobulinaemia. Bone marrow shows cells with features of lymphocytes and plasma cells.

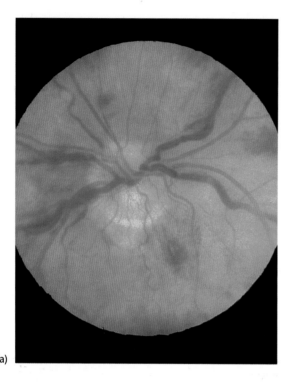

(a)

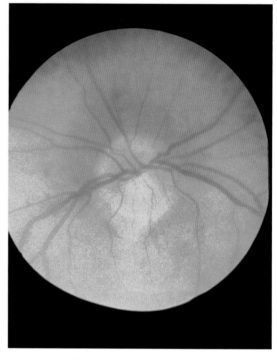

(b)

Fig. 16.8 Waldenström's macroglobulinaemia: hyperviscosity syndrome. (a) The retina before plasmapheresis shows distension of retinal vessels, particularly the veins which show bulging and constriction (the 'linked sausage' effect) and areas of haemorrhage; (b) following plasmapheresis the vessels have returned to normal and the areas of haemorrhage have cleared.

or lymph node infiltration with lymphoplasma-cytoid cells. The ESR is raised and there may be a peripheral blood lymphocytosis.

Treatment

Specific
No therapy is needed for patients without symptoms, significant hepatosplenomegaly or adenopathy or anaemia. Chlorambucil or cyclophosphamide have been the mainstay of therapy but fludarabine or 2-chlorodeoxyadeno-sine are also useful for initial therapy or relapsed

cases. Combination chemotherapy, for example CHOP (see p. 194) may be used in advanced disease.

Supportive
Acute hyperviscosity syndrome is treated with repeated plasmapheresis. As IgM is mainly intravascular, plasmapheresis is more effective than with IgG or IgA paraproteins when much of the protein is extravascular and so rapidly replenishes the plasma compartment. Regular transfusions may be required for chronic anaemia.

MONOCLONAL GAMMOPATHY OF UNDETERMINED SIGNIFICANCE

A paraprotein may be found in the serum, particularly of older subjects, with no definite evidence of myeloma, macroglobulinaemia or lymphoma and no other underlying disease. There are no bone lesions, no Bence Jones proteinuria, and the proportion of plasma cells in the marrow is normal (<4%) or only slightly raised (<10%). The concentration of monoclonal immunoglobulin in serum is usually less than 20 g/l and remains stationary when followed over a period of 2 or 3 years. Other serum immunoglobulins are not depressed. After many years of follow-up, however, a substantial proportion of these patients develop overt myeloma or lymphoma.

The distinguishing features of benign and malignant paraproteinaemia are listed in Table 16.2.

AMYLOIDOSIS

The amyloidoses are a heterogeneous group of disorders characterized by the extracellular deposition of protein in an abnormal fibrillar form. Amyloidosis may be hereditary or acquired and

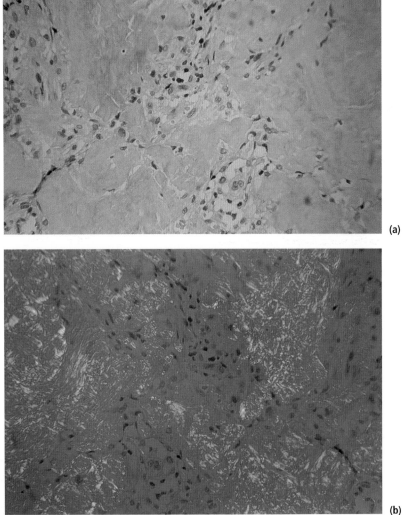

(a)

(b)

Fig. 16.9 Amyloidosis: (a) Congo red staining and (b) blue–green birefringence under polarized light.

Table 16.2 Features of benign and malignant paraproteinaemia

	Benign	Malignant
Bence Jones proteinuria	Absent	May be present
Serum paraprotein concentration	Usually < 20 g/l and stationary	Usually > 20 g/l and rising
Immuneparesis	Absent	Present
Underlying lymphoproliferative disease or myeloma	Absent	Present
Bone lesions	Absent	Present
Plasma cells in marrow	<10%	>10%

deposits may be focal, localized or systemic in distribution. The amyloid is made from different amyloid fibril precursor proteins in each type of disease. Except for intracerebral amyloid plaques, all amyloid deposits contain a non-fibrillary glycoprotein amyloid P which is derived from a normal serum precursor structurally related to C-reactive protein. The classic diagnostic test is red–green birefringence after staining with Congo red and viewing under polarized light (Fig. 16.9).

Amyloidosis is classified in Table 16.3.

Systemic AL amyloidosis

In this, amyloid disease is associated with clonal

Table 16.3 Classification of amyloidosis: types, structure and organ involvement. Other forms include hereditary amyloidosis and localized amyloid such as occurs in the central nervous system, endocrine tumours or skin

Type	Chemical nature	Organs involved
Systemic AL amyloidosis Associated with myeloma, Waldenström's macroglobulinaemia or MGUS May also occur on its own as primary amyloidosis (associated with an occult plasma cell proliferation) May also occur in localized form with local 'immunocyte' proliferation	Immunoglobulin light chains and/or parts of their variable regions (AL)	Tongue Skin Heart Nerves Connective tissue Kidneys Liver Spleen
Reactive systemic AA amyloidosis Rheumatoid arthritis, tuberculosis, bronchiectasis, chronic osteomyelitis, Hodgkin's disease, carcinomas, familial Mediterranean fever	Protein A (acute reactive, AA)	Liver Spleen Kidneys Bone marrow
Familial amyloidosis	e.g. Transthyretin abnormalities	Nerves Heart Eyes
Localised amyloidosis Central nervous system Endocrine Senile	β-amyloid protein Peptic hormones Various	Alzheimer's disease Endocrine tumours Heart, brain, joints, prostate, etc.

AA, AL, these are defined by their chemical nature as in the table; MGUS, monoclonal gammopathy of undetermined significance.

plasma cell proliferation. There is deposition of monoclonal light chain components which may be associated with a detectable paraproteinaemia. The clinical features are caused by involvement of the heart, tongue (Fig. 16.10), peripheral nerves and kidneys (Fig. 16.11), and the patient may present with heart failure, macroglossia, peripheral neuropathy, carpal tunnel syndrome or renal failure. Treatment is with similar chemotherapy to that used in myeloma, possibly with autologous stem cell transplantation, and may improve prognosis.

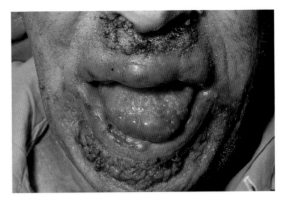

Fig. 16.10 Multiple myeloma: the tongue and lips are enlarged because of nodular and waxy deposits of amyloid.

Fig. 16.11 Serial anterior whole body ^{123}I-labelled serum amyloid P component (SAP) scans of a 52-year-old-woman who presented with renal failure due to systemic AL amyloidosis. (a) The initial scan demonstrates a large amyloid load with hepatic, splenic, renal and bone marrow deposits. Her underlying plasma cell dyscrasia responded to high-dose melphalan followed by autologous stem cell rescue. (b) Follow-up SAP scintigraphy 3 years after chemotherapy showed greatly reduced uptake of tracer indicating substantial regression of her amyloid deposits. (Courtesy of Professor P.N. Hawkins, National Amyloidosis Centre, Royal Free Hospital, London.)

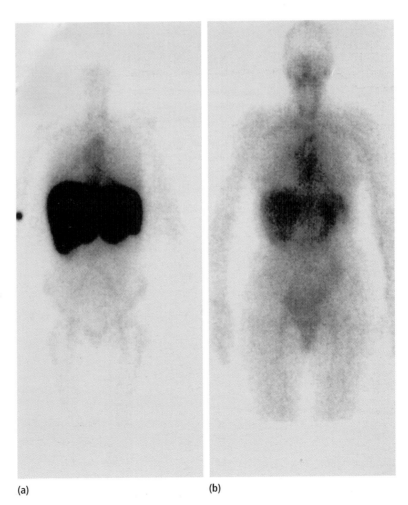

(a)   (b)

HYPERVISCOSITY SYNDROME

The most common cause is polycythaemia (p. 228). Hyperviscosity may also occur in patients with myeloma or Waldenström's macroglobulin-aemia or in patients with chronic or acute leukaemias associated with very high white cell counts. Rarely, haemophiliac patients with circulating inhibitors, being treated with massive doses of cryoprecipitate, have developed hyperviscosity because of the large volumes of fibrinogen infused.

The clinical features of the hyperviscosity syndrome include visual disturbances, lethargy, confusion, muscle weakness, nervous system symptoms and signs, and congestive heart failure. The retina may show a variety of changes: engorged veins, haemorrhages, exudates and a blurred disc (Fig. 16.8).

Emergency treatment varies with the cause: venesection or isovolaemic exchange of a plasma substitute for red cells in a polycythaemic patient; plasmapheresis in myeloma, Waldenström's disease or hyperfibrinogenaemia; and leucopheresis or chemotherapy in leukaemias associated with high white counts. The long-term treatment depends on control of the primary disease with specific therapy.

BIBLIOGRAPHY

Barlogie B., Jaganath S., Desikan K.R. *et al.* (1999) Total therapy with tandem transplants for newly diagnosed multiple myeloma. *Blood* **93**, 55–65.

Falk R.H., Comenzo R.L. and Skinner M. (1997) The systemic amyloidoses. *N. Engl. J. Med.* **337**, 898–909.

Gillmore J.D. *et al.* (1997) Amyloidosis: a review of recent diagnostic and therapeutic developments. *Br. J. Haematol.* **99**, 245–56.

Halek M., Bersagel P.L. and Anderson K.C. (1998) Multiple myeloma: increasing evidence for a multistep transformation process. *Blood* **91**, 3–21.

Jantunen E. *et al.* (1996) Bisphosphonates in multiple myeloma: current status; future perspectives. *Br. J. Haematol.* **93**, 501.

Kyle R.A. (2000) The role of high-dose chemotherapy in the treatment of multiple myeloma: a controversy. *Ann. Oncol.* **2**, Suppl. 1, S55–8.

Lokhorst H.M. (1999) Intensive treatment for multiple myeloma: where do we stand? *Br. J. Haematol.* **106**, 18–27.

Reece D.E. (1998) New advances in multiple myeloma. *Curr. Opin. Haematol.* **5**, 460–4.

Samson D. (1998) Current perspectives in the management of multipe myeloma. *CME Bull. Haematol.* **1**, 46–50.

Singal S., Mehta J. and Desikan R. (1999) Antitumour activity of thalidomide in refractory myeloma. *N. Engl. J. Med.* **341**, 1565–71.

Sjak-Shia N.N., Vescio R.A. and Berenson J.R. (2000) Recent advances in multiple myeloma. *Curr. Opin. Hematol.* **7**, 241–6.

Myeloproliferative disorders

The term myeloproliferative disorders describes a group of conditions arising from marrow stem cells and characterized by clonal proliferation of one or more haemopoietic components in the bone marrow and, in many cases, the liver and spleen. Four disorders are included in this classification:

1 Polycythaemia rubra vera.
2 Essential thrombocythaemia.
3 Myelofibrosis.
4 Chronic myeloid leukaemia.

These disorders are closely related to each other. Indeed, transitional forms occur and in many patients an evolution from one entity into another occurs during the course of the disease (Fig. 17.1). Polycythaemia rubra vera (PRV), essential thrombocythaemia and myelofibrosis are collectively known as the non-leukaemic myeloproliferative disorders and are discussed here; chronic myeloid leukaemia is discussed in Chapter 13.

POLYCYTHAEMIA

Polycythaemia (erythrocytosis) is defined as an increase in the haemoglobin concentration above the upper limit of normal for the patient's age and sex.

Classification of polycythaemia

Polycythaemia is classified according to its pathophysiology but the major subdivision is into absolute polycythaemia, in which the red cell mass (volume) is raised, and relative or pseudo-polycythaemia in which the red cell volume is normal but the plasma volume is reduced (Table 17.1). Absolute polycythaemia can then be subdivided into primary polycythaemia (polycythaemia rubra vera) or secondary polycythaemia (Table 17.2).

POLYCYTHAEMIA (RUBRA) VERA

In PRV, the increase in red cell volume is caused by a clonal malignancy of a marrow stem cell. Although the increase in red cells is the diagnostic finding, in many patients there is also an overproduction of granulocytes and platelets.

The disease is associated with a number of chromosomal changes, of which deletions of chromosome 20q are the most frequent.

Diagnosis

Making the diagnosis of PRV in a patient who presents with polycythaemia can be difficult and the diagnostic criteria of the Polycythaemia Vera Study Group are very valuable (Table 17.3).

Clinical features

This is a disease of older subjects with an equal sex incidence. Clinical features are the result of hyperviscosity, hypervolaemia or hypermetabolism.

1 Headaches, dyspnoea, blurred vision and night sweats. Pruritus, characteristically after a hot bath, can be a severe problem.

2 Plethoric appearance—ruddy cyanosis (Fig. 17.2), conjunctival suffusion and retinal venous engorgement.

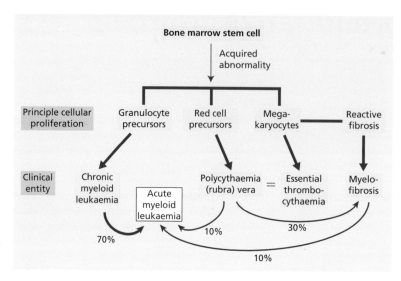

Fig. 17.1 Relationship between the various myeloproliferative diseases. They may all arise by somatic mutation in the pluripotential stem and progenitor cells. Many transitional cases occur showing features of two conditions and, in other cases, the disease transforms during its course from one of these diseases to another or to acute myeloid leukaemia. Chronic myeloid leukaemia may also transform into acute lymphoblastic leukaemia.

Table 17.1 Radiodilution methods for measuring red cell and plasma volume

	Normal	Primary or secondary polycythaemia	Relative polycythaemia
Total red cell volume (TRCV) (^{51}Cr)	Men 25–35 ml/kg Women 22–32 ml/kg	Increased	Normal
Total plasma volume (^{125}I-albumin)	40–50 ml/kg	Increased or normal	Decreased

Table 17.2 Causes of polycythaemia

Primary
Polycythaemia (rubra) vera

Secondary
Caused by compensatory erythropoietin increase in
　high altitudes
　pulmonary disease and alveolar hypoventilation
　cardiovascular disease, especially congenital with cyanosis
　increased affinity haemoglobin (familial polycythaemia)
　　(Chapter 6)
　heavy cigarette smoking
Caused by inappropriate erythropoietin increase in
　renal diseases, e.g. hydronephrosis, vascular impairment, cysts,
　　carcinoma
　tumours such as uterine fibromyoma, hepatocellular carcinoma,
　　cerebellar haemangioblastoma

Relative
Stress or pseudopolycythaemia
Cigarette smoking
Dehydration: water deprivation, vomiting
Plasma loss: burns, enteropathy

Table 17.3 Criteria for diagnosis of polycythaemia (rubra) vera

Category A
Total red cell mass
　male > 35 ml/kg
　female > 32 ml/kg
Arterial oxygen saturation > 92%
Splenomegaly

Category B
Platelets > 400×10^9/l
White cells > 12×10^9/l
Increased NAP score
Raised serum vitamin B_{12} level

NAP, neutrophil alkaline phosphatase.

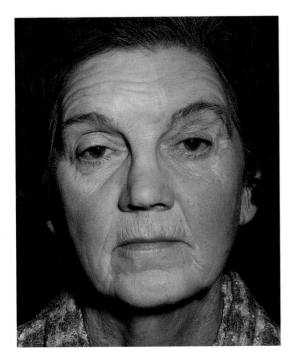

Fig. 17.2 Polycythaemia vera: facial plethora and conjunctival suffusion in a 63-year-old woman. Haemoglobin 18 g/dl; total red cell volume 45 ml/kg.

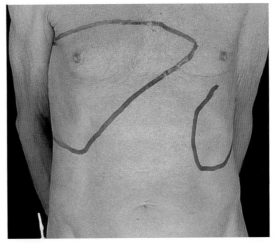

(a)

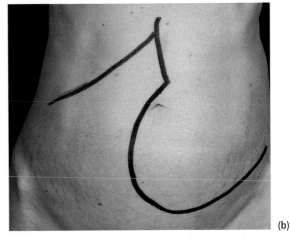

(b)

Fig. 17.3 Splenomegaly: enlarged spleens in male patients with (a) polycythaemia vera and (b) myelofibrosis.

3 Splenomegaly in 75% of patients (Fig. 17.3a).

4 Haemorrhage (e.g. gastrointestinal, uterine, cerebral) or thrombosis either arterial (e.g. cardiac, cerebral, peripheral) or venous (e.g. deep or superficial leg veins, cerebral, portal or hepatic veins) are frequent.

5 Hypertension in one-third of patients.

6 Gout (as a result of raised uric acid production) (Fig. 17.4a).

7 Peptic ulceration occurs in 5–10% of patients.

Laboratory findings

1 The haemoglobin, haematocrit and red cell count are increased. The total red cell volume (TRCV) (Table 17.1) is increased.

2 A neutrophil leucocytosis is seen in over half the patients, and some have increased circulating basophils.

3 A raised platelet count is present in about half the patients.

4 The neutrophil alkaline phosphatase (NAP) score is usually increased (see Table 13.2).

5 Increased serum vitamin B_{12} and vitamin B_{12}-binding capacity because of an increase in transcobalamin I.

6 The bone marrow is hypercellular with prominent megakaryocytes, best assessed by a trephine biopsy (Fig. 17.5a). Clonal cytogenetic abnormalities may occur, but there is no single characteristic change.

7 Blood viscosity is increased.

8 Plasma urate is often increased.

9 Circulating erythroid progenitors (erythroid colony-forming unit, CFU_E, and erythroid burst-

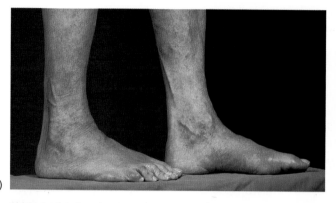

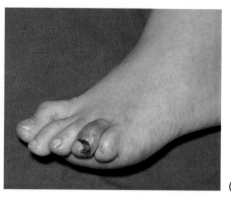

(a)

(b)

Fig. 17.4 (a) The feet of a 72-year-old man with polycythaemia rubra vera. There is inflammation of the right metatarsophalangeal and other joints caused by uric acid deposits. (b) Gangrene of the left fourth toe in essential thrombocythaemia.

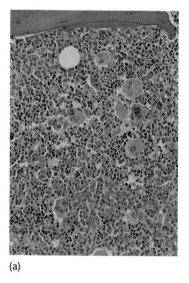

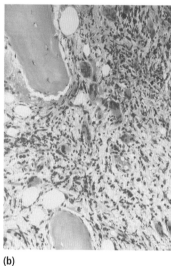

(a)   (b)

Fig. 17.5 Iliac crest trephine biopsies. (a) Polycythaemia vera: fat spaces are almost completely replaced by hyperplastic haemopoietic tissue. All haemopoietic cell lines are increased with megakaryocytes particularly prominent. (b) Myelofibrosis: normal marrow architecture is lost and haemopoietic cells are surrounded by increased fibrous tissue and intercellular substance.

forming unit, BFU_E) (p. 2) are increased compared to normal and grow *in vitro* independently of added erythropoietin.

Treatment

Treatment is aimed at maintaining a normal blood count. The haematocrit should be maintained at about 0.45 and the platelet count below $400 \times 10^9/l$.

Venesection
This form of therapy is particularly useful when a rapid reduction of red cell volume is required, e.g. at the start of therapy. It is especially indicated in younger patients and those with mild disease. The resulting iron deficiency may limit erythropoiesis. Unfortunately, venesection does not control the platelet count.

Cytotoxic myelosuppression
Daily hydroxyurea is valuable in controlling the blood count and may need to be continued for years (Fig. 17.6). Busulphan, which can be used intermittently, is sometimes used in older patients. The concern with cytotoxic drugs, especially busulphan, is that they may be associated

with an increased rate of progression to leukaemia. This is very low for hydroxyurea, but the exact risk is not yet clear.

Phosphorus-32 therapy

This is excellent therapy for older patients with severe disease. ^{32}P is a β-emitter, with a half-life of 14.3 days. It is concentrated in bone and is a most effective myelosuppressive agent. The usual remission time after a single dose is 2 years. Concern about late development of leukaemia limits its use.

Interferon

Clinical trials of interferon-α have shown good haematological responses. Longer trials are needed to determine whether this therapy alters the natural history of the disease. The therapy is less convenient and side-effects frequent. It may be particularly valuable in controlling itching.

Course and prognosis

Typically the prognosis is good with a median survival of 10–16 years. Thrombosis and haemorrhage are the major clinical problems. Increased viscosity, vascular stasis and high platelet levels may all contribute to thrombosis whereas defective platelet function may promote haemorrhage.

Transition from PRV to myelofibrosis occurs in about 30% of patients and around 5% of patients progress to acute leukaemia. ^{32}P and busulphan are generally avoided in younger subjects as they may increase this risk.

SECONDARY POLYCYTHAEMIA

The causes of secondary polycythaemia are listed in Table 17.2. Hypoxia caused by chronic obstruc-

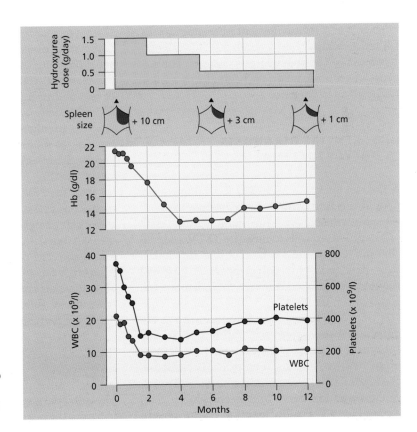

Fig. 17.6 Haematological response to therapy with hydroxyurea in polycythaemia vera. Hb, haemoglobin; WBC, white blood cells.

tive airways disease is one of the most common causes, and measurement of arterial oxygen saturation is a valuable test. Renal and tumour causes of inappropriate erythropoietin secretion are rare. Patients with a high affinity haemoglobin often have a family history of polycythaemia and present at a young age. There is debate as to whether or not patients with polycythaemia secondary to hypoxia and cyanotic heart disease should have their haematocrit reduced but values above 0.55–0.6 impair tissue oxygen delivery.

RELATIVE POLYCYTHAEMIA

Relative polycythaemia, also known as apparent polycythaemia or pseudopolycythaemia, is the result of plasma volume contraction. By definition, the TRCV is normal. The cause is uncertain but it is far more common than PRV. It occurs particularly in young or middle-aged men and may be associated with cardiovascular problems, e.g. hypertension (Gaisbock syndrome), myocardial ischaemia or cerebral transient ischaemic attacks. Diuretic therapy, heavy smoking and alcohol consumption are frequent associations. Trials of venesection to maintain an haematocrit around 0.45–0.47 are in progress.

DIFFERENTIAL DIAGNOSIS OF POLYCYTHAEMIA

A rational approach is needed to evaluate a patient presenting with a high haemoglobin. If the polycythaemia is consistent, studies with ^{51}Cr-labelled red cells to measure TRCV and ^{125}I-albumin to measure plasma volume are vital. If these confirm absolute polycythaemia the patient should be investigated for PRV. As well as the full blood count, the NAP score, bone marrow aspirate trephine biopsy, and ultrasound of the abdomen to assess spleen size and to detect renal abnormalities are most useful (Table 17.3). If these prove negative look for lung or cardiac disease, check arterial Po_2 and consider a check of the oxygen dissociation curve and haemoglobin (Hb) electrophoresis. Finally, look for erythropoietin

secreting tumours by renal and splenic ultrasound, computed tomography (CT) or magnetic resonance imaging (MRI). The serum erythropoietin level is also useful in screening for tumours.

ESSENTIAL THROMBOCYTHAEMIA

In this condition there is a sustained increase in platelet count because of megakaryocyte proliferation and overproduction of platelets. A persisting platelet count of $> 600 \times 10^9/l$ is the central diagnostic feature but other causes of a raised platelet count need to be excluded before the diagnosis can be made.

Clinical and laboratory findings

The dominant clinical features are thrombosis and haemorrhage. Many cases are symptomless and diagnosed on routine blood counts. Thrombosis may occur in the venous or arterial systems (Fig. 17.4b) whereas haemorrhage, as a result of abnormal platelet function, may cause either chronic or acute bleeding. A characteristic symptom is erythromelalgia, a burning sensation felt in the hands or feet and promptly relieved by aspirin. Up to 40% of patients will have palpable splenomegaly whereas in others there may be splenic atrophy because of infarction. Abnormal large platelets and megakaryocyte fragments may be seen in the blood film (Fig. 17.7). The bone marrow is similar to that in PRV but an excess of abnormal megakaryocytes is typical. Cytogenetics and molecular analysis for the *BCR-ABL* fusion gene are analysed to exclude chronic myeloid leukaemia. The condition must be distinguished from other causes of a raised platelet count (Table 17.4). Platelet function tests (p. 259) are consistently abnormal, failure of aggregation with adrenaline being particularly characteristic.

Treatment

The principle is to control the platelet count so as to reduce the risk of thrombosis which is the major

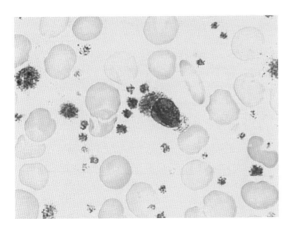

Fig. 17.7 Peripheral blood film in essential thrombocythaemia showing increased numbers of platelets and a nucleated megakaryocytic fragment.

Table 17.4 Causes of a raised platelet count

Reactive
Haemorrhage, trauma, postoperative
Chronic iron deficiency
Malignancy
Chronic infections
Connective tissue diseases, e.g. rheumatoid arthritis
Postsplenectomy

Endogenous
Essential thrombocythaemia
In some cases of polycythaemia vera, myelofibrosis and chronic myeloid leukaemia

clinical problem. The patients may be placed in risk groups according to age, size of platelet count and previous episodes of thrombosis or haemorrhage. The thrombotic risk depends on other risk factors such as smoking history and hypertension, and the treatment should take account of these risks. In those with a high risk, the aim is to keep the platelet count below $600 \times 10^9/l$. Hydroxyurea is probably the most widely used treatment although α-interferon is also valuable in younger patients. The role of anagrelide, which is highly effective in reducing the platelet count, is being assessed in clinical trials. Busulphan and ^{32}P were used but are not now favoured because of possible long-term complications. Platelet pheresis may be helpful in short-term management. Aspirin is commonly used to reduce thrombotic risk and in patients younger than 60 years with no previous thrombosis or haemorrhage and platelets $<1000 \times 10^9/l$ it may be the treatment of choice.

Course

Often the disease is stationary for 10–20 years or more. Patients may transform after a number of years to myelofibrosis; the risk of transformation to acute leukaemia is relatively low ($<5\%$).

MYELOFIBROSIS

The predominant feature of myelofibrosis is a progressive generalized fibrosis of the bone marrow in association with the development of haemopoiesis in the spleen and liver (known as myeloid metaplasia). Clinically this leads to anaemia and massive hepatosplenomegaly. Confusingly, the condition has many names—idiopathic myelofibrosis; myelosclerosis; agnogenic myeloid metaplasia; or myelofibrosis with myeloid metaplasia (MMM).

The fibrosis of the bone marrow is secondary to hyperplasia of abnormal megakaryocytes. It is thought that fibroblasts are stimulated by platelet-derived growth factor and other proteins secreted by megakaryocytes and platelets.

One-third or more of the patients have a previous history of PRV and some patients present with clinical and laboratory features of both disorders.

Clinical features

1 An insidious onset in older people is usual with symptoms of anaemia.
2 Symptoms resulting from massive splenomegaly (e.g. abdominal discomfort, pain or indigestion) are frequent; splenomegaly is the main physical finding (Fig. 17.3b).
3 Hypermetabolic symptoms such as loss of weight, anorexia, fever and night sweats are common.

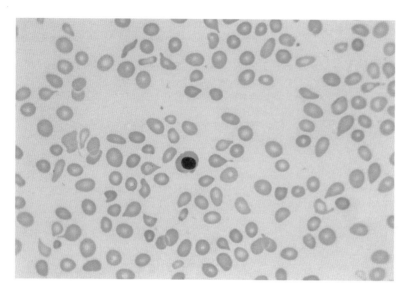

Fig. 17.8 Peripheral blood film in myelofibrosis. Leucoerythroblastic change with 'tear-drop' cells and an erythroblast.

4 Bleeding problems, bone pain or gout occur in a minority of patients.

Myelofibrosis and chronic myeloid leukaemia are responsible for most cases of massive (> 20 cm) splenic enlargement in the UK and North America (see Table 22.6).

Laboratory findings

1 Anaemia is usual but a normal or increased haemoglobin level may be found in some patients.
2 The white cell and platelet counts are frequently high at the time of presentation. Later in the disease leucopenia and thrombocytopenia are common.
3 A leucoerythroblastic blood film is found. The red cells show characteristic 'tear-drop' poikilocytes (Fig. 17.8).
4 Bone marrow is usually unobtainable by aspiration. Trephine biopsy (Fig. 17.5b) shows a fibrotic, hypercellular marrow. Increased megakaryocytes are frequently seen. In 10% of cases there is increased bone formation with increased bone density on X-ray.
5 Low serum and red cell folate, raised serum vitamin B_{12} and vitamin B_{12}-binding capacity, and an increased Neutrophil alkaline phosphatase (NAP) score are usual.
6 High serum urate, lactate dehydrogenase (LDH) and hydroxybutyrate dehydrogenase levels reflect the increased but largely ineffective turnover of haemopoietic cells. The serum LDH is normal in PRV.
7 Transformation to acute myeloid leukaemia occurs in 10–20% of patients.

Treatment

This is palliative and aimed at reducing the effects of anaemia and splenomegaly. Blood transfusions and regular folic acid therapy are used in severely anaemic patients. Hydroxyurea may help to reduce splenomegaly and hypermetabolic symptoms. Splenectomy is considered for patients with severe symptomatic splenomegaly—mechanical discomfort, thrombocytopenia, portal hypertension, excessive transfusion requirements or hypermetabolic symptoms. Splenic irradiation is an alternative but usually provides relief only for 3–6 months. Allopurinol is indicated in virtually all patients to prevent gout and urate nephropathy from hyperuricaemia. Allogeneic stem cell transplantation is currently experimental but may be curative for young patients.

The median survival is around 3.5 years and causes of death include heart failure, infection and leukaemic transformation. A haemoglobin level of less than 10 g/dl, a white cell count of less than 4 or greater than $30\times10^9/l$ and the presence of abnormal chromosome are associated with a worse prognosis.

Systemic mastocytosis

This disease results from a chronic neoplastic proliferation of mast cells involving usually the bone marrow, heart, spleen, lymph nodes and skin. The skin usually shows urticaria pigmentosa. Symptoms are related to histamine and prostaglandin release and include flushing, pruritus, abdominal pain and bronchospasm. It may pursue an indolent or aggressive course. It may terminate as acute myeloid leukaemia. Treatment is with H_1 and H_2 histamine antagonists. Control of mast cell proliferation with, for example α-interferon, hydroxyurea and 2-chlorodeoxyadenosine may also be helpful in some cases.

BIBLIOGRAPHY

Bain B.J. (1999) Systemic mastocytosis and other mast cell neoplasms. *Br. J. Haematol.* **106**, 9–17.

Dupriez B. *et al.* (1996) Prognostic factors in agnogenic myeloid metaplasia: a report on 195 cases with a new scoring system. *Blood* **88**, 1013–18.

Harrison C.N., Gale R.E., Machin S.J. and Linch D.C. (1999) A large proportion of patients with a diagnosis of essential thrombocythemia do not have a clonal disorder and may be at lower risk of thrombotic complications. *Blood* **93**, 417–24.

Michiels J.J. (1996) The myeloproliferative disorders. *Leuk. Lymph.* **22S**, 1–4.

Najean Y. and Rai J.D. (1997) Treatment of polycythaemia vera—the use of hydroxyurea and pipobroman in 292 patients under the age of 65 years. *Blood* **90**, 3370–7.

Radia D. and Pearson T.C. (1999) The management of primary thrombocythaemia. *CME Bull. Haematol.* **2**, 35–9.

Reilly J.T. (1997) Idiopathic myelofibrosis: pathogenesis, natural history and management. *Blood Rev.* **11**, 233.

Silver R.T. (1997) Interferon-α: effects of long-term treatment for polycythaemia vera. *Semin. Haematol.* **34**, 40–50.

Tefferi A. (2000) Myelofibrosis with myeloid metaplasia. *N. Engl. J. Med.* **342**, 1255–65.

Tefferi A., Mesa R.A., Nagorney D.M. *et al.* (2000) Splenectomy in myelofibrosis with myeloid metaplasia: a single institution experience with 223 patients. *Blood* **95**, 2226–33.

Platelets, blood coagulation and haemostasis

An efficient and rapid mechanism for stopping bleeding from sites of blood vessel injury is clearly essential for survival. Nevertheless, such a response needs to be tightly controlled to prevent extensive clots developing and to break down such clots once damage is repaired. The haemostatic system thus represents a delicate balance between procoagulant and anticoagulant mechanims allied to a process for fibrinolysis. The five major components involved are platelets, coagulation factors, coagulation inhibitors, fibrinolysis and blood vessels.

PLATELETS

Platelet production

Platelets are produced in the bone marrow by fragmentation of the cytoplasm of megakaryocytes. The precursor of the megakaryocyte—the megakaryoblast—arises by a process of differentiation from the haemopoietic stem cell (Fig. 18.1). The megakaryocyte matures by endomitotic synchronous nuclear replication, enlarging the cytoplasmic volume as the number of nuclear lobes increase in multiples of two. At a variable stage in development, most commonly at the eight nucleus stage, the cytoplasm becomes granular and platelets are liberated (Fig. 18.1). A mature polyploid megakaryocyte is shown in Fig. 18.2. Platelet production follows formation of microvesicles in the cytoplasm of the cell which coalesce to form platelet demarcation membranes.

Each megakaryocyte is responsible for the production of about 4000 platelets. The time interval from differentiation of the human stem cell to the production of platelets averages at about 10 days.

Thrombopoietin is the major regulator of platelet production and is constitutively produced by the liver and kidneys. Platelets have receptors (C-MPL) for thrombopoietin and remove it from the circulation. Therefore levels are high in thrombocytopenia due to marrow aplasia and vice versa. Thrombopoietin increases the number and rate of maturation of megakaryocytes. Trials of thrombopoietin have been carried out. Platelet levels start to rise 6 days after the start of therapy and remain high for 7–10 days. Interleukin-11 (IL-11) can also increase the circulating platelet count and is entering clinical trials. Neither drug is yet available for routine clinical practice.

The normal platelet count is about $250 \times 10^9/l$ (range $150–400 \times 10^9/l$) and the normal platelet lifespan is 7–10 days. Up to one-third of the marrow output of platelets may be trapped at any one time in the normal spleen but this rises to 90% in cases of massive splenomegaly (p. 257).

Platelet structure

The ultrastructure of platelets is represented in Fig. 18.3. The glycoproteins of the surface coat are particularly important in the platelet reactions of adhesion and aggregation which are the initial events leading to platelet plug formation during haemostasis. Adhesion to collagen is facilitated by glycoprotein Ia (GPIa). Glycoproteins Ib

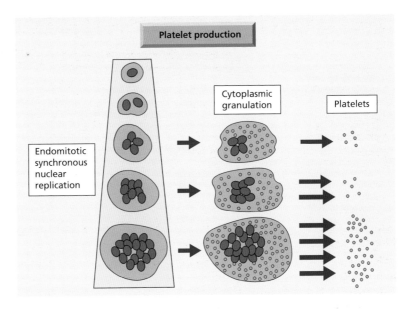

Fig. 18.1 Simplified diagram to illustrate platelet production from megakaryocytes.

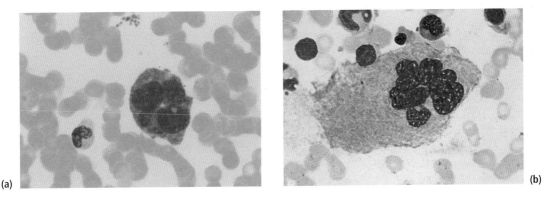

(a)   (b)

Fig. 18.2 Megakaryocytes: (a) immature form with basophilic cytoplasm; (b) mature form with many nuclear lobes and pronounced granulation of the cytoplasm.

(defective in Bernard–Soulier syndrome) and IIb/IIIa (defective in thrombasthenia) are important in the attachment of platelets to von Willebrand factor (VWF) and hence to vascular subendothelium (Fig. 18.4). The binding site for IIb/IIIa is also the receptor for fibrinogen which is important in platelet–platelet aggregation.

The plasma membrane invaginates into the platelet interior to form an open membrane (canalicular) system which provides a large reactive surface to which the plasma coagulation proteins may be selectively absorbed. The membrane phospholipids (previously known as platelet factor 3) are of particular importance in the conversion of coagulation factor X to Xa and prothrombin (factor II) to thrombin (factor IIa) (see Fig. 18.6).

In the platelet interior calcium, nucleotides (particularly adenosine diphosphate (ADP) and adenosine triphosphate (ATP)) and serotonin are contained in electron-dense granules. The more frequent specific α granules contain a heparin antagonist, platelet-derived growth factor (PDGF), β-thromboglobulin, fibrinogen,

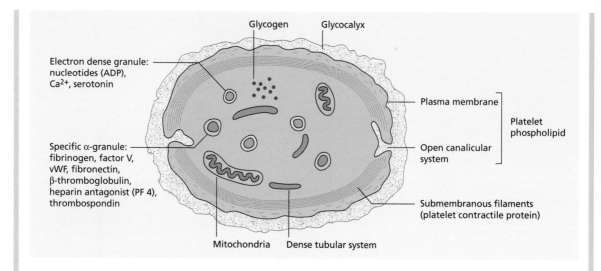

Fig. 18.3 The ultrastructure of platelets. ADP, adenosine diphosphate; PF, platelet factor; vWF, von Willebrand factor.

vWF and other clotting factors. Dense granules are less common and contain ADP, ATP, 5-hydroxytryptamine (5-HT) and calcium. Other specific organelles include lysosomes which con-

Fig. 18.4 Platelet adhesion. The binding of glycoprotein (GP) Ib (which consists of four proteins GPIbα, GPIbβ, GPIX, GPV) to von Willebrand factor leads to adhesion to the subendothelium and also exposes the GPIIb/IIIa ($\alpha_{IIb}\beta_3$ integrin) binding sites to fibrinogen and von Willebrand factor leading to platelet aggregation. The GPIa site permits direct adhesion to collagen.

tain hydrolytic enzymes, and peroxisomes which contain catalase. During the release reaction described below, the contents of the granules are discharged into the open canalicular system.

Platelet antigens

Several platelet surface proteins have been found to be important antigens in platelet-specific autoimmunity and they have been termed human platelet antigens (HPA). In most cases two different alleles exist, termed a or b alleles, e.g. HPA-1a. Platelets also express ABO and human leucocyte antigen (HLA) class I but not class II antigens.

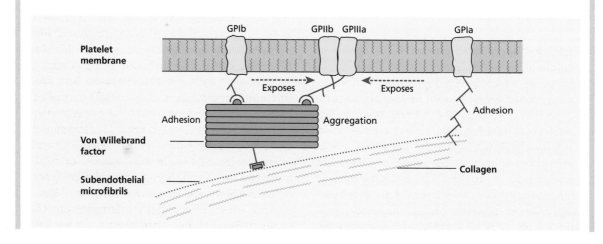

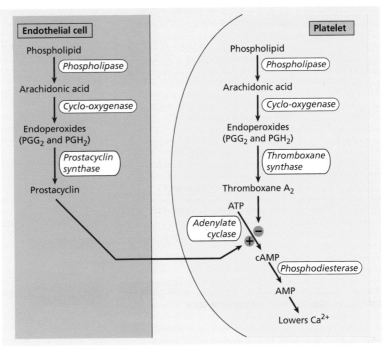

Fig. 18.5 The synthesis of prostacyclin and thromboxane. The opposing effects of these agents are mediated by changes in the concentration of cyclic adenosine monophosphate (cAMP) in platelets via stimulation or inhibition of the enzyme adenylate cyclase. cAMP controls the concentration of free calcium ions in the platelet which are important in the processes which cause adhesion and aggregation. High levels of cAMP lead to low free calcium ion concentrations and prevent aggregation and adhesion. ATP, adenosine triphosphate; Ca, calcium; PG, prostaglandin (G_2 and H_2).

Platelet function

The main function of platelets is the formation of mechanical plugs during the normal haemostatic response to vascular injury. In the absence of platelets spontaneous leakage of blood through small vessels may occur. Central to their function are the platelet reactions of adhesion, secretion, aggregation and fusion as well as their procoagulant activity.

Platelet adhesion and aggregation in response to vessel injury

Following blood vessel injury, platelets adhere to the exposed subendothelial connective tissues. Subendothelial microfibrils bind the larger multimers of VWF which bind to platelet membrane Ib complex (Fig. 18.4). Under the influence of shear stress platelets move along the surface of vessels until the platelet surface GPIa/IIa (integrin $\alpha_2\beta_1$) engages collagen and halts translocation. Following adhesion, platelets become more spherical and extrude long pseudopods which enhance interaction between adjacent platelets. Platelet activation is then achieved by glycoprotein IIb/IIIa ($\alpha_{IIb}\beta_3$ integrin) binding fibrinogen to produce platelet aggregation. The IIb–IIIa receptor complex also forms a secondary binding site with VWF further promoting adhesion.

Von Willebrand Factor VWF is involved in platelet adhesion to the vessel wall and to other platelets (aggregation). It also carries factor VIII (see below) and used to be referred to as factor VIII-related antigen (VIII-Rag). It is a large complex multimeric molecule (molecular weight (MW) $0.8–20 \times 10^6$) made up of several subunit chains ranging from dimers (MW 5×10^5) to multimers (MW 20×10^6) linked by disulphide bonds. VWF is encoded by a gene on chromosome 12 and is synthesized by endothelial cells and megakaryocytes. It is stored in Weibel–Palade bodies in endothelial cells and in specific platelet α granules. Release of VWF from endothelial cells occurs under the influence of several hormones. Stress and exercise or infusion of either adrenaline or desmopressin (1-deamino-8-D-arginine vasopressin, DDAVP)

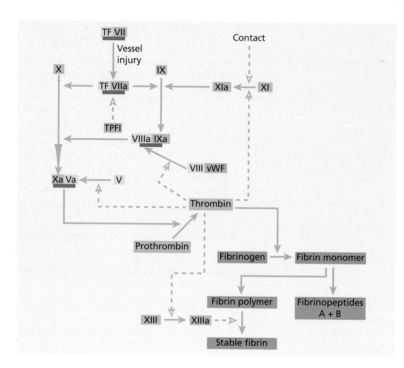

Fig. 18.6 The pathway of blood coagulation initiated by tissue factor (TF) on the cell surface. When plasma comes into contact with TF, factor VII binds to TF. The complex of TF and activated VII (VIIa) activates X and IX. TF pathway inhibitor (TFPI) is an important inhibitor of TF/VIIa. VIIIa–IXa complex greatly amplifies Xa production from X. The generation of thrombin from prothrombin by the action of Xa–Va complex leads to fibrin formation. Thrombin also activates XI (dashed line), V and XIII. Thrombin cleaves VIII from its carrier von Willebrand factor (vWF) greatly increasing the formation of VIIIa–IXa and hence of Xa–Va. Pale green, serine proteases; yellow, cofactors.

produces considerable increase in the level of circulating VWF.

Platelet release reaction

Collagen exposure or thrombin action results in the secretion of platelet granule contents which include ADP, serotonin, fibrinogen, lysosomal enzymes, β thromboglobulin and heparin neutralizing factor (platelet factor 4). Collagen and thrombin activate platelet prostaglandin synthesis. There is membrane release of diacylglycerol (which activates protein phosphorylation via protein kinase C) and inositol triphosphate (which causes release of intracellular calcium ions). There is also arachidonate release from the cell membrane leading to the formation of a labile substance, thromboxane A_2, which lowers platelet cyclic adenosine monophosphate (cAMP) levels and initiates the release reaction (Fig. 18.5). Thromboxane A_2 not only potentiates platelet aggregation but also has powerful vasoconstrictive activity. The release reaction is inhibited by substances which increase the level of platelet cAMP. One such substance is the prostaglandin prosta-

cyclin (PGI_2) which is synthesized by vascular endothelial cells. It is a potent inhibitor of platelet aggregation and prevents their deposition on normal vascular endothelium.

Platelet aggregation

Released ADP and thromboxane A_2 cause additional platelets to aggregate at the site of vascular injury. ADP causes platelets to swell and encourages the platelet membranes of adjacent platelets to adhere to each other. As they do so further release reactions occur liberating more ADP and thromboxane A_2 causing secondary platelet aggregation. This positive feedback process results in the formation of a platelet mass large enough to plug the area of endothelial injury.

Platelet procoagulant activity

After platelet aggregation and release the exposed membrane phospholipid (platelet factor 3) is available for two reactions in the coagulation cascade. Both phospholipid-mediated reactions are calcium-ion dependent. The first (tenase) involves factors IXa, VIIIa and X in the formation of factor

Xa (Fig. 18.6). The second (prothrombinase) results in the formation of thrombin from the interaction of factors Xa, Va and prothrombin (II). The phospholipid surface forms an ideal template for the crucial concentration and orientation of these proteins.

Irreversible platelet aggregation

High concentrations of ADP, the enzymes released during the release reaction, and platelet contractile proteins contribute to irreversible fusion of platelets aggregated at the site of vascular injury. Thrombin also encourages fusion of platelets, and fibrin formation reinforces the stability of the evolving platelet plug.

Growth factor

PDGF found in the specific granules of platelets stimulates vascular smooth muscle cells to multiply and this may hasten vascular healing following injury.

BLOOD COAGULATION

The coagulation cascade

Blood coagulation involves a biological amplification system in which relatively few initiation substances sequentially activate by proteolysis a cascade of circulating precursor proteins (the coagulation factor enzymes) which culminates in the generation of thrombin; this, in turn, converts soluble plasma fibrinogen into fibrin (Fig. 18.6). Fibrin enmeshes the platelet aggregates at the sites of vascular injury and converts the unstable primary platelet plugs to firm, definitive and stable haemostatic plugs. A list of the coagulation factors appears in Table 18.1.

The operation of this enzyme cascade requires local concentration of circulating coagulation factors at the site of injury.

Surface-mediated reactions occur on exposed collagen, platelet phospholipid and tissue factor. With the exception of fibrinogen, which is the fibrin clot subunit, the coagulation factors are either enzyme precursors or cofactors (Table 18.1). All the enzymes, except factor XIII, are serine proteases, i.e. their ability to hydrolyse peptide bonds depends upon the amino acid serine at their active centre (Fig. 18.7). The scale of amplification achieved in this system is dramatic, e.g. 1 mol of activated factor XI through sequential activation

Table 18.1 The coagulation factors

Factor number	Descriptive name	Active form
I	Fibrinogen	Fibrin subunit
II	Prothrombin	Serine protease
III	Tissue factor	Receptor/cofactor*
V	Labile factor	Cofactor
VII	Proconvertin	Serine protease
VIII	Antihaemophilic factor	Cofactor
IX	Christmas factor	Serine protease
X	Stuart–Prower factor	Serine protease
XI	Plasma thromboplastin antecedent	Serine protease
XII	Hageman (contact) factor	Serine protease
XIII	Fibrin-stabilizing factor	Transglutaminase
	Prekallikrein (Fletcher factor)	Serine protease
	HMWK (Fitzgerald factor)	Cofactor*

*Active without proteolytic modification.
HMWK, high molecular weight kininogen.

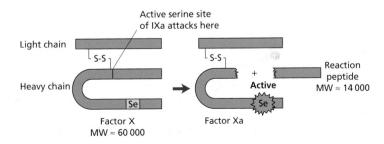

Fig. 18.7 Serine (Se) protease activity. This example shows the activation of factor X by factor IX.

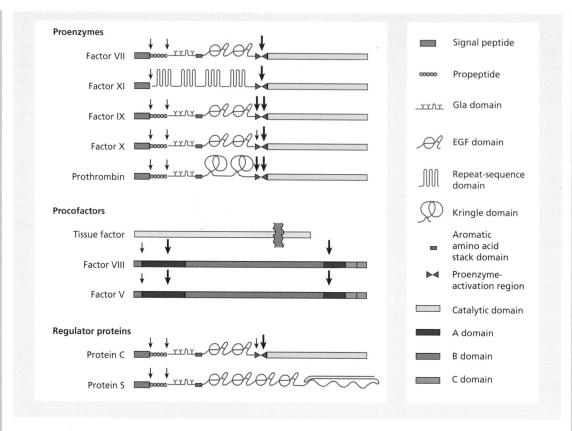

Fig. 18.8 Domains of the enzymes, receptors and cofactors involved in blood coagulation and regulation. The components of blood coagulation are proenzymes, procofactors and regulator proteins. The proenzymes, including protein C, contain a catalytic domain, an activation region and a signal peptide. The vitamin K-dependent proteins include a propeptide and a γ-carboxyglutamic acid (Gla) domain. Other important domains include the epidermal growth factor-like (EGF) domain, the kringle domain and the repeat-sequence domain. Tissue factor is an integral membrane protein unrelated to other known proteins. Factor V and VIII have marked similarities in structure. Sites of intracellular peptide bonds cleaved during synthesis are indicated by thin arrows, and sites of peptide bonds cleaved during protein activation are indicated by thick arrows. The transmembrane domain of tissue factor is shown within the phospholipid bilayer. (From B. Furie and B.C. Furie 1992, courtesy of the *New England Journal of Medicine*.)

of factors IX, X and prothrombin may generate up to 2×10^8 mol of fibrin.

Coagulation is thought to be initiated *in vivo* by tissue factor, found on the surface of perivascular tissue, binding to coagulation factor VII (Fig. 18.6). This activates factor VII which then activates both factor IX and X. Activation of factor X leads to generation of small amounts of thrombin which amplify the coagulation process by activating cofactors V and VIII (Fig. 18.6). This amplification pathway involving factors VIII and IX assumes the dominant role of consolidating the production of activated factor X. Thrombin also activates

factor XI which increases production of activated factor IX.

Coagulation factor VIII is a single chain protein with MW 350 000 (Fig. 18.8). It is coded by a 186-kb gene located in the long arm (q2.8 region) of the X chromosome. Factor VIII is bound in plasma to VWF. It is synthesized in the liver by hepatocytes.

In the 'classical' pathway formulated to explain *in vitro* coagulation testing, initiation of the pathway required contact reactions between factor XII, kallikrein and high molecular weight kininogen (HMWK) leading to the activation of factor XI. However, the lack of abnormal bleeding in individuals with hereditary deficiencies of these contact factors suggests that these reactions are not required for physiological coagulation *in vivo*.

Factor XI does not seem to have a role in the physiological initiation of coagulation. It has a supplementary role in the activation of factor IX (see above) and may be important at major sites of trauma or for operations.

Activated factor X, in association with cofactor V on the phospholipid surface and calcium, converts prothrombin into thrombin. Thrombin hydrolyses fibrinogen, releasing fibrinopeptides A and B to form fibrin monomers (Fig. 18.9). Fibrin monomers link spontaneously by hydrogen bonds to form a loose, insoluble fibrin polymer. Factor XIII is also activated by thrombin together with calcium. Activated factor XIII stabilizes the fibrin polymers with the formation of covalent bond cross links.

Fibrinogen has a MW 340 000 and consists of two identical subunits, each containing three dissimilar polypeptide chains (Aα, Bβ and γ) which are linked by disulphide bonds. After cleavage by thrombin of fibrinopeptides A and B, fibrin monomer consists of three paired α, β and γ chains.

Some of the properties of the coagulation factors are listed in Table 18.2. The activity of factors II, VII, IX and X is dependent upon vitamin K which is responsible for carboxylation of a num-

ber of terminal glutamic acid residues on each of these molecules (see Fig. 20.7).

The serine protease coagulation factors along with those of the fibrinolytic system (see below) have a high degree of homology and contain characteristic structural domains (Fig. 18.8), such as the kringles which are concerned with substrate binding and the carboxylated glutamic acid (Gla) residues which bind to phospholipid. There are also regions of homology with fibronectin (finger regions) and with epidermal growth factor. Although factor VIII and V cofactors are not protease enzymes they circulate in a precursor form that requires limited cleavage by thrombin for expression of full cofactor activity.

Physiological limitation of blood coagulation

Unchecked blood coagulation would lead to dangerous occlusion of blood vessels (thrombosis) if the following protective mechanisms were not in operation.

Coagulation factor inhibitors
It is important that the effect of thrombin is limited to the site of injury. The first inhibitor to act is tissue factor pathway inhibitor (tFPI) which is present in plasma and platelets and accumulates at

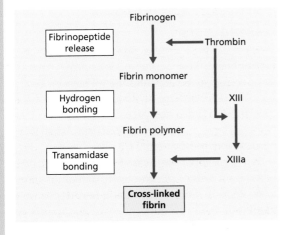

Fig. 18.9 The formation and stabilization of fibrin.

Table 18.2 The coagulation factors

Factor	Plasma half-life (h)	Plasma concentration (mg/l)	Comments
II	65	100	Prothrombin group: vitamin K needed for synthesis; require Ca^{2+} for activation; stable
VII	5	0.5	
IX	25	5	
X	40	10	
I	90	3000	Thrombin interacts with them; increase in inflammation, pregnancy, oral contraceptives
V	15	10	
VIII	10	0.1	
XI	45	5	
XII	50	30	

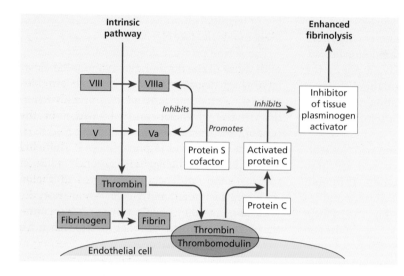

Fig. 18.10 Activation and action of protein C by thrombin which has bound to thrombomodulin on the endothelial cell surface. Protein S is a cofactor which facilitates binding of activated protein C to the platelet surface. The inactivation of factors Va and VIIIa results in the inhibition of blood coagulation. The inactivation of tissue plasminogen activator inhibitor (PAI) enhances fibrinolysis.

the site of injury caused by local platelet activation. This inhibits Xa and VIIa and tissue factor to limit the main *in vivo* pathway. There is direct inactivation of thrombin and other serine protease factors by other circulating inhibitors of which antithrombin is the most potent. It inactivates serine proteases by combining with them by peptide bonding to form high molecular weight stable complexes. Heparin potentiates its action markedly. Another protein, heparin cofactor II, also inhibits thrombin. α_2-macroglobulins, α_2-antiplasmin, C_1 esterase inhibitor and α_1-antitrypsin also exert inhibitory effects on circulating serine proteases.

Protein C and protein S

There are also inhibitors of coagulation cofactors V and VIII. Thrombin binds to an endothelial cell surface receptor thrombomodulin. The resulting complex activates the vitamin K-dependent serine protease protein C which is able to destroy activated factors V and VIII, thus preventing further thrombin generation. The action of protein C is enhanced by another vitamin K-dependent protein, S, which binds protein C to the platelet surface (Fig. 18.10). In addition, activated protein C enhances fibrinolysis (see below).

Blood flow

At the periphery of a damaged area of tissue,

blood flow rapidly achieves a dilution and dispersal of activated factors before fibrin formation has occurred. Activated factors are destroyed by liver parenchymal cells and particulate matter is removed by liver Kupffer cells and other reticuloendothelial cells.

Plasmin and fibrin split products

Plasmin generation at the site of injury also limits the extent of the evolving thrombus (see below). The split products of fibrinolysis are competitive inhibitors of thrombin and fibrin polymerization. Normally α_2-antiplasmin inhibits any local free plasmin.

FIBRINOLYSIS

Fibrinolysis (like coagulation) is a normal haemostatic response to vascular injury. Plasminogen, a β-globulin proenzyme in blood and tissue fluid, is converted to the serine protease plasmin by activators either from the vessel wall (intrinsic activation) or from the tissues (extrinsic activation) (Fig. 18.11). The most important route follows the release of tissue plasminogen activator (tPA) from endothelial cells. tPA is a serine protease that binds to fibrin. This enhances its capacity to convert thrombus-bound plasminogen into plasmin. This fibrin dependence of tPA action strongly

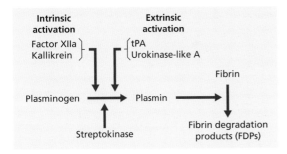

Fig. 18.11 The fibrinolytic system. tPA, tissue plasminogen activator.

localizes plasmin generation by tPA to the fibrin clot. Release of tPA occurs after such stimuli as trauma, exercise or emotional stress. Activated protein C stimulates fibrinolysis by destroying plasma inhibitors of tPA (Fig. 18.10). On the other hand thrombin inhibits fibrinolysis by activating thrombin-activated fibrinolysis inhibitor (TAFI).

Fibrinolytic agents are widely used in clinical practice. Therapeutic tPA has been synthesized using recombinant DNA technology. The bacterial agent streptokinase is a peptide produced by haemolytic streptococci and forms a complex with plasminogen, which converts other plasminogen molecules to plasmin. Urokinase is a tPA initially isolated from human urine.

Plasmin is capable of digesting fibrinogen, fibrin, factors V and VIII and many other proteins. Cleavage of peptide bonds in fibrin and fibrinogen produces a variety of split (degradation) products (Fig. 18.11). Large amounts of the smallest fragments D and E can be detected in the plasma of patients with disseminated intravascular coagulation (see p. 268).

Inactivation of plasmin

Tissue plasminogen activator is inactivated by plasminogen activator inhibitor (PAI). Circulating plasmin is inactivated by potent inhibitors α_2-antiplasmin and α_2-macroglobulin.

Endothelial cells

The endothelial cell has an active role in the maintenance of vascular integrity. This cell provides the basement membrane which normally separates collagen, elastin and fibronectin of the subendothelial connective tissue from the circulating blood. Loss or damage to the endothelial lining results in both haemorrhage and activation of the haemostatic mechanism. The endothelial cell also has a potent inhibitory influence on the haemostatic response, largely through the synthesis of PGI_2 and nitric oxide (NO) which have vasodilatory properties and inhibit platelet aggregation. In contrast, endothelins are a family of vasoactive peptides that can activate fibrinolysis via the release of tPA. Synthesis of tissue factor which initiates haemostasis only occurs in endothelial cells following activation and its natural inhibitor, TFPI, is also synthesized. Synthesis of prostacyclin, VWF, plasminogen activator, antithrombin and thrombomodulin, the surface protein responsible for activation of protein C, provides agents which are vital to both platelet reactions and blood coagulation (Fig. 18.12).

HAEMOSTATIC RESPONSE

The normal haemostatic response to vascular damage depends on closely linked interaction between the blood vessel wall, circulating platelets and blood coagulation factors (Fig. 18.13).

Vasoconstriction

An immediate vasoconstriction of the injured vessel and reflex constriction of adjacent small arteries and arterioles is responsible for an initial slowing of blood flow to the area of injury. When there is widespread damage this vascular reaction prevents exsanguination. The reduced blood flow allows contact activation of platelets and coagulation factors. The vasoactive amines and thromboxane A_2 liberated from platelets, and the

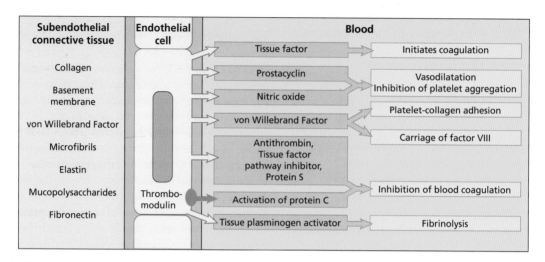

Fig. 18.12 The endothelial cell forms a barrier between platelets and plasma clotting factors and the sub-endothelial connected tissues. Endothelial cells produce substances which can initiate coagulation, cause vasodilatation, inhibit platelet aggregation or haemostasis or activate fibrinolysis.

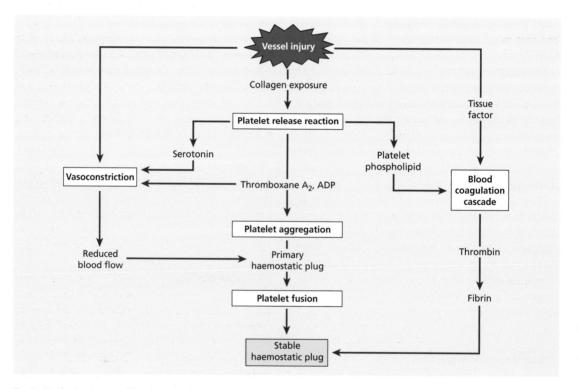

Fig. 18.13 The involvement of blood vessels, platelets and blood coagulation in haemostasis. ADP, adenosine diphosphate.

fibrinopeptides liberated during fibrin formation, also have vasoconstrictive activity.

Platelet reactions and primary haemostatic plug formation

Following a break in the endothelial lining, there is an initial adherence of platelets to exposed connective tissue, potentiated by VWF. Collagen exposure and thrombin produced at the site of injury cause the adherent platelets to release their granule contents and also activate platelet prostaglandin synthesis leading to the formation of thromboxane A_2. Released ADP causes platelets to swell and aggregate. Additional platelets from the circulating blood are drawn to the area of injury. This continuing platelet aggregation promotes the growth of the haemostatic plug which soon covers the exposed connective tissue. The unstable primary haemostatic plug produced by these platelet reactions in the first minute or so following injury is usually sufficient to provide temporary control of bleeding. It seems likely that prostacyclin, produced by endothelial and smooth muscle cells in the vessel wall adjacent to the area of damage, is important in limiting the extent of the initial platelet plug.

Stabilization of the platelet plug by fibrin

Definitive haemostasis is achieved when fibrin formed by blood coagulation is added to the platelet mass and by platelet-induced clot retraction/compaction.

Following vascular injury, activation of tissue factor activates factor VII to start the coagulation cascade. Platelet aggregation and release reactions accelerate the coagulation process by providing abundant membrane phospholipid. Thrombin generated at the injury site converts soluble plasma fibrinogen into fibrin, potentiates platelet aggregation and secretion and also activates factor XI and XIII and cofactors V and VIII. The fibrin component of the haemostatic plug increases as the fused platelets autolyse and after a

few hours the entire haemostatic plug is transformed into a solid mass of cross-linked fibrin. Nevertheless, because of incorporation of plasminogen and tPA (p. 245) this plug begins to autodigest during the same time frame.

TESTS OF HAEMOSTATIC FUNCTION

Defective haemostasis with abnormal bleeding may result from:
1 a vascular disorder;
2 thrombocytopenia or a disorder of platelet function; or
3 defective blood coagulation.

A number of simple tests are employed to assess the platelet, vessel wall and coagulation components of haemostasis.

Blood count and blood film examination

As thrombocytopenia is a common cause of abnormal bleeding, patients with suspected bleeding disorders should initially have a blood count including platelet count and blood film examination. In addition to establishing the presence of thrombocytopenia, the cause may be obvious, e.g. acute leukaemia.

Screening tests of blood coagulation

Screening tests provide an assessment of the 'extrinsic' and 'intrinsic' systems of blood coagulation and also the central conversion of fibrinogen to fibrin (Table 18.3).

The prothrombin time (PT) measures factors VII, X, V, prothrombin and fibrinogen. Tissue thromboplastin (a brain extract) and calcium are added to citrated plasma. The normal time for clotting is 10–14 s. It may be expressed as the international normalized ratio (INR) (p. 286).

The activated partial thromboplastin time (APTT) measures factors VIII, IX, XI and XII in addition to factors X, V, prothrombin and fibrinogen. Three substances—phospholipid, a surface activator (e.g. kaolin) and calcium—are added to

Table 18.3 Screening tests used in the diagnosis of coagulation disorders

Screening tests	Abnormalities indicated by prolongation	Most common cause of disorder
Thrombin time (TT)	Deficiency or abnormality of fibrinogen or inhibition of thrombin by heparin or FDPs	Disseminated intravascular coagulation Heparin therapy
Prothrombin time (PT)	Deficiency or inhibition of one or more of the following coagulation factors: VII, X, V, II, fibrinogen	Liver disease Warfarin therapy (+ conditions above)
Activated partial thromboplastin time (APTT or PTTK)	Deficiency or inhibition of one or more of the following coagulation factors: XII, XI, IX (Christmas disease), VIII (haemophilia), X, V, II, fibrinogen	Haemophilia, Christmas disease (+ conditions above)

FDPs, fibrin degradation products.

citrated plasma. The normal time for clotting is about 30–40 s.

Prolonged clotting times in the PT and APTT because of factor deficiency are corrected by the addition of normal plasma to the test plasma. If there is no correction or incomplete correction with normal plasma the presence of an inhibitor of coagulation is suspected.

The thrombin (clotting) time (TT) is sensitive to a deficiency of fibrinogen or inhibition of thrombin. Diluted bovine thrombin is added to citrated plasma at a concentration giving a clotting time of 14–16 s with normal subjects.

Specific assays of coagulation factors

Most factor assays are based on an APTT or PT in which all factors except the one to be measured are present in the substrate plasma. This usually requires a supply of plasma from patients with hereditary deficiency of the factor in question or artificially produced factor-deficient plasma. The corrective effect of the unknown plasma on the prolonged clotting time of the deficient substrate plasma is then compared with the corrective effect of normal plasma. Results are expressed as a percentage of normal activity.

A number of chemical, chromogenic and immunological methods are available for quantification of other proteins such as fibrinogen, VWF and factor VIII. Factor XIII activity can be assessed by testing for clot solubility in urea.

Bleeding time

The bleeding time is a useful test for abnormal platelet function including the diagnosis of VWF deficiency. It will also be prolonged in thrombocytopenia but is normal in vascular causes of abnormal bleeding. The test involves the application of pressure to the upper arm with a blood pressure cuff, after which small incisions are made in the flexor surface forearm skin. Bleeding stops normally in 3–8 min.

Tests of platelet function

The most valuable investigation is platelet aggregometry which measures the fall in light absorbance in platelet-rich plasma as platelets aggregate. Initial (primary) aggregation is caused by an external agent, the secondary response to aggregating agents released from the platelets themselves. The five external aggregating agents most commonly used are ADP, collagen, ristocetin, arachidonic acid and adrenaline. The pattern of response to each agent helps to make the diagnosis (see Fig. 19.11). Flow cytometry is now increasingly used in routine practice to identify platelet glyoprotein defects.

Test of fibrinolysis

Increased levels of circulating plasminogen activator may be detected by demonstrating shortened euglobulin clot lysis times. A number of immunological methods are available to detect fibrinogen or fibrin degradation products in serum. In patients with enhanced fibrinolysis, low levels of circulating plasminogen may be detected.

BIBLIOGRAPHY

Bloom A.L., Forbes C.D., Thomas D.P. and Tuddenham E.G.D. (eds) (1994) *Haemostasis and Thrombosis*. 3rd edn. Churchill-Livingstone, Edinburgh.

Coleman R.W., Hirsh J., Marder V.J., Clowes A.W. and George J.N. (eds) (2000) *Hemostasis and Thrombosis: Basic Principles and Clinical Practice*, 4th edn. Lipincott, Williams & Wilkins, Hagerstown.

Cramer E.M. (1999) Megakaryocyte structure and function. *Curr. Opin. Hematol.* **6**, 354–61.

Dahlbäck B (2000) Blood coagulation. *Lancet* **355**, 1627–32.

Furie B. and Furie B.C. (1992) Molecular and cellular biology of blood and coagulation. *N. Engl. J. Med.* **326**, 800–6.

George J.N. (2000) Platelets. *Lancet* **355**, 1531–9.

Hutton R.A., Laffan M.A. and Tuddenham E.G.D. (1999) Normal haemostasis. In: *Postgraduate Haematology*, 4th edn (eds A.V. Hoffbrand, S.M. Lewis and E.G.D. Tuddenham). Butterworth-Heinemann, Oxford, pp. 550–80.

Kaushansky K. (1998) Thrombopoietin. *N. Engl. J. Med.* **339**, 746–54.

Ratnoff O.D. and Forbes C.D. (eds) (1996) *Disorders of Haematosis*, 3rd edn. W.B. Saunders, Philadelphia.

Bleeding disorders caused by vascular and platelet abnormalities

Abnormal bleeding may result from:
1 vascular disorders;
2 thrombocytopenia;
3 defective platelet function; or
4 defective coagulation.

The pattern of bleeding is relatively predictable depending on the aetiology. Vascular and platelet disorders tend to be associated with bleeding from mucous membranes and into the skin whereas in coagulation disorders the bleeding is often into joints or soft tissue.

The first three categories are discussed in this chapter and the disorders of blood coagulation follow in Chapter 20.

VASCULAR BLEEDING DISORDERS

The vascular disorders are a heterogeneous group of conditions characterized by easy bruising and spontaneous bleeding from the small vessels. The underlying abnormality is either in the vessels themselves or in the perivascular connective tissues. Most cases of bleeding caused by vascular defects alone are not severe. Frequently the bleeding is mainly in the skin causing petechiae, ecchymoses or both (Fig. 19.1). In some disorders there is also bleeding from mucous membranes. In these conditions the standard screening tests are normal. The bleeding time is normal and the other tests of haemostasis are also normal. Vascular defects may be inherited or acquired.

Inherited vascular disorders

Hereditary haemorrhagic telangiectasia
In this uncommon disorder, which is transmitted as an autosomal dominant trait, there are dilated microvascular swellings which appear during childhood and become more numerous in adult life. These telangiectasia develop in the skin, mucous membranes (Fig. 19.1a) and internal organs. Pulmonary arteriovenous malformations are seen in around 10% of cases. Recurrent gastrointestinal tract haemorrhage may cause chronic iron deficiency anaemia. Treatment is with embolization, laser treatment, oestrogens, tranexamic acid and iron supplementation.

Connective tissue disorders
In the Ehlers–Danlos syndrome there are hereditary collagen abnormalities with purpura due to defective platelet aggregation, hyperextensibility of joints and hyperelastic friable skin. Pseudoxanthoma elasticum is associated with arterial haemorrhage and thrombosis. Mild cases may present with superficial bruising and purpura following minor trauma.

Acquired vascular defects

1 Simple easy bruising is a common benign disorder which occurs in otherwise healthy women, especially those of child-bearing age.
2 Senile purpura caused by atrophy of the supporting tissues of cutaneous blood vessels is seen

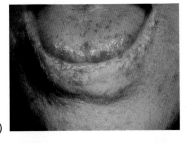

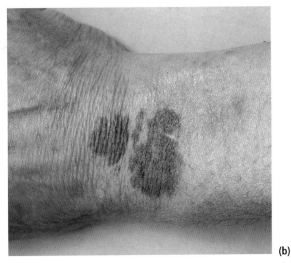

(a)

(b)

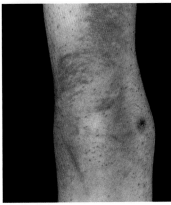

(c)

Fig. 19.1 (a) Hereditary haemorrhagic telangiectasia: the characteristic small vascular lesions are obvious on the lips and tongue. (b) Senile purpura. (c) Characteristic perifollicular petechiae in vitamin C deficiency (scurvy).

mainly on dorsal aspects of the forearms and hands (Fig. 19.1b).

3 Purpura associated with infections. Many bacterial, viral or rickettsial infections may cause purpura from vascular damage by the organism or as a result of immune complex formation, e.g. measles, dengue fever or meningococcal septicaemia.

4 The Henoch–Schönlein syndrome is usually seen in children and often follows an acute infection. It is an immunoglobulin A (IgA)-mediated vasculitis. The characteristic purpuric rash accompanied by localized oedema and itching is usually most prominent on the buttocks and extensor surfaces of the lower legs and elbows (Fig. 19.2). Painful joint swelling, haematuria and abdominal pain may also occur. It is usually a self-limiting condition but occasional patients develop renal failure.

5 Scurvy. In vitamin C deficiency, defective collagen may cause perifollicular petechiae, bruising and mucosal haemorrhage (Fig. 19.1c).

6 Steroid purpura. The purpura which is associated with long-term steroid therapy or

Cushing's syndrome is caused by defective vascular supportive tissue.

Tranexamic acid and aminocaproic acid are useful antifibrinolytic drugs which may reduce bleeding due to vascular disorders or thrombocytopenia but are contraindicated in the presence of haematuria since they might lead to clots obstructing the renal tract.

THROMBOCYTOPENIA

Abnormal bleeding associated with thrombocytopenia or abnormal platelet function is characterized by spontaneous skin purpura (Fig. 19.3) and mucosal haemorrhage and prolonged bleeding after trauma. The main causes of thrombocytopenia are listed in Tables 19.1 and 19.2.

Failure of platelet production

This is the most common cause of thrombocytopenia and is usually part of a generalized bone mar-

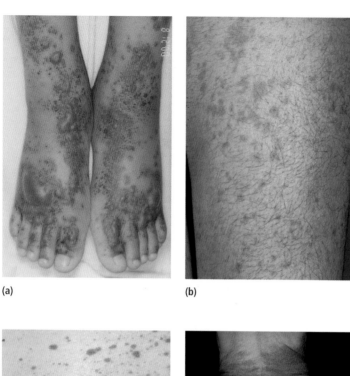

(a)　　　　　　(b)

Fig. 19.2 Henoch–Schönlein purpura: (a) unusually severe purpura on legs with bullous formation in a 6-year-old child; and (b) early urticarial lesions.

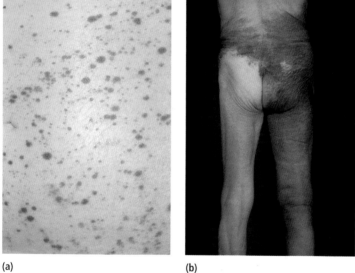

(a)　　　　　　(b)

Fig. 19.3 (a) Typical purpura; and (b) massive subcutaneous haemorrhage in a patient with drug-induced thrombocytopenia.

row failure (Table 19.1). Selective megakaryocyte depression may result from drug toxicity or viral infection. Rarely, it is congenital due to mutation of the c-MPL thrombopoietin receptor, in association with absent radii, or in May-Hegglin or Wiskott-Aldrich syndrome. Diagnosis of these causes of thrombocytopenia is made from the clinical history, peripheral blood count, the blood film and bone marrow examination.

Increased destruction of platelets

Autoimmune (idiopathic) thrombocytopenic purpura

Autoimmune (idiopathic) thrombocytopenic purpura (ITP) may be divided into chronic and acute forms.

Table 19.1 Causes of thrombocytopenia

Failure of platelet production
Selective megakaryocyte depression
  rare congenital defects
  drugs, chemicals, viral infections
Part of general bone marrow failure
  cytotoxic drugs
  radiotherapy
  aplastic anaemia
  leukaemia
  myelodysplastic syndromes
  myelofibrosis
  marrow infiltration, e.g. carcinoma, lymphoma
  multiple myeloma
  megaloblastic anaemia
  HIV infection

Increased consumption of platelets
Immune
  autoimmune (idiopathic)
  associated with systemic lupus erythematosus, chronic
    lymphocytic leukaemia or lymphoma
  infections: HIV, other viruses, malaria
  drug-induced
  heparin
  post-transfusional purpura
  feto-maternal alloimmune thrombocytopenia
Disseminated intravascular coagulation
Thrombotic thrombocytopenic purpura

Abnormal distribution of platelets
Splenomegaly

Dilutional loss
Massive transfusion of stored blood to bleeding patients

HIV, human immunodeficiency virus.

Table 19.2 Thrombocytopenia as a result of drugs or toxins

Bone marrow suppression
Predictable (dose-related)
  ionizing radiation, cytotoxic drugs, ethanol
Occasional
  chloramphenicol, co-trimoxazole, idoxuridine, penicillamine,
    organic arsenicals, benzene, etc.

Immune mechanisms (proven or probable)
Analgesics, anti-inflammatory drugs,
  gold salts, rifampicin
Antimicrobials
  penicillins, sulphonamides, trimethoprim, para-aminosalicylate
Sedatives, anticonvulsants
  diazepam, sodium valproate, carbamazepine
Diuretics
  acetazolamide, chlorathiazides, frusemide
Antidiabetics
  chlorpropamide, tolbutamide
Others
  digitoxin, heparin, methyldopa, oxyprenolol, quinine, quinidine

Platelet aggregation
Ristocetin, heparin (p. 283)

Chronic ITP

This is a relatively common disorder. The highest incidence has been considered to be in women aged 15–50 years although some reports suggest an increasing incidence with age. It is the most common cause of thrombocytopenia without anaemia or neutropenia. It is usually idiopathic but may be seen in association with other diseases such as systemic lupus erythematosus (SLE), human immunodeficiency virus (HIV) infection, chronic lymphocytic leukaemia (CLL), Hodgkin's disease or autoimmune haemolytic anaemia (Table 19.1).

Pathogenesis

Platelet sensitization with autoantibodies (usually IgG) results in their premature removal from the circulation by macrophages of the reticuloendothelial system, especially the spleen (Fig. 19.4). In many cases the antibody is directed against antigen sites on the glycoprotein IIb–IIIa or Ib complex. The normal lifespan of a platelet is about 7 days but in ITP this is reduced to a few hours. Total megakaryocyte mass and platelet turnover are increased in parallel to about five times normal.

Clinical features

The onset is often insidious with petechial haemorrhage, easy bruising and, in women, menorrhagia. Mucosal bleeding, e.g. epistaxes or gum bleeding, occurs in severe cases but fortunately intracranial haemorrhage is rare. The severity of bleeding in ITP is usually less than that seen in patients with comparable degrees of thrombocytopenia from bone marrow failure; this is attributed to the circulation of predominantly young,

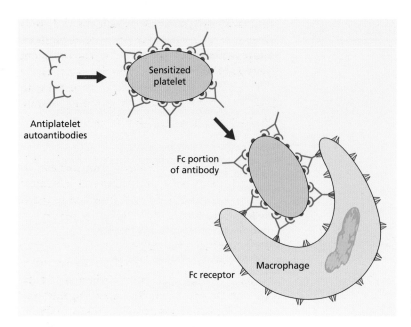

Fig. 19.4 The pathogenesis of thrombocytopenia in autoimmune thrombocytopenic purpura.

functionally superior platelets in ITP. Chronic ITP tends to relapse and remit spontaneously so the course may be difficult to predict. Many asymtomatic cases are discovered by a routine blood count.

The spleen is not palpable unless there is an associated disease causing splenomegaly.

Diagnosis
1 The platelet count is usually $10–50 \times 10^9/l$. The haemoglobin concentration and white cell count are typically normal unless there is iron deficiency anaemia because of blood loss.
2 The blood film shows reduced numbers of platelets, those present often being large.
3 The bone marrow shows normal or increased numbers of megakaryocytes.
4 Sensitive tests are able to demonstrate specific antiglycoprotein GPIIb/IIIa or GPIb antibodies on the platelet surface or in the serum in most patients. Platelet-associated IgG assays are less specific.

Treatment
As this is a chronic disease the aim of treatment should be to maintain a platelet count above the level at which spontaneous bruising or bleeding occurs with the minimum of intervention. In general, a platelet count above $50 \times 10^9/l$ does not require treatment.
1 Corticosteroids. Eighty per cent of patients remit on high-dose corticosteroid therapy. Prednisolone 1 mg/kg daily is the usual initial therapy in adults and the dosage is gradually reduced after 10–14 days. In poor responders the dosage is reduced more slowly but splenectomy or alternative immunosuppression is considered.
2 Splenectomy (Fig. 19.5). This operation is recommended in patients who still have platelets $<30 \times 10^9/l$ after 3 months of steroid therapy or who require unacceptably high doses of steroids to maintain a platelet count above $30 \times 10^9/l$. Good results occur in most of the patients, but in patients with ITP refractory to steroids or immunoglobulin there may be little benefit. Splenunculi must be removed otherwise subsequent relapse of ITP can occur.
3 High-dose intravenous immunoglobulin therapy is able to produce a rapid rise in platelet count in the majority of patients. A dosage of 400 mg/kg/day for 5 days or 1 g/kg/day for 2 days is recommended. It is particularly useful in

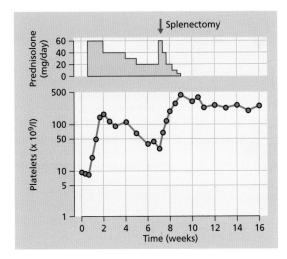

Fig. 19.5 Response to prednisolone in chronic immune thrombocytopenic purpura with subsequent relapse and response to splenectomy.

patients with life-threatening haemorrhage, in steroid-refractory ITP, during pregnancy or prior to surgery. The mechanism of action may be blockage of Fc receptors on macrophages or modification of autoantibody production.

4 Immunosuppressive drugs, e.g. vincristine, cyclophosphamide, azathioprine or cyclosporin alone or in combination, are usually reserved for those patients who do not respond sufficiently to steroids and splenectomy.

5 Other treatments which may elicit a remission include danazol (an androgen which may virilize in women) and anti-D immunoglobulin.

6 Platelet transfusions. Platelet concentrates are beneficial in patients with acute, life-threatening bleeding. Their benefit will only last a few hours.

Acute ITP
This is most common in children. In about 75% of patients the episode follows vaccination or an infection such as chicken pox or infectious mononucleosis. Most cases are due to non-specific immune complex attachments. Spontaneous remissions are usual but in 5–10% of cases the disease becomes chronic (lasting >6 months). Fortunately, morbidity and mortality in acute ITP is very low.

The diagnosis is one of exclusion and there is debate as to the need for bone marrow aspiration. If the platelet count is over $30 \times 10^9/l$ no treatment is necessary unless the bleeding is severe. Those with counts below $20 \times 10^9/l$ may be treated with steroids and/or intravenous immunoglobulin, especially if there is significant bleeding.

Infections
It seems likely that the thrombocytopenia associated with many viral and protozoal infections is immune-mediated. In HIV infection reduced platelet production is also involved (p. 143).

Post-transfusion purpura
Thrombocytopenia occurring about 10 days after a blood transfusion has been attributed to antibodies in the recipient developing against the human platelet antigen-1a (HPA-1a) (absent from the patient's own platelets) on transfused platelets. The reason why the patient's own platelets are then destroyed is unknown. Treatment is with intravenous immunoglobulin, plasma exchange or corticosteroids.

Drug-induced immune thrombocytopenia
An immunological mechanism has been demonstrated as the cause of many drug-induced thrombocytopenias (Fig. 19.6). Quinine (including that in tonic water), quinidine and heparin are particularly common causes (Table 19.2).

The platelet count is often less than $10 \times 10^9/l$, and the bone marrow shows normal or increased numbers of megakaryocytes. Drug-dependent antibodies against platelets may be demonstrated in the sera of some patients. The immediate treatment is to stop all suspected drugs but platelet concentrates should be given to patients with dangerous bleeding.

Thrombotic thrombocytopenic purpura and haemolytic uraemic syndrome
Thrombotic thrombocytopenic purpura (TTP) occurs in familial or acquired forms. There is deficiency of a metalloprotease (caspase) which breaks down high molecular weight multimers of von Willebrand factor (VWF) (Fig. 19.7). In familial forms this is because of a genetic defect

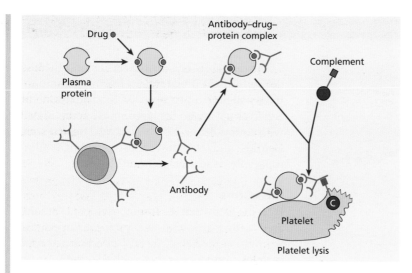

Fig. 19.6 Usual type of platelet damage caused by drugs in which an antibody–drug–protein complex is deposited on the platelet surface. If complement is attached and the sequence goes to completion, the platelet may be lysed directly. Otherwise it is removed by reticuloendothelial cells because of opsonization with immunoglobulin and/or the C3 component of complement.

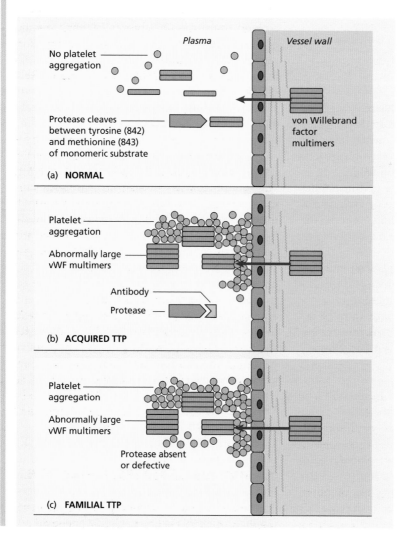

Fig. 19.7 Proposed pathogenesis of thrombotic thrombocytopenic purpura (TTP). Von Willebrand factor (vWF) consists of a series of vWF multimers each of molecular weight (MW) 250 kDa which are covalently linked. (a) Under physiological circumstances a metalloprotease cleaves high molecular weight multimers at a Tyr-842–Met-843 bond and the resulting vWF has an MW of 500–20 000 kDa. (b) In non-familial TTP an antibody develops to the metalloprotease which blocks cleavage of VWF multimers. (c) In congenital forms of TTP the protease appears to be absent. In both cases the resultant unusually large vWF multimers can bind platelets under high shear stress conditions and lead to platelet aggregation.

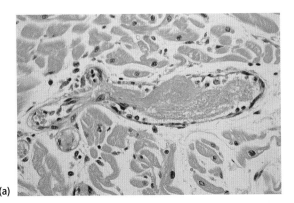

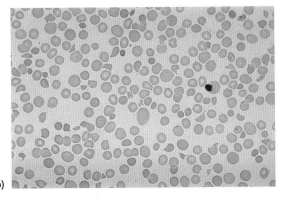

Fig. 19.8 Thrombotic thrombocytopenic purpura: (a) platelet thrombus in a small cardiac vessel with minor endothelial and inflammatory reaction (courtesy of Dr J.E. McLaughlin); and (b) peripheral blood film showing red cell fragmentation.

whereas in acquired forms it follows the development of an inhibitory antibody, the presence of which may be stimulated by infection. High molecular weight vWF multimers in plasma induce platelet aggregation, resulting in microthrombi formation in small vessels. In the closely related haemolytic uraemic syndrome (HUS) caspase levels are normal.

TTP is characterized by fever, severe thrombocytopenia, microangiopathic haemolytic anaemia and neurological symptoms (Fig. 19.8). Jaundice is usually present. Treatment is with plasma exchange, using fresh frozen plasma (FFP) or cryosupernatant. This removes the large molecular weight VWF multimers and the antibody. The platelet count and lactate dehydrogenase (LDH) are useful for monitoring the response to treatment. In refractory cases high-dose corticosteroids, vincristine, aspirin and immunosuppressive therapy with azathioprine or cyclophosphamide have been used. In untreated cases mortality may approach 90%. Relapses are frequent.

HUS in children has many common features but organ damage is limited to the kidneys. Fits are frequent. Many cases are associated with *Escherichia coli* infection with verotoxin 0157 or with other organisms, especially *Shigella*. Supportive renal dialysis and control of hypertension and fits are the mainstays of treatment. Platelet transfusions are contraindicated in HUS and TTP.

Disseminated intravascular coagulation

Thrombocytopenia may result from an increased rate of platelet destruction through consumption of platelets because of their participation in disseminated intravascular coagulation (DIC) (p. 268).

Increased splenic pooling

The major factor responsible for thrombocytopenia in splenomegaly is platelet 'pooling' by the spleen. In splenomegaly, up to 90% of platelets may be sequestered in the spleen whereas normally this accounts for about one-third of the total platelet mass (Fig. 19.9). Platelet lifespan is normal and in the absence of additional haemostatic defects, the thrombocytopenia of splenomegaly is not usually associated with bleeding.

Massive transfusion syndrome

Platelets are unstable in blood stored at 4°C and the platelet count rapidly falls in blood stored for more than 24 h. Patients transfused with massive amounts of stored blood (more than 10 units over a 24-h period) frequently show abnormal clotting and thrombocytopenia. These should be corrected by the use of platelet transfusions and FFP.

DISORDERS OF PLATELET FUNCTION

Disorders of platelet function are suspected in patients who show skin and mucosal haemorrhage

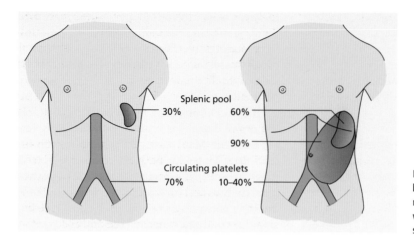

Splenic pool
30%   60%

90%

Circulating platelets
70%   10–40%

Fig. 19.9 The platelet distribution between the circulation and spleen in normal individuals (left), and in patients with moderate or massive splenomegaly (right).

and in whom the bleeding time is prolonged despite a normal platelet count. These disorders may be hereditary or acquired.

Hereditary disorders

Rare inherited disorders may produce defects at each of the different phases of the platelet reactions leading to the formation of the haemostatic platelet plug.

Thrombasthenia (Glanzmann's disease) This autosomal recessive disorder leads to failure of primary platelet aggregation because of a deficiency of membrane glycoproteins IIb and IIIa. It usually presents in the neonatal period and, characteristically, platelets fail to aggregate *in vitro* to any agonist.

Bernard–Soulier syndrome In this disease the platelets are larger than normal and there is a deficiency of glycoprotein Ib. There is defective binding to VWF, defective adherence to exposed subendothelial connective tissues and platelets do not aggregate with ristocetin. There is a variable degree of thrombocytopenia.

Storage pool diseases In the rare grey platelet syndrome, the platelets are larger than normal and there is a virtual absence of α granules with

deficiency of their proteins. In the more common β-storage pool disease there is a deficiency of dense granules.

Platelet function is abnormal in von Willebrand's disease due to an inherited defect in von Willebrand factor (see p. 267).

Acquired disorders

Antiplatelet drugs Aspirin therapy is the most common cause of defective platelet function. It produces an abnormal bleeding time and, although purpura may not be obvious, the defect may contribute to the associated gastrointestinal haemorrhage. The cause of the aspirin defect is inhibition of cyclo-oxygenase with impaired thromboxane A_2 synthesis (see Fig. 21.8). There is consequent impairment of the release reaction and aggregation with adrenaline and adenosine diphosphate (ADP). After a single dose the defect lasts 7–10 days. Dipyridamole inhibits platelet aggregation by blocking reuptake of adenosine and is usually used as an adjunct to oral anticoagulants. Clopidogrel inhibits binding of ADP to its platelet receptor and is used for prevention of thrombotic events (e.g. after coronary stenting or angioplasty) in patients with a history of symptomatic atherosclerotic disease. Abciximab, eptifibatide and tirofiban are inhibitors of glycoprotein GPIIb/IIIa receptor sites and may be used in patients undergoing percutaneous coronary intervention and unstable angina.

Hyperglobulinaemia Hyperglobulinaemia associated with multiple myeloma or Waldenström's disease may cause interference with platelet adherence, release and aggregation.

Myeloproliferative and myelodysplastic disorders Intrinsic abnormalities of platelet function occur in many patients with essential thrombocythaemia and other myeloproliferative and myelodysplastic diseases and in paroxysmal nocturnal haemoglobinuria.

Uraemia This is associated with various abnormalities of platelet function. Heparin, dextrans, alcohol and radiographic contrast agents may also cause defective function.

DIAGNOSIS OF PLATELET DISORDERS

Patients with suspected platelet or blood vessel abnormalities should initially have a blood count and blood film examination (Fig. 19.10). Bone marrow examination is essential in thrombocytopenic patients to determine whether or not there is a failure of platelet production. The marrow may also reveal one of the conditions associated with defective production (Table 19.1). In

patients with thrombocytopenia, a negative drug history, normal or excessive numbers of marrow megakaryocytes and no other marrow abnormality or splenomegaly, ITP is the usual diagnosis. Tests for platelet antibodies may confirm this. Screening tests for DIC are also useful, as are tests for an underlying disease, e.g. SLE or HIV infection.

When the blood count, including platelet count and blood film examination, are normal the bleeding time is assessed to detect abnormal platelet function. In most patients with abnormal platelet function demonstrated by prolonged bleeding time, the defect is acquired and associated either with systemic disease (e.g. uraemia) or with aspirin therapy. The very rare hereditary defects of platelet function require more elaborate *in vitro* tests to define the specific abnormality. These include platelet aggregation studies (Fig. 19.11) and nucleotide pool measurements. If von Willebrand's disease is suspected, assay of VWF and coagulation factor VIII are required.

PLATELET TRANSFUSIONS

Transfusion of platelet concentrates are indicated in the following circumstances.

1 Thrombocytopenia or abnormal platelet function when bleeding or before invasive procedures and there is no alternative therapy (e.g. steroids

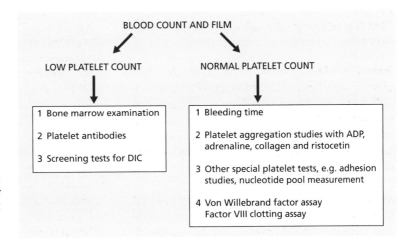

Fig. 19.10 Laboratory tests for platelet disorders. NB. Some intrinsic platelet functional disorders are associated with thrombocytopenia, e.g. Bernard–Soulier syndrome. ADP, adenosine diphosphate; DIC, disseminated intravascular coagulation.

BLOOD COUNT AND FILM

LOW PLATELET COUNT

NORMAL PLATELET COUNT

1 Bone marrow examination
2 Platelet antibodies
3 Screening tests for DIC

1 Bleeding time
2 Platelet aggregation studies with ADP, adrenaline, collagen and ristocetin
3 Other special platelet tests, e.g. adhesion studies, nucleotide pool measurement
4 Von Willebrand factor assay
  Factor VIII clotting assay

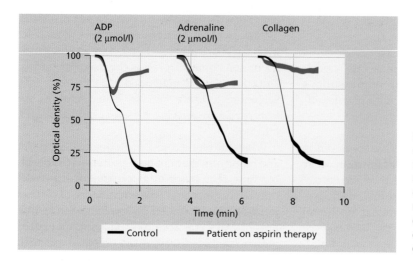

Fig. 19.11 Defective platelet aggregation in a patient on aspirin therapy. There is no secondary phase aggregation with adenosine diphosphate (ADP) and reduced responses to both adrenaline and collagen. Similar results are obtained in α-storage granule deficiency and cyclo-oxygenase deficiency.

or high-dose immunoglobulin) available. The platelet count should be above $50 \times 10^9/l$ before, for example, liver biopsy or lumbar puncture.

2 Prophylactically in patients with platelet counts $<5–10 \times 10^9/l$. If there is infection, potential bleeding sites or coagulopathy the count should be kept $>20 \times 10^9/l$).

The indications for transfusion of platelet concentrates are discussed further on p. 316.

BIBLIOGRAPHY

Blanchette V.S., Johnson J. and Rand M. (2000) The management of alloimmune neonatal thrombocytopenia *Clin. Haematol.* **13**, 365–90.

British Committee for Standards in Haematology, Working Party of Blood Transfusion Task Force (1992) Guidelines for platelet transfusions. *Transfus. Med.* **2**, 1777–80.

Furlan M., Robles R., Galbusera M. *et al.* (1998) Von Willebrand factor cleaving protease in thrombotic thrombocytopenic purpura and hemolytic uremic syndrome. *N. Engl. J. Med.* **339**, 1578–84.

George J.N. (2000) How I treat patients with thrombotic thrombocytopenic purpura/hemolytic uremic syndrome. *Blood* **96**, 1223–9.

George J.N. *et al.* (1998) Drug induced thrombocytopenia: a systemic review of published case reports. *Am. Intern. Med.* **129**, 886–90.

George J.N. *et al.* (1996) Idiopathic thrombocytopenic purpura: a practice guideline developed by explicit methods for the American Society of Haematology. *Blood* **88**, 3–40.

Kelton J.G. and Bussel J.B. (2000) Idiopathic thrombocytopenic purpura. *Semin. Hematol.* **37**, 219–314.

Lilleyman J. (2000) Chronic childhood idiopathic thrombocytopenic purpura. *Clin. Haematol.* **13**, 469–83.

Mannucci P.M. (1998) Hemostatic drugs. *N. Engl. J. Med.* **339**, 245–53.

Neild G.H. (1994) Haemolytic–uraemic syndrome in practice. *Lancet* **343**, 398–401.

Rock G. (2000) Management of thrombotic thrombocytopenic purpura. *Br. J. Haematol.* **109**, 496–507.

Tsai H.M. and Lian E.C.Y. (1998) Antibodies to von Willebrand factor-cleaving protease in acute thrombotic thrombocytopenic purpura. *N. Engl. J. Med.* **339**, 1584–94.

Coagulation disorders

HEREDITARY COAGULATION DISORDERS

Hereditary deficiencies of each of the coagulation factors have been described. Haemophilia A (factor VIII deficiency), haemophilia B (Christmas disease, factor IX deficiency) and von Willebrand's disease (VWD) are the most common; the others are rare.

HAEMOPHILIA A

Haemophilia A is the most common of the hereditary clotting factor deficiencies. The prevalence is of the order of 30–100 per million population. The inheritance is sex-linked (Fig. 20.1) but up to 33% of patients have no family history and result from spontaneous mutation. The factor VIII gene is situated near the tip of the long arm of the X chromosome (Xq2.6 region). It is extremely large and consists of 26 exons. The factor VIII protein includes a triplicated region $A_1A_2A_3$ with 30% homology with each other, a duplicated homology region C_1C_2 and a heavy glycosylated B domain which is removed when factor VIII is activated by thrombin.

The defect is an absence or low level of plasma factor VIII. Approximately half of the patients have missense or frameshift mutations or deletions in the factor VIII gene. In others a characteristic 'flip-tip' inversion is seen in which the factor VIII gene is broken by an inversion at the end of the X chromosome (Fig. 20.2). This mutation leads to a severe clinical form of haemophilia A.

Clinical features

Infants may suffer from profuse postcircumcision haemorrhage or develop joint and soft tissue bleeds and excessive bruising when they start to be active. Recurrent painful haemarthroses and muscle haematomas dominate the clinical course of severely affected patients and if poorly treated may lead to progressive joint deformity and disability (Figs 20.3–20.6). Prolonged bleeding occurs after dental extractions. Spontaneous haematuria and gastrointestinal haemorrhage can also occur. The clinical severity of the disease correlates with the extent of the factor VIII deficiency (Table 20.1). Operative and post-traumatic haemorrhage are life-threatening both in severely and mildly affected patients. Although not common, spontaneous intracerebral haemorrhage occurs more frequently than in the general population and is an important cause of death in patients with severe disease.

Haemophilic pseudotumours may occur in the long bones, pelvis, fingers and toes. These result from repeated subperiosteal haemorrhages with bone destruction, new bone formation, expansion of the bone and pathological fractures.

As a result of human immunodeficiency virus (HIV) present in concentrates made from human plasma during the early 1980s, over 50% of haemophiliacs treated in the USA or Western Europe became infected with HIV. Acquired immune deficiency syndrome (AIDS) has been a common cause of death in severe haemophilia. Thrombocytopenia from HIV infection may exacerbate bleeding episodes. Donor testing and viral inactivation steps during concentrate preparation now prevent HIV transmission. Factor VIII made by recombinant DNA techniques is also free of infection risk.

Many patients were infected with hepatitis C virus before testing of donors and blood products became possible. This is causing an increasing amount of morbidity including chronic hepatitis, cirrhosis and hepatoma. Hepatitis B transmission may also be a risk.

Laboratory findings (Table 20.2)
The following tests are abnormal.
1 Activated partial thromboplastin time (APTT).
2 Factor VIII clotting assay.

The bleeding time and prothrombin time (PT) tests are normal.

Carrier detection and antenatal diagnosis
Until recently, carrier detection and antenatal diagnosis were limited to measuring plasma levels of factor VIII and von Willebrand factor (VWF).

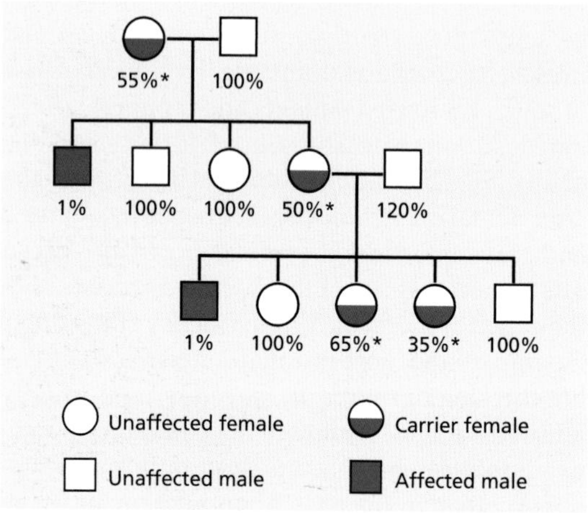

Fig. 20.1 A typical family tree in a family with haemophilia. Note the variable levels of factor VIII activity in carriers (*) because of random inactivation of X chromosome (Lyonization). The percentages show the degree of factor VIII activity as a percentage of normal.

Table 20.1 Correlation of coagulation factor activity and disease severity in haemophilia A or haemophilia B

Coagulation factor activity (percentage of normal)	Clinical manifestations
<1	Severe disease
	Frequent spontaneous bleeding episodes from early life
	Joint deformity and crippling if not adequately treated
1–5	Moderate disease
	Post-traumatic bleeding
	Occasional spontaneous episodes
5–20	Mild disease
	Post-traumatic bleeding

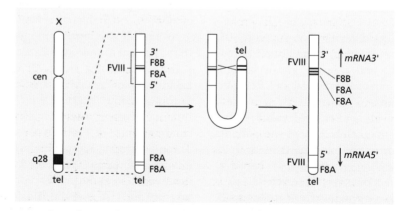

Fig. 20.2 The mechanism of the flip-tip inversion leading to disruption of the factor VIII gene. (Left) The orientation of the factor VIII gene is shown with the three copies of gene A in this region in (one within in intron 22 and two near the telomere). (Middle) During spermatogenesis at meiosis, the single X pairs with the Y chromosome in the homologous regions. The X chromosome is longer than the Y and there is nothing to pair with most of the long arm of X. The chromosome undergoes homologous recombination between the A genes. (Right) The final result is that the factor VIII gene is disrupted. cen, centromeric end; tel, telomere; the arrows indicate the direction of transcription from the A gene.

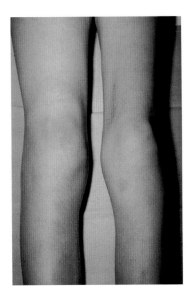

Fig. 20.3 Haemophilia A: acute haemarthrosis of the right knee joint with swelling of the suprapatellar region. There is wasting of the quadriceps muscles, particularly on the left.

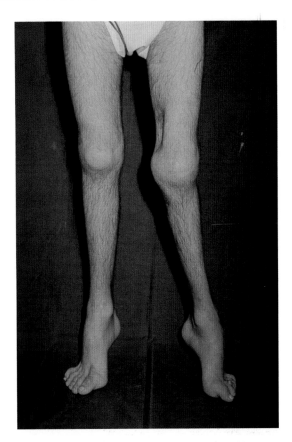

Fig. 20.4 Haemophilia A showing severe disability. The left knee is swollen with posterior subluxation of the tibia on the femur. The ankles and feet show residual deformities of talipes equinus, with some cavus and associated toe clawing. There is generalized muscle wasting. The scar on the medial side of the left lower thigh is the site of a previously excised pseudotumour.

Carriers are now better detected with DNA probes. A known specific mutation can be identified or restriction fragment length polymorphisms (p. 88) within or close to the factor VIII gene allows the mutant allele to be tracked. Chorionic biopsies at 8–10 weeks of gestation provide sufficient fetal DNA for analysis. Antenatal diagnosis is also possible following the demonstration of low levels of factor VIII in fetal blood obtained at 16–20 weeks' gestation from the umbilical vein by ultrasound-guided needle aspiration.

Treatment

Most patients attend specialized haemophilia centres where there is a multidisciplinary team dedicated to their care. Bleeding episodes are treated with factor VIII replacement therapy and spontaneous bleeding is usually controlled if the patient's factor VIII level is raised above 20% of normal. For major surgery, serious post-traumatic bleeding or when haemorrhage is occurring at a dangerous site, however, the factor VIII level should be elevated to 100% and then maintained above 50% when acute bleeding has stopped, until healing has occurred.

Recombinant factor VIII and immunoaffinity-purified factor VIII preparations are now available for clinical use and eliminate the risk of viral transmission.

DDAVP (desmopressin) provides an alternative means of increasing the plasma factor VIII level in milder haemophiliacs. Following the intravenous administration of this drug there is a moderate rise in the patient's own factor VIII by release from endothelial cells and this rise is proportional to the resting level. DDAVP may also be taken nasally—this has been used as immediate treatment for mild haemophilia after accidental trauma or haemorrhage.

Local supportive measures used in treating haemarthroses and haematomas include resting

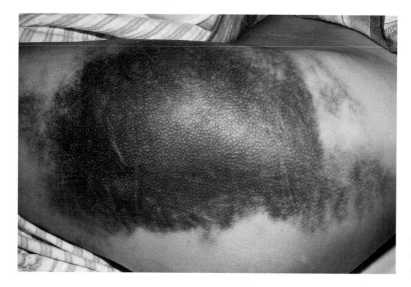

Fig. 20.5 Haemophilia A: massive haemorrhage in the area of the right buttock.

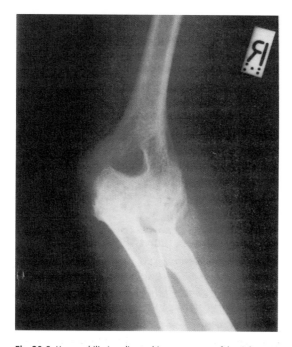

Fig. 20.6 Haemophilia A: radiographic appearances of the right elbow joint in a 25-year-old male. The joint space has been destroyed and there is bony ankylosis. Subchondral cystic areas are prominent.

the affected part and the prevention of further trauma.

Prophylactic treatment

The increased availability of factor VIII concentrates which may be stored in domestic refrigerators has dramatically altered haemophilia treatment. At the earliest suggestion of bleeding the haemophilic child may be treated at home. This advance has reduced the occurrence of crippling haemarthroses and the need for inpatient care. Severely affected patients are now reaching adult life with little or no arthritis. There is a continuing debate as to whether or not patients should be offered regular prophylactic treatment with factor VIII in an attempt to prevent bleeding episodes occurring. Prophylaxis begun before the age of 3 years aimed at keeping factor VIII (or factor IX) levels above 1% has been recommended in the USA.

Haemophiliacs are advised to have regular conservative dental care. Haemophilic children and their parents often require extensive help with social and psychological matters. With modern treatment the lifestyle of a haemophilic child can be almost normal but certain activities such as body contact sports are to be avoided.

Table 20.2 Main clinical and laboratory findings in haemophilia A, factor IX deficiency (haemophilia B, Christmas disease) and von Willebrand's disease

	Haemophilia A	Factor IX deficiency	Von Willebrand's disease
Inheritance	Sex-linked	Sex-linked	Dominant (incomplete)
Main sites of haemorrhage	Muscle, joints, post-trauma or postoperative	Muscle, joints, post-trauma or postoperative	Mucous membranes, skin cuts, post-trauma or postoperative
Platelet count	Normal	Normal	Normal
Bleeding time	Normal	Normal	Prolonged
Prothrombin time	Normal	Normal	Normal
Partial thromboplastin time	Prolonged	Prolonged	Prolonged or normal
Factor VIII	Low	Normal	May be moderately reduced
Factor IX	Normal	Low	Normal
VWF	Normal	Normal	Low
Ristocetin-induced platelet aggregation	Normal	Normal	Impaired

VWF, von Willebrand factor.

Gene therapy

Since it is only necessary to maintain factor levels >1% to prevent most of the mortality and morbidity of factor VIII or factor IX deficiency, there is great interest in gene-based therapy and clinical trials are underway. Various viral vectors (retroviral, lentiviral, adeno-associated) as well as non-viral vectors are being explored.

Inhibitors

One of the most serious complications of haemophilia is the development of antibodies (inhibitors) to infused factor VIII which occurs in 5–10% of patients. This renders the patient refractory to further replacement therapy so that tremendous doses have to be given to achieve a significant rise in plasma factor VIII activity. Immunosuppression has been used in an attempt to reduce formation of the antibody. Porcine factor VIII concentrates, recombinant factor VIIa and activated prothrombin complex concentrates (also known as FEIBA—factor *e*ight *i*nhibitor *by*-passing *a*ctivity) can be useful in the treatment of bleeding episodes.

Factor IX deficiency

The inheritance and clinical features of factor IX deficiency (Christmas disease, haemophilia B) are identical to those of haemophilia A. Indeed the two disorders can only be distinguished by specific coagulation factor assays. The incidence is one-fifth that of haemophilia A. Factor IX is coded by a gene close to the gene for factor VIII near the tip of the long arm of the X chromosome. Carrier detection and antenatal diagnosis is performed as for haemophilia A. The principles of replacement therapy are similar to those of haemophilia A. Bleeding episodes are treated with factor IX concentrates. Because of its longer biological half-life, infusions do not have to be given as frequently as factor VIII concentrates in haemophilia A. Recombinant factor IX is now available. Higher doses are needed compared with plasma-derived factor IX.

Laboratory findings (Table 20.2)
The following tests are abnormal.
1 APTT.
2 Factor IX clotting assay.

As in haemophilia A, the bleeding time and PT tests are normal.

von Willebrand's disease

In this disorder there is either a reduced level or abnormal function of vWF due to a point mutation or major deletion. vWF is a protein that has two roles. It promotes platelet adhesion to damaged endothelium and it is the carrier molecule for factor VIII, protecting it from premature destruction. The latter property explains the occasional reduced factor VIII levels found in vWD.

VWF is synthesized as a large 300-kDa protein which then forms multimers up to 10^6 Da in weight. Three types of vWD have been described. Type 1 and 3 vWD are associated with a reduction in the level of otherwise normal vWF, whereas type 2 is due to an abnormal form of the protein. Type 1 is a partial reduction in vWF whereas type 3 is a total lack of protein. Four subtypes of type 2 vWF are described, 2A associated with loss of high molecular weight multimers and type 2B is associated with abnormally high affinity for platelets, type 2M having a defective GP1b binding site and type 2N having reduced affinity for factor VIII.

vWD is the most common inherited bleeding disorder. Usually the inheritance is autosomal dominant with varying expression. The severity of the bleeding is variable. Typically there is mucous membrane bleeding (e.g. epistaxes, menorrhagia), excessive blood loss from superficial cuts and abrasions, and operative and post-traumatic haemorrhage. The severity is variable in the different types. Haemarthroses and muscle haematomas are rare, except in type 3 disease.

Laboratory findings (Table 20.2)
1 The bleeding time can be prolonged.
2 Factor VIII levels are often low and the APTT may be prolonged.
3 VWF levels are usually low.
4 There is defective platelet aggregation with ristocetin. (Abnormal sensitivity to ristocetin is seen in type 2B disease.) Aggregation to other agents (adenosine diphosphate (ADP), collagen, thrombin or adrenaline) is usually normal.

5 The platelet count is normal except for type 2B disease (where it is low).
6 Multimer analysis is useful for diagnosing different subtypes.

Treatment
Options are as follows:
1 Local measures and antifibrinolytic agent, e.g. tranexamic acid for mild bleeding.
2 DDAVP infusion for those with type 1 vWD.
3 Intermediate-purity factor VIII concentrates (which contain both vWF and factor VIII) for patients with very low vWF levels.

Hereditary disorders of other coagulation factors

All these disorders are rare. In most the inheritance is autosomal recessive. Factor XI deficiency is seen mainly in Ashkenazi Jews. It usually causes excess bleeding only after trauma such as surgery, and is treated by factor XI concentrate. Factor XIII deficiency produces a severe bleeding tendency, characteristically with umbilical stump bleeding. Specific concentrates or recombinant preparation of factors XI, XIII and VII are now available.

ACQUIRED COAGULATION DISORDERS

The acquired coagulation disorders (Table 20.3) are more common than the inherited disorders. Unlike the inherited disorders, multiple clotting factor deficiencies are usual.

Vitamin K deficiency

Fat-soluble vitamin K is obtained from green vegetables and bacterial synthesis in the gut. Deficiency may present in the newborn (haemorrhagic disease of the newborn) or in later life.

Deficiency of vitamin K is caused by an inadequate diet, malabsorption or inhibition of vitamin K by drugs such as warfarin which act as vitamin K antagonists. Warfarin is associated with a decrease in the functional activity of factors II, VII,

IX and X and proteins C and S, but immunological methods show normal levels of these factors. The non-functional proteins are called PIVKA (proteins formed in vitamin K absence). Conversion of PIVKA factors to their biologically active forms is a post-translational event involving carboxylation of glutamic acid residues in the N-terminal region where these factors show strong sequence homology (Fig. 20.7). Gamma-carboxylated glutamic acid binds calcium ions through which it forms a complex with phospholipid. In the

Table 20.3 The acquired coagulation disorders

Deficiency of vitamin K-dependent factors
Haemorrhagic disease of the newborn
Biliary obstruction
Malabsorption of vitamin K, e.g. sprue, gluten-induced enteropathy
Vitamin K-antagonist therapy, e.g. coumarins, indandiones

Liver disease

Disseminated intravascular coagulation

Inhibition of coagulation
Specific inhibitors, e.g. antibodies against factor VIII components
Non-specific inhibitors, e.g. antibodies found in systemic lupus erythematosus, rheumatoid arthritis

Miscellaneous
Diseases with M-protein production
L-Asparaginase
Therapy with heparin, defibrinating agents or thrombolytics
Massive transfusion syndrome

process of carboxylation, vitamin K is converted to vitamin K epoxide which is cycled back to the reduced form by reductases. Warfarin interferes with the reduction of vitamin K epoxide leading to a functional vitamin K deficiency.

Haemorrhagic disease of the newborn
Vitamin K-dependent factors are low at birth and fall further in breast-fed infants in the first few days of life. Liver cell immaturity, lack of gut bacterial synthesis of the vitamin and low quantities in breast milk may all contribute to a deficiency which may cause haemorrhage, usually on the second to fourth day of life, but occasionally during the first 2 months.

Diagnosis
The PT and APTT are both abnormal. The platelet count and fibrinogen are normal with absent fibrin degradation products.

Treatment
1 Prophylaxis. For many years vitamin K has been given to all newborn babies as a single intramuscular injection of 1 mg. This remains the most appropriate and safest treatment. Following epidemiological evidence suggesting a possible link between intramuscular vitamin K and an increased risk of childhood tumours (which has not been substantiated), some centres recommended an oral regimen but this is less effective in prevention.

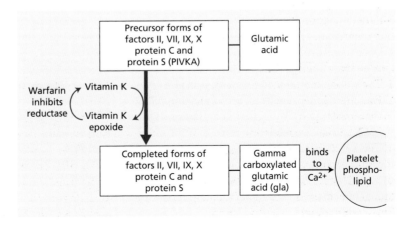

Fig. 20.7 The action of vitamin K in γ-carboxylation of glutamic acid in coagulation factors which are then able to bind Ca²⁺ and attach to the platelet phospholipid.

2 In bleeding infants: vitamin K 1 mg intramuscularly is given every 6 h with, initially, fresh frozen plasma if haemorrhage is severe.

Vitamin K deficiency in children or adults

Deficiency resulting from obstructive jaundice, pancreatic or small bowel disease occasionally causes a bleeding diathesis in children or adults.

Diagnosis

Both PT and APTT are prolonged. There are low plasma levels of factors II, VII, IX and X.

Treatment

1 Prophylaxis: vitamin K 5mg orally each day.
2 Active bleeding or prior to liver biopsy: vitamin K 10 mg slowly intravenously. Some correction of PT is usual within 6 h. The dose should be repeated on the next 2 days after which optimal correction is usual.

Liver disease

Multiple haemostatic abnormalities contribute to a bleeding tendency and may exacerbate haemorrhage from oesophageal varices.

1 Biliary obstruction results in impaired absorption of vitamin K and therefore decreased synthesis of factors II, VII, IX and X by liver parenchymal cells.
2 With severe hepatocellular disease, in addition to a deficiency of these factors, there are often reduced levels of factor V and fibrinogen and increased amounts of plasminogen activator.
3 Functional abnormality of fibrinogen (dysfibrinogenaemia) is found in many patients.
4 Decreased thrombopoietin production from the liver contributes to thrombocytopenia.
5 Hypersplenism associated with portal hypertension frequently results in thrombocytopenia.
6 Disseminated intravascular coagulation (DIC, see below) may be related to release of thromboplastins from damaged liver cells and reduced concentrations of antithrombin, protein C and α_2-antiplasmin. In addition there is impaired removal of activated clotting factors and increased fibrinolytic activity.

Disseminated intravascular coagulation

Widespread intravascular deposition of fibrin with consumption of coagulation factors and platelets occurs as a consequence of many disorders which release procoagulant material into the circulation or cause widespread endothelial damage or platelet aggregation (Table 20.4). It may be associated with a fulminant haemorrhagic or thrombotic syndrome or run a less severe and more chronic course.

Table 20.4 Causes of disseminated intravascular coagulation

Infections
Gram-negative and meningococcal septicaemia
Clostridium welchii septicaemia
Severe Falciparum malaria
Viral infection — varicella, HIV, hepatitis, cytomegalovirus

Malignancy
Widespread mucin-secreting adenocarcinoma
Acute promyelocytic leukaemia

Obstetric complications
Amniotic fluid embolism
Premature separation of placenta
Eclampsia; retained placenta
Septic abortion

Hypersensitivity reactions
Anaphylaxis
Incompatible blood transfusion

Widespread tissue damage
Following surgery or trauma
After severe burns

Vascular abnormalities
Kasabach–Merritt syndrome
Leaking prosthetic valves
Cardiac bypass surgery

Miscellaneous
Liver failure
Snake and invertebrate venoms
Hypothermia
Heat stroke
Acute hypoxia

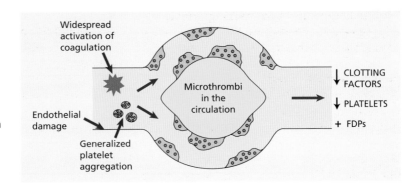

Fig. 20.8 The pathogenesis of disseminated intravascular coagulation and the changes in clotting factors, platelets and fibrin degradation products (FDPs) that occur in this syndrome.

Pathogenesis (Fig. 20.8)

1 DIC may be triggered by the entry of procoagulant material into the circulation in the following situations: amniotic fluid embolism, premature separation of the placenta, widespread mucin-secreting adenocarcinomas, acute promyelocytic leukaemia (AML type M_3), liver disease, severe falciparum malaria, haemolytic transfusion reaction and some snake bites.

2 DIC may also be initiated by widespread endothelial damage and collagen exposure (e.g. endotoxaemia, Gram-negative and meningococcal septicaemia, septic abortion), certain virus infections and severe burns or hypothermia.

In addition to its role in the deposition of fibrin in the microcirculation, intravascular thrombin formation produces large amounts of circulating fibrin monomers which form complexes with fibrinogen. Intense fibrinolysis is stimulated by thrombi on vascular walls and the release of split products interferes with fibrin polymerization, thus contributing to the coagulation defect. The combined action of thrombin and plasmin normally causes depletion of fibrinogen, prothrombin and factors V and VIII. Intravascular thrombin also causes widespread platelet aggregation and deposition in the vessels. The bleeding problems which may be a feature of DIC are compounded by thrombocytopenia caused by consumption of platelets.

Clinical features

These are dominated by bleeding, particularly from venepuncture sites or recent wounds (Fig.

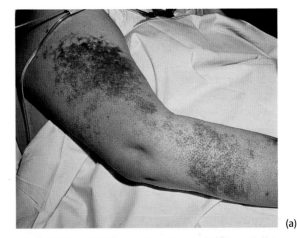

(a)

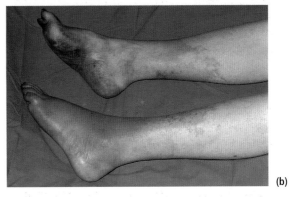

(b)

Fig. 20.9 Clinical features of disseminated intravascular coagulation: (a) indurated and confluent purpura of the arm; (b) peripheral gangrene with swelling and discoloration of the skin of the feet in fulminant disease.

Table 20.5 Haemostasis tests: typical results in acquired bleeding disorders

	Platelet count	Prothrombin time	Activated partial thromboplastin time	Thrombin time
Liver disease	Low	Prolonged	Prolonged	Normal (rarely prolonged)
Disseminated intravascular coagulation	Low	Prolonged	Prolonged	Grossly prolonged
Massive transfusion	Low	Prolonged	Prolonged	Normal
Oral anticoagulants	Normal	Grossly prolonged	Prolonged	Normal
Heparin	Normal (rarely low)	Mildly prolonged	Prolonged	Prolonged
Circulating anticoagulant	Normal	Normal or prolonged	Prolonged	Normal

20.9). There may be generalized bleeding in the gastrointestinal tract, the oropharynx, into the lungs, urogenital tract and in obstetric cases vaginal bleeding may be particularly severe. Less frequently microthrombi may cause skin lesions, renal failure, gangrene of the fingers or toes or cerebral ischaemia.

Laboratory findings (Table 20.5)

In many acute syndromes the blood may fail to clot because of gross fibrinogen deficiency.

Tests of haemostasis
1 The platelet count is low.
2 Fibrinogen screening tests, titres or assays indicate deficiency.
3 The thrombin time is prolonged.
4 High levels of fibrinogen (and fibrin) degradation products such as D-dimers are found in serum and urine.
5 The PT and APTT are prolonged in the acute syndromes.

Blood film examination
In many patients there is a haemolytic anaemia ('microangiopathic') and the red cells show prominent fragmentation because of damage caused when passing through fibrin strands in small vessels (pp. 68 and 291).

Treatment
1 Treatment of the underlying cause is most important.
2 Supportive therapy with fresh frozen plasma

Table 20.6 Indications for the use of fresh frozen plasma (National Institutes of Health Consensus Guidelines)

Coagulation factor deficiency (where specific or combined factor concentrate is not available)
Reversal of warfarin effect
Multiple coagulation defects, e.g. in patients with liver disease, DIC
Massive blood transfusion with coagulopathy and clinical bleeding
Thrombotic thrombocytopenic purpura
Deficiencies of antithrombin, protein C or protein S
Some patients with immunedeficiency syndromes

DIC, disseminated intravascular coagulation.

(Table 20.6) and platelet concentrates is indicated in patients with dangerous or extensive bleeding. Cryoprecipitate provides a more concentrated source of fibrinogen and red cell transfusions may be required.

The use of heparin or antiplatelet drugs to inhibit the coagulation process is usually not indicated because bleeding may, in some cases, be aggravated. Fibrinolytic inhibitors should not be considered because failure to lyse thrombi in organs such as the kidney may have adverse effects. The use of antithrombin and protein C concentrates to inhibit DIC in severe cases (e.g. meningococcal septicaemia) appears promising.

Coagulation deficiency caused by antibodies

Circulating antibodies to coagulation factors are occasionally seen with an incidence of approximately 1 per millon per year. Alloantibodies to factor VIII occur in 5–10% of haemophiliacs. Factor VIII autoantibodies may also result in a bleeding syndrome. These immunoglobulin G (IgG) antibodies occur rarely post-partum, in certain immunological disorders (e.g. rheumatoid arthritis) and in old age. Treatment usually consists of a combination of immunosuppression and treatment with factor replacement, usually as human or porcine factor VIII, recombinant VIIa or activated prothrombin complex concentrate (FEIBA).

Another protein known as the lupus anticoagulant interferes with lipoprotein-dependent stages of coagulation and is usually detected by prolongation of the APTT test (Table 20.5). This inhibitor is detected in 10% of patients with systemic lupus erythematosus (SLE) and in patients with other autoimmune diseases who frequently have anti-bodies to other lipid-containing antigens, e.g. cardiolipin. The antibody is not associated with a bleeding tendency but there is an increased risk of thrombosis and, as with other causes of thrombophilia, an association with recurrent miscarriage (Chapter 21).

Massive transfusion syndrome

Many factors may contribute to a bleeding disorder following massive transfusion. Blood loss results in reduced levels of platelets, coagulation factors and inhibitors. Further dilution of these factors occurs during replacement with stored blood. After 24-h storage at 4°C platelets aggregate and function poorly and the platelet count falls progressively. The labile coagulation factors

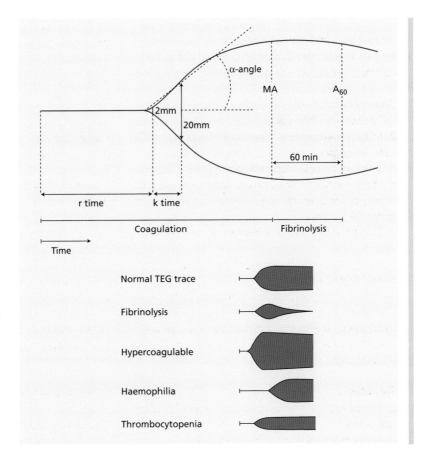

Fig. 20.10 Thromboelastography (TEG): normal trace and appearances in different pathological states. α angle, speed of solid clot formation; A$_{60}$, measure of clot lysis or retraction at 60 min; k, clot formation time; r, rate of initial fibrin formation; MA, absolute strength of fibrin clot. (Redrawn from S.V. Mallett and D.J.A. Cox 1992. Thromboelastography. *Br. J. Anaesth.* **69**, 307–13.)

V and VIII are also poorly preserved after a few days of storage. Minor activation of coagulation factors, microaggregates and degenerate cells may initiate or aggravate DIC. Some patients may have a pre-existing bleeding defect. Management is discussed on p. 270.

The results of haemostasis screening tests in acquired bleeding disorders are shown in Table 20.5 and a summary of the indications for use of fresh frozen plasma in Table 20.6.

THROMBOELASTOGRAPHY

Thromboelastography (TEG) is a technique for a global assessment of haemostatic function of a single blood sample in which the reaction of platelets with the protein coagulation cascade is made from the time of the initial platelet fibrin interaction through platelet aggregation, clot strengthening and fibrin cross-linkage to eventual clot lysis. It is suited as a monitor of haemostasis in surgery, e.g. of the liver or heart associated with haemostatic defects. Freshly drawn blood is placed in a cuvette which is oscillated, the motion being transferred to a pin which writes on heat-sensitive paper. As fibrin strands form the fibrin clot affects movement of the pin. The normal trace shows the rate of initial fibrin formation, the time to formation of a clot (coagulation time), strength of the fibrin clot, clot lysis index or retraction. Typical patterns showing results in fibrinolysis, hypercoagulability, haemophilia and thrombocytopenia are shown in Fig. 20.10.

BIBLIOGRAPHY

Astermark J., Petrini P., Tenbotn L., Shulman S., Ljung R. and Bentorp E. (1999) Primary prophylaxis in severe hemophilia should be started early but can be individualized. *Int. J. Haematol.* **105**, 1109–13.

Collins P.W. (1998) Disseminated intravascular coagulation. *CME Bull. Hematol.* **1**, 86–8.

Hedner U. and Ingenslev J. (1998) Clinical use of recombinant FVIIa (rFVIIa). *Transfus. Sci.* **19**, 163–76.

Herzog R.W. and High K.A. (1998) Problems and prospects for gene therapy for haemophilia. *Curr. Opin. Haematol.* **5**, 321–6.

High K.A. (2000) Gene therapy for hemophilia. Hematology 2000. *Am. Soc. Hematol. Educ. Prog.* Book 525–30.

Lakich D. *et al.* (1993) Inversions disrupting the factor VIII gene are a common cause of severe haemophilia A. *Nature Genet.* **5**, 236–41.

Ljung R.C.R. (1998) Can haemophilic arthropathy be prevented? *Br. J. Haematol.* **101**, 215–19.

Ljung R.C.R. (1999) Prophylactic infusion regimens in the management of hemophilia. *Thromb. Hemost.* **82**, 525–30.

Lusher J.M.N. (2000) First and second generation recombinant factor VIII concentrates in previously untreated patients: recovery, safety, efficacy and inhibition development. *Sem. Thromb. Hemost.* (in press).

Mannucci P.M. (1998) Hemostatic drugs. *N. Engl. J. Med.* **339**, 245–53.

Mannuci P.M. (2001) How I treat patients with von Willebrand disease. *Blood.* **97**, 1915–19.

Mannucci P.M. and Giangrande P.L.F. (2000) Choice of replacement therapy for hemophilia, recombinant products only? *Hematol. J.* **1**, 72–6.

Pamphilon D. (2000) Review: viral inactivaton of fresh frozen plasma. *Br. J. Haematol.* **109**, 680–93.

Thrombosis and antithrombotic therapy

Thrombi are solid masses or plugs formed in the circulation from blood constituents. Platelets and fibrin form the basic structure. Their clinical significance results from ischaemia from local vascular obstruction or distant embolization. Thrombi are involved in the pathogenesis of myocardial infarction, cerebrovascular disease, peripheral arterial disease and deep vein occlusion.

Thrombosis, both arterial and venous, is more common as age increases and is frequently associated with risk factors, e.g. operations or pregnancy. The term thrombophilia is used to describe the inherited or acquired disorders of the haemostatic mechanism which predispose to thrombosis.

ARTERIAL THROMBOSIS

Pathogenesis

Atherosclerosis of the arterial wall, plaque rupture and endothelial injury expose blood to subendothelial collagen and tissue factor. This initiates the formation of a platelet nidus on which platelets adhere and aggregate.

Platelet deposition and thrombus formation are important in the pathogenesis of atherosclerosis. Platelet-derived growth factor (PDGF) stimulates the migration and proliferation of smooth muscle cells and fibroblasts in the arterial intima. Regrowth of endothelium and repair at the site of arterial damage and incorporated thrombus result in thickening of the vessel wall.

As well as blocking arteries locally, emboli of platelets and fibrin may break away from the primary thrombus to occlude distal arteries. Examples are carotid artery thrombi leading to cerebral thrombosis and transient ischaemic attacks (TIAs) and heart valve and chamber thrombi leading to systemic emboli and infarcts (Fig. 21.1).

Clinical risk factors

The risk factors for arterial thrombosis are related to the development of atherosclerosis and are listed in Table 21.1. The identification of patients at risk is largely based on clinical assessment. A number of epidemiological studies have resulted in the construction of coronary artery thrombosis risk profiles based on sex, age, elevated blood pressure, high levels of serum cholesterol, glucose intolerance, cigarette smoking and electrocardiogram (ECG) abnormalities. These profiles have allowed presymptomatic assessment of young and apparently fit subjects and are valuable in counselling a change in lifestyle or for recommending medical therapy in individuals at risk. The Northwick Park heart study showed that elevated plasma levels of factor VII and fibrinogen are the strongest independent predictors of coronary events. Hyperhomocysteinaemia has been recognized more recently as a risk factor for peripheral and coronary arterial disease and stroke.

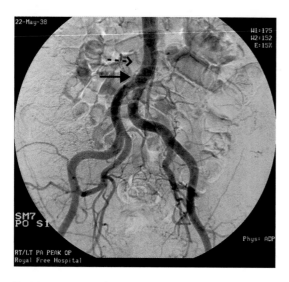

Fig. 21.1 Arteriogram showing saddle embolus at the aortic bifurcation (dotted arrow) and embolus in the left common iliac artery (solid arrow).

Table 21.1 Risk factors in arterial thrombosis (atherosclerosis)

Positive family history
Male sex
Hyperlipidaemia
Hyperhomocysteinaemia
Low serum folate, vitamin B_{12}, vitamin B_6
Hypertension
Diabetes mellitus
Gout
Polycythaemia
Cigarette smoking
ECG abnormalities
Elevated factor VII
Elevated fibrinogen
Lupus anticoagulant
Collagen vascular diseases
Behçet's disease

ECG, electrocardiogram.

VENOUS THROMBOSIS

Pathogenesis and risk factors

Virchow's triad suggests that there are three components that are important in thrombus formation:
1 slowing down of blood flow;
2 hypercoagulability of the blood; and
3 vessel wall damage.

For venous thrombosis, increased systemic co-agulability and stasis are most important, vessel wall damage being less important than in arterial thrombosis, although it may be important in patients with sepsis and in-dwelling catheters. Stasis allows the completion of blood coagulation at the site of initiation of the thrombus, e.g. behind the valve pockets of the leg veins in immobile patients.

Table 21.2 lists a number of recognized risk factors.

Hereditary disorders of haemostasis

The prevalence of inherited disorders associated with increased risk of thrombosis is at least as high as that of hereditary bleeding disorders. A hereditary 'thrombophilia' should be particularly suspected in young patients who suffer from spontaneous thrombosis, recurrent deep vein thromboses (Fig. 21.2); or an unusual site of thrombosis, e.g. axillary, splanchnic veins, sagittal sinus. Several abnormalities are now well characterized (Table 21.2).

Factor V Leiden gene mutation (activated protein C resistance)

This is the most common inherited cause of an increased risk of venous thrombosis. It occurs in about 4% of Caucasian factor V alleles. It was first recognized because of a failure to see prolongation in the activated partial thromboplastin time (APTT) test when activated protein C was added to the plasma of certain patients. Protein C breaks down activated factor V so activated protein C should slow the clotting reaction and prolong the APTT. In 1994 the underlying reason for this phenomenon was recognized to be a genetic polymorphism in the factor V gene (replacement of arginine at position 506 with glutamine—Arg-506-Gln) which makes factor V less susceptible to cleavage by activated protein C (Fig. 21.3). This is

Table 21.2 Risk factors for venous thrombosis

Related to coagulation abnormality	Related to stasis
Hereditary haemostatic disorders	Cardiac failure
factor V Leiden	Stroke
prothrombin G20210 A variant	Prolonged immobility
protein C deficiency	Pelvic obstruction
antithrombin deficiency	Nephrotic syndrome
protein S deficiency	Dehydration
abnormal fibrinogen	Hyperviscosity, polycythaemia
abnormal plasminogen	Varicose veins
Hereditary or acquired haemostatic disorders	**Related to unknown factors**
raised plasma levels of factor VII, VIII, IX or XI	Age
raised plasma levels of fibrinogen	Obesity
raised plasma levels of homocysteine	Sepsis
glucosylceramide deficiency	Paroxysmal nocturnal haemoglobinuria
coagulation factor IX concentrates	Behçet's disease
lupus anticoagulant	
oestrogen therapy (oral contraceptive and HRT)	
heparin-induced thrombocytopenia	
pregnancy and puerperium	
surgery, especially abdominal and hip	
major trauma	
malignancy	
myocardial infarct	
thrombocythaemia	

HRT, hormone replacement therapy.

called the factor V Leiden mutation. The frequency of factor V Leiden in the general population in Western countries means that it cannot be regarded as a rare mutation but as a genetic polymorphism that is maintained in the population (Fig. 21.4). Presumably individuals with this allele have been 'selected', probably because of reduced bleeding tendency. It does not increase the risk of arterial thrombosis.

Patients who are heterozygous for factor V Leiden are at an approximately fivefold increased risk of thrombosis compared to the general population. Individuals who are homozygous have around a 50-fold risk. Following venous thrombosis they have a higher risk of re-thrombosis compared to individuals with deep vein thrombosis (DVT) but normal factor V.

The incidence of factor V Leiden in patients with venous thrombosis is around 20–40%. Polymerase chain reaction (PCR) screening for the mu-

tation is relatively simple and the test is widely performed. The absolute risk of thrombosis will depend on many other factors and it is difficult to advise individual patients of their risk. At present it is not recommended to start anticoagulation therapy in individuals with the Leiden mutation, even if homozygous, with no history of thrombosis. A small minority of patients with activated protein C resistance do not have factor V Leiden and presumably have other mutations of factor V.

Antithrombin deficiency

Inheritance is autosomal dominant. There are recurrent venous thromboses usually starting in early adult life. Arterial thrombi occur occasionally. Antithrombin concentrates are available and are used to prevent thrombosis during surgery or childbirth. Many molecular variants of antithrombin have been categorized and are associated with varying degrees of risk of thrombosis.

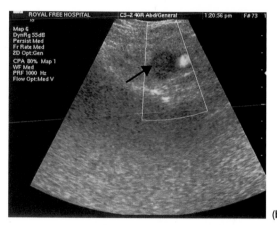

(a)

(b)

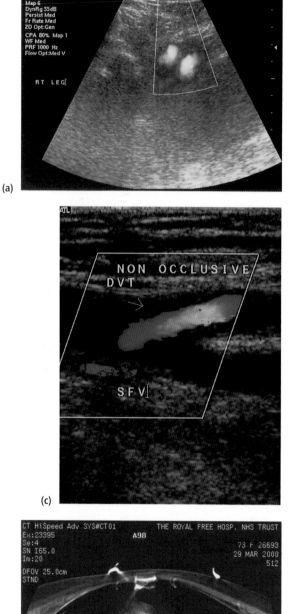

(c)

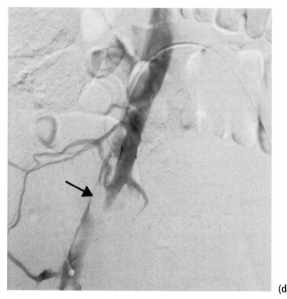

(d)

(e)

Fig. 21.2 Power Doppler ultrasound examination at the level of the common femoral vessels in both groins. (a) Normal flow in both the right common femoral vein and artery; (b) absence of flow in the left common femoral vein (arrow) with normal flow in the artery. The common femoral vein is non-compressible and filled with thrombus. (Courtesy of Dr A. Watkinson.) (c) Colour duplex study demonstrating non-occlusive thrombosis of the superficial femoral vein (SFV) (arrowed hypoechoic area). The colour (red/blue) represents blood flow (courtesy of Vascular Unit, Royal Free Hospital). (d) Deep vein thrombosis: a femoral venogram demonstrating extensive thrombus within the right external iliac vein (courtesy of Drs I.S. Francis and A.F. Watkinson). (e) Contrast-enhanced CT pulmonary angiogram showing bilateral pulmonary emboli (arrowed) within the (R) + (L) pulmonary trunk. (Courtesy of Dr I.S. Francis).

Protein C deficiency

Inheritance is autosomal dominant with variable penetrance. Protein C levels in heterozygotes are around 50% of normal. Characteristically, many patients develop skin necrosis as a result of dermal vessel occlusion when treated with warfarin, thought to be caused by reduction of protein C levels even further in the first day or two of warfarin therapy before reduction in the levels of the vitamin K-dependent clotting factors, especially factor VII. Rarely infants may be born with homozygous deficiency and characteristically present with severe disseminated intravascular coagulation (DIC) or purpura fulminans in infancy. Protein C concentrates are available.

Protein S deficiency

Protein S deficiency has been found in a number of families with a thrombotic tendency. It is a cofactor for protein C and the clinical features are similar to protein C deficiency, including a tendency to skin necrosis with warfarin therapy. The inheritance is autosomal dominant.

Prothrombin allele G20210 A

Prothrombin allele G20210 A is a variant (prevalence 2–3% in the population) which leads to increased plasma prothrombin levels and increases thrombotic risk by at least twofold. It is probable

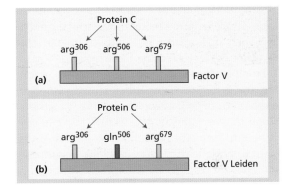

Fig. 21.3 The genetic basis of factor V Leiden. (a) Activated protein C inactivates factor Va by proteolytic cleavage at three sites in the Va heavy chain. (b) In the factor V Leiden mutation the Arg-506-Gln polymorphism leads to glutamine at position 506 with less efficient inactivation of factor V and increased risk of thrombosis.

Fig. 21.4 The incidence of carriers of factor V Leiden in different countries.

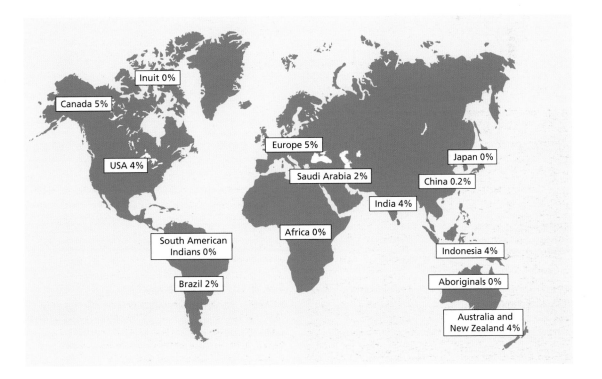

that the cause of venous thrombosis with this mutation and with high levels of factor VIII, IX and XI is that sustained generation of thrombin results in prolonged down-regulation of fibrinolysis through activation of thrombin-activated fibrinolysis inhibitor (see p. 244).

Hyperhomocyst(e)inaemia

Higher levels of plasma homocysteine may be genetic or acquired and are associated with increased risk for both venous and arterial thrombosis. There is, however, no evidence in 2001 that lowering the levels reduces these risks.

Homocysteine is derived from dietary methionine and is removed by either remethylation to methionine or conversion to cysteine via a trans-sulphuration pathway (Fig. 21.5). Classic homocysteinuria is a rare autosomal recessive disorder caused by deficiency of cystathione β-synthase, the enzyme responsible for trans-sulphuration. Vascular disease and thrombosis are major features of the disease. Heterozygous cystathione β-synthase deficiency is present in around 0.5% of the population and leads to a moderate increase in homocysteine. Methylene tetrahydrofolate reductase (MTHR) is involved in the remethylation pathway and a common thermolabile variant of the enzyme may be responsible for mild homocysteinaemia (above 15 μmol/l) although this may only be seen in the presence of folate deficiency (p. 50). Acquired risk factors for hyperhomocysteinaemia include deficiencies of folate, vitamin B_{12} or vitamin B_6, drugs (e.g. cyclosporin), renal damage and smoking. The levels also increase with age and are higher in men and post-menopausal females.

Defects of fibrinogen

Defects of fibrinogen are usually clinically silent or cause excess bleeding. Thrombosis is a rare association.

Hereditary or acquired disorders of haemostasis

High factor VII or fibrinogen levels are also associated arterial thrombosis.

The combination of multiple risk factors is associated with increased risk of thrombosis. If these are persistent they may represent a reason for extended anticoagulation.

Acquired risk factors

These may cause thrombosis in patients without another identifiable abnormality but are most

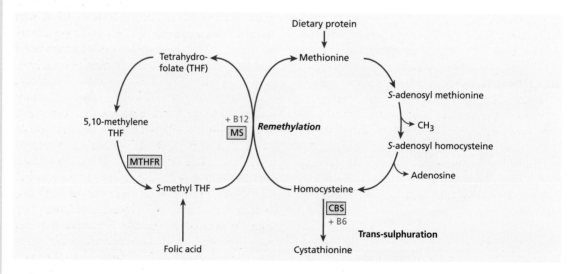

Fig. 21.5 The metabolism of homocysteine. Homocysteine is derived from dietary methionine and is metabolized either by the trans-sulphuration or remethylation pathways. Trans-sulphuration proceeds using the cystathionine β-synthase (CBS) enzyme with vitamin B_6 as a cofactor. Remethylation involves the action of methionine synthase (MS) on 5-methyl-THF with vitamin B_{12} as a cofactor. In addition, methylene-tetrahydrofolate reductase (MTHFR) is involved in this cycle.

likely to do so if an inherited predisposing abnormality, e.g. factor V Leiden, is also present.

Postoperative venous thrombosis

This is more likely to occur in the elderly, obese, those with a previous or family history of venous thrombosis, and in those in whom major abdominal or hip operations are performed.

Venous stasis and immobility

These factors are probably responsible for the high incidence of postoperative venous thrombosis and for venous thrombosis associated with congestive cardiac failure, myocardial infarction and varicose veins. In atrial fibrillation, thrombin generation from accumulation of activated clotting factors leads to a high risk of systemic embolization. The use of muscle relaxants during anaesthesia may also contribute to venous stasis. Venous thrombosis also has a higher frequency after prolonged aeroplane journeys.

Malignancy

Patients with carcinoma of the breast, lung, prostate, pancreas or bowel have an increased risk of venous thrombosis. Mucin-secreting adenocarcinomas may be associated with DIC.

Blood disorders

Increased viscosity, thrombocytosis, altered platelet membrane receptors and responses are possible factors for the high incidence of thrombosis in patients with polycythaemia vera and essential thrombocythaemia. There is a high incidence of venous thrombosis, including thrombi in large veins, e.g. the hepatic vein, in patients with paroxysmal nocturnal haemoglobinuria. An increased tendency to venous thrombosis has been observed in patients with sickle cell disease and patients with postsplenectomy thrombocytosis.

Oestrogen therapy

Oestrogen therapy, particularly high-dose therapy, is associated with increased plasma levels of factors II, VII, VIII, IX and X and depressed levels of antithrombin and tissue plasminogen activator in the vessel wall. There is a high incidence of postoperative venous thrombosis in women on high-dose oestrogen therapy and full-dose oestrogen-containing oral contraceptives. The risk is much less with low-dose oestrogen contraceptive preparations. Hormone replacement therapy also increases the risk of thrombosis, largely obviated by the use of low oestrogen preparations.

The antiphospholipid syndrome

This may be defined as the occurrence of thrombosis or recurrent miscarriage in association with laboratory evidence of persistent antiphospholipid antibody. One antiphospholipid antibody is the 'lupus anticoagulant' (LA) which was initially detected in patients with systemic lupus erythematosus (SLE), and is identified by a prolonged plasma APTT which does not correct with a 50 : 50 mixture of normal plasma. A second test dependent on limiting quantities of phospholipid, e.g. the dilute Russell's viper venom test, is also used in diagnosis. It represents part of the spectrum of antiphospholipid antibody syndrome (APS) and whereas lupus anticoagulants are reactive in the fluid phase the other antiphospholipid antibodies (APAs), such as anticardiolipin antibodies (ACA) and antibodies to β_2-glycoprotein (β_2-GPI), are identified by solid phase immunoassay. Both solid phase assays and coagulation tests for LA should be used in the diagnosis of APS. As well as patients with SLE, APS is also found in other autoimmune disorders particularly of connective tissues, lymphoproliferative diseases, postviral infections, with certain drugs including phenothiazines and as an 'idiopathic' phenomenon in otherwise healthy subjects. Paradoxically, in view of its name, it is associated with venous and arterial thrombosis. The arterial thrombosis may cause peripheral limb ischaemia, stroke or myocardial infarct. As with other causes of thrombophilia, recurrent abortion caused by placental infarction is also associated (Table 21.3). Thrombocytopenia may be present and livedo reticularis is a frequent dermal manifestation. Treatment is with anticoagulation where indicated. It is usual to maintain an international normalized ratio (INR) of between 2.0 and 3.0 with warfarin but higher levels may be needed if previous arterial or major DVT has

Table 21.3 Clinical associations of lupus anticoagulant and anticardiolipin antibodies

---

Venous thrombosis
   deep venous thrombosis/pulmonary embolism
   renal, hepatic, retinal veins
Arterial thrombosis
Recurrent fetal loss
Thrombocytopenia
Livedo reticularis

---

occurred or recurrence of thrombosis occurs on warfarin therapy. Low-dose heparin and aspirin are useful in the management of recurrent miscarriage.

Collagen vascular diseases and Behçet's syndrome are also associated with arterial and venous thrombosis, whether or not the lupus anticoagulant is present.

Factor IX concentrates

Venous thrombosis may complicate the use of factor IX concentrates which contain trace amounts of activated coagulation factors. Patients with liver disease who are unable to clear these activated factors are especially at risk.

Glucosylceramide deficiency

Reduced plasma levels of the glycolipid glucosylceramide are a potential risk factor for venous thrombosis particularly in young male patients. The glycolipid modulates the protein C pathway.

INVESTIGATION OF THROMBOPHILIA

Many of the conditions associated with an increased thrombotic risk are obvious following clinical examination. A full assessment is indicated particularly in patients who have recurrent or spontaneous DVT or pulmonary emboli, in patients who have thrombosis at a young age and in those patients with a familial tendency to thrombosis or thrombosis at an unusual site. With the increasing recognition of systemic causes of thrombophilia, the indications for thrombophilia screening are widening. The following laboratory tests are used in diagnosis.

Screening tests

1 Blood count and erythrocyte sedimentation rate (ESR)—to detect elevation in haematocrit, white cell count, platelet count, fibrinogen and globulins.
2 Blood film examination—may provide evidence of myeloproliferative disorder; leucoerythroblastic features may indicate malignant disease.
3 Prothrombin time (PT) and APTT—a shortened APPT is often seen in thrombotic states and may indicate the presence of activated clotting factors. A prolonged APTT test, not corrected by the addition of normal plasma, suggests a 'lupus anticoagulant' or an acquired inhibitor to a coagulation factor.
4 Thrombin time and reptilase time—prolongation suggests an abnormal fibrinogen.
5 Fibrinogen assay.
6 Activated protein C (APC) resistance test and DNA analysis for factor V Leiden.
7 Antithrombin—immunological and functional assays.
8 Protein C and protein S—immunological and functional assays.
9 Prothrombin gene analysis for the G20210 A variant.
10 Plasma homocysteine estimation.
   In many patients even full investigation yields no abnormalities and treatment with oral anticoagulants may remain empirical.
11 Acid lysis test and test for CD59 and CD55 expression (paroxysmal nocturnal haemoglobinuria) are preferred if paroxysmal nocturnal haemoglobinuria is suspected.

DIAGNOSIS OF VENOUS THROMBOSIS

Deep vein thrombosis

Serial compression ultrasound This is the most reliable and practical method for patients with first suspicion of DVT in the legs and other sites (Fig. 21.2a,b). It can be combined with spectral, colour (Fig. 21.2c) or power Doppler (Duplex) scanning which improves accuracy by focusing on individual veins. It does not distinguish between acute and chronic thrombi.

Contrast venography Iodinated contrast medium is injected into a vein peripheral to the suspected DVT. This permits direct demonstration by X-ray of the site, size and extent of the thrombus (Fig. 21.2d). It is, however, a painful, invasive technique with a risk of contrast reaction and procedure-induced DVT.

Plasma D-dimer concentration The concentration of these fibrin breakdown products are raised when there is a fresh venous thrombosis. It is a useful assay when recurrent thrombosis is suspected and also may be combined with the tests above for diagnosis of a first event.

Magnetic resonance imagining (MRI) This may also be used but is expensive. Impedance plethysmography is less sensitive and accurate and is falling out of use.

Pulmonary embolus

Chest X-ray This is often normal but may show evidence of pulmonary infarction or pleural effusion.

Ventilation perfusion (VQ) scintigraphy This detects areas of the lung being ventilated but not perfused.

Computed tomography (CT) pulmonary angiography Fine slices of the lung are scanned by spiral CT so that filling defects in the pulmonary arteries are visualized (Fig. 21.2e).

Magnetic resonance pulmonary angiography Gadolinium-enhanced MRI is a relatively new, expensive but accurate technique.

Pulmonary angiography This is the traditional reference method but is invasive with complications, albeit uncommon, such as arrhythmia or contrast reaction.

Electrocardiogram This is performed to determine whether there is right heart 'strain' which occurs only in relatively severe cases.

ANTICOAGULANT DRUGS

Anticoagulant drugs are used widely in the treatment of venous thromboembolic disease. Their value in the treatment of arterial thrombosis is less well established.

HEPARIN

This acidic, unfractionated mucopolysaccharide of average molecular weight 15 000–18 000 is an inhibitor of blood coagulation because of its action in potentiating the activity of antithrombin (see below). As it is not absorbed from the gastrointestinal tract it must be given by injection. It is inactivated by the liver and excreted in the urine. The effective biological half-life is about 1 h (Table 21.4).

Table 21.4 Comparison of unfractionated heparin with low molecular weight heparin

	Unfractionated heparin	Low molecular weight heparin
Mean molecular weight in kilodaltons (range)	15 (4–30)	4.5 (2–10)
Anti-Xa : anti-IIa	1 : 1	2 : 1 to 4 : 1
Inhibits platelet function	Yes	No
Bioavailability	50%	100%
Half-life		
intravenous	1 h	2 h
subcutaneous	2 h	4 h
Elimination	Renal and hepatic	Renal
Monitoring	APTT	Xa assay (usually not needed)
Frequency of heparin-induced thrombocytopenia	High	Low
Osteoporosis	Yes	Less frequent

APTT, activated partial thromboplastin time.

Mode of action

Heparin dramatically potentiates the formation of complexes between antithrombin and activated serine protease coagulation factors, thrombin (IIa) and factors IXa, Xa and XIa (Fig. 21.6). This complex formation inactivates these factors irreversibly. In addition, heparin impairs platelet function.

Low molecular weight heparin (LMWH) preparations (MW 2000–10000) are produced by enzymatic or chemical depolymerization of unfractionated heparin. They have a greater ability to inhibit factor Xa than to inhibit thrombin and interact less with platelets compared with standard heparin, and so may have a lesser tendency to cause bleeding. They also have greater bioavailability and a more prolonged half-life in plasma making once-daily administration in prophylaxis or treatment feasible (Table 21.4).

Indications

Heparin is routinely used in deep vein thrombosis, pulmonary embolism and unstable angina pectoris. It is also widely used in the prophylaxis of venous thrombosis and is the drug of choice for women requiring anticoagulation in pregnancy because it does not cross the placenta. It is also used during cardiopulmonary bypass surgery, for maintaining the patency of in-dwelling venous lines and in some case of DIC if the manifestations are predominantly vaso-occlusive.

Administration and laboratory control

Standard heparin

Continuous intravenous infusion This provides the smoothest control of heparin therapy and is commonly used in treatment of acute DVT or pulmonary embolus. In an adult, dosage of 30000–40000 units over 24h (1000–2000 units/h with a loading dose of 5000 units) is usually satisfactory. Therapy is monitored by maintaining the APTT at between 1.5 and 2.5 times the normal value. It is usual to start warfarin therapy within 2 days of starting heparin therapy and to discontinue heparin when the INR has been above 2.0 on two successive days. For acute coronary syndromes both unfractionated heparin and low molecular weight heparin are of benefit when used with aspirin in the prevention of mural thrombosis, systemic embolization and venous thrombosis.

Subcutaneous heparin Intermittent subcutaneous injections are preferred when heparin is given as prophylaxis against venous thrombosis, e.g. for surgical procedures. The usual dosage is 5000 units 12-hourly preoperatively followed by this dosage 8–12-hourly for 7 days or until the patient is mobile. Low molecular weight heparin (see below) is usually perferred as it can be given once daily.

Low molecular weight heparin

Low molecular weight heparin is given by subcutaneous injection and as it has a longer half-life than standard heparin it can be given once a day in prophylaxis, or once or twice a day in treatment (Table 21.4). APTT monitoring is not required. Typical dosage is tinzaparin 175 anti-Xa units/kg or dalteparin 200 anti-Xa units/kg subcutaneously each day. Low molecular weight heparin is beginning to replace unfractionated heparin for therapy of DVT including pulmonary embolism and many patients with uncomplicated DVTs may now be managed at home with regular low

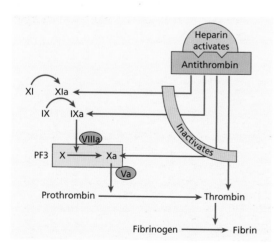

Fig. 21.6 The action of heparin. This activates antithrombin which then forms complexes with activated serine protease coagulation factors (thrombin, Xa, IXa and XIa) and so inactivates them.

molecular weight heparin injections once or twice daily according to the preparation. This shorter stay in hospital compensates for the higher cost of low molecular weight heparin.

Complications

Unfractionated heparin is associated with a number of side-effects. The risk of these complications appears to be reduced by around 50% by the use of low molecular weight heparin.

Bleeding during heparin therapy

Bleeding may be because of excessive prolonged anticoagulation or to an antiplatelet functional effect of heparin. Intravenous heparin has a half-life of less than 1 h and it is usually only necessary to stop the infusion. Protamine is able to inactivate heparin immediately and, for severe bleeding a dose of 1 mg/100 units of heparin provides effective neutralization. However, protamine itself may act as an anticoagulant when in excess.

Heparin-induced thombocytopenia

A mild lowering of the platelet count may occur in the first 24 h as a result of platelet clumping. This is of no clinical consequence (heparin-induced thombocytopenia, HIT, type 1). The important HIT, type 2, may occur in up to 5% of patients who are treated with unfractionated heparin and paradoxically presents with thrombosis. It results from the binding of heparin to platelets followed by the generation of an immunoglobulin G (IgG) antibody to the heparin–platelet factor 4 (PF4) complex which leads to platelet activation (Fig. 21.7). Typically it presents as a fall of > 50% in the platelet count 5 or more days after starting heparin treatment or earlier if heparin has been given previously. Diagnosis is difficult but assays have recently been developed to allow the detection of antibodies to immobilized heparin–PF4 complex. Heparin therapy must be discontinued. Thrombin inhibitors such as hirudin or lepirudin appear promising as alternatives and the heparinoid danaparoid may also be used. Low molecular weight heparin is less likely than unfractionated heparin to cause HIT but there is cross-reactivity of the antibody. Warfarin therapy in some cases causes skin necrosis and should be delayed until alternative anticoagulation has been achieved.

Osteoporosis

This occurs with long-term (>2 months) heparin therapy, especially in pregnancy. The drug complexes minerals from the bones but the exact pathogenesis is unknown.

Direct thrombin inhibitors

Hirudins, hirudin fragments and other low molecular weight direct inhibitors of thrombin have potential as antithrombotic agents, but are not yet in routine clinical use.

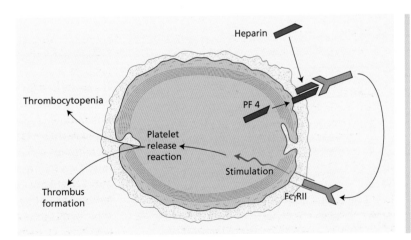

Fig. 21.7 Mechanism of heparin-induced thrombocytopenia (HIT). Platelet factor 4 (PF4) is released from α granules and forms a complex on the platelet surface with heparin. Immunoglobulin G antibodies (usually IgG₂) develop against this complex and once bound can activate the platelet through the platelet immunoglobulin receptor Fc-γRII. This leads to platelet stimulation, further release of PF4 and the platelet release reaction with consequent thrombocytopenia and thrombus development.

ORAL ANTICOAGULANTS

These are derivatives of coumarin or indandione. Warfarin, a coumarin, is most widely used. The drugs are vitamin K antagonists (p. 267) and so treatment results in decreased biological activity of the vitamin K-dependent factors II, VII, IX and X. Oral anticoagulants block the postribosomal γ-carboxylation of glutamic acid residues of these proteins (Fig. 20.7). After warfarin is given, factor VII levels fall considerably within 24 h but prothrombin has a longer plasma half-life and only falls to 50% of normal at 3 days; the patient is fully anticoagulated only after this period.

Principles of oral anticoagulation

A typical starting regime for warfarin would be 10 mg on day 1, 10 mg on day 2 and then 5 mg on the third day. After this the dosage should be adjusted according to the PT. The usual maintenance dosage of warfarin is 3–9 mg daily but individual responses vary greatly. Lower dosage is recommended for the very elderly or those with liver disease.

The indications and recommended ranges for International Normalized Ratio (INR) with warfarin treatment are summarized in Table 21.5. The effect of oral anticoagulants is monitored by the PT. The INR is used and is based on the ratio of the patient's PT to a mean normal PT with correction

for the 'sensitivity' of the thromboplastin used. This is calibrated against a primary World Health Organization (WHO) standard thromboplastin.

Warfarin crosses the placenta and is teratogenic. Heparin is preferred for pregnant patients because it does not cross the placenta and its action is short-lived.

It is usual to continue warfarin in the short to medium term (up to 6 months) for established DVT, pulmonary embolism and following xenograft heart valves or coronary bypass surgery. Long-term therapy is given for recurrent venous thrombosis, for embolic complications of rheumatic heart disease or atrial fibrillation, and with prosthetic valves and arterial grafts. It is also given long term in patients with a severe cause of thrombophilia, e.g. the lupus anticoagulant and a history of thrombosis.

Drug interactions

About 97% of warfarin in the circulation is bound to albumin and only a small fraction of warfarin is free and can enter the liver parenchymal cells. It is this free fraction which is active. In the liver cells, warfarin is degraded in microsomes to an inactive water-soluble metabolite which is conjugated and excreted in the bile and partially reabsorbed to be also excreted in urine. Drugs which affect the albumin binding or excretion of warfarin (or of other oral anticoagulants) or those which decrease the absorption of vitamin K will interfere with the control of therapy (Table 21.6).

Management of warfarin overdose

If the INR is in excess of 4.5 without bleeding warfarin should be stopped for 1 or 2 days and the dose adjusted according to the INR. The long half-life of warfarin (40 h) delays the full impact of dose changes for 4–5 days. Mild bleeding usually only needs an INR assessment, drug withdrawal and subsequent dosage adjustment (Table 21.7). More serious bleeding may need cessation of therapy, vitamin K therapy or the infusion of fresh frozen plasma or factor concentrates. The latter, however,

Table 21.5 Oral anticoagulant control tests. Target levels recommended by the British Society for Haematology (2000)

Target INR	Clinical state
2.5 (2.0–3.0)	Treatment of DVT, pulmonary embolism, atrial fibrillation, recurrent DVT off warfarin; symptomatic inherited thrombophilia, cardiomyopathy, mural thrombus, cardioversion
3.5 (3.0–4.0)	Recurrent DVT while on warfarin, mechanical prosthetic heart valves, antiphospholipid syndrome (some cases)

DVT, deep vein thrombosis; INR, international normalized ratio.

Table 21.6 Drugs and other factors which interfere with the control of anticoagulant therapy

Potentiation of oral anticoagulants	Inhibition of oral anticoagulants
Drugs which increase the effect of coumarins	**Drugs which depress the action of coumarins**
Reduced coumarin binding to serum albumin	*Acceleration of hepatic microsomal degradation of coumarin*
sulphonamides	barbiturates
Inhibition of hepatic microsomal degradation of coumarin	rifampicin
cimetidine	*Enhanced synthesis of clotting factors*
allopurinol	oral contraceptives
tricyclic antidepressants	
metronidazole	**Hereditary resistance to oral anticoagulants**
sulphonamides	
Alteration of hepatic receptor site for drug	**Pregnancy**
thyroxine	
quinidine	
Decreased synthesis of vitamin K factors	
high doses of salicylates	
some cephalosporins	
Liver disease	
Decreased synthesis of vitamin K factors	
Decreased absorption of vitamin K	
e.g. malabsorption, antibiotic therapy, laxatives	

NB. Patients are also more likely to bleed if taking antiplatelet agents (e.g. NSAIDs, dipyridamole or aspirin); alcohol in large amounts enhances warfarin action.

carry the risks of DIC and both may transmit viruses. Vitamin K is the specific antidote; an oral or intravenous dose of 2.5 mg is usually effective but higher doses result in resistance to further warfarin therapy for 2–3 weeks.

FIBRINOLYTIC AGENTS

A number of fibrinolytic agents are able to lyse fresh thrombi (Table 21.8). They may be used systemically for patients with acute myocardial infarction, major pulmonary embolism or iliofemoral thrombosis, and locally in patients with acute peripheral arterial occlusion.

Administration of thrombolytic agents has been simplified with standardized dosage regimens. The therapy is most effective in the first 6 h after symptoms begin but is still of benefit up to 24 h. Streptokinase is given in a loading dose of 250 000 units followed by a maintenance dose 100 000 units hourly for 12–48 h. In acute myocardial infarction, streptokinase is given as a single dose of 1 500 000 units over 60 min. Aspirin therapy is also given and the value of additional heparin therapy is under study.

The use of laboratory tests for monitoring and control of short-term thrombolytic therapy is now considered unnecessary. However, certain clinical complications exclude the use of thrombolytic agents (Table 21.9).

Recombinant tissue plasminogen activator (tPA) has a particularly high affinity for fibrin and this allows lysis of thrombi with less systemic activation of fibrinolysis. Acylated plasminogen streptokinase activator complex (APSAC) and single-chain urokinase-type plasminogen activator (SCU-PA) are two other fibrinolytic agents.

Table 21.7 Recommendations on the management of bleeding and excessive anticoagulation by the British Committee for Standards in Haematology (2000)

INR 3.0–6.0 (target INR 2.5)	Reduce warfarin dose or stop
INR 4.0–6.0 (target INR 3.5)	Restart warfarin when INR < 5.0
INR 6.0–8.0 No bleeding or minor bleeding	Stop warfarin* Restart when INR < 5.0
INR > 8.0 No bleeding or minor bleeding	Stop warfarin Restart warfarin when INR < 5.0 If other risk factors for bleeding give 0.5–2.5 mg of vitamin K orally
Major bleeding	Stop warfarin Give prothrombin complex concentrate 50 units/kg or FFP 15 ml/kg Give 5 mg vitamin K (oral or i.v.)

FFP, fresh frozen plasma; INR, international normalized ratio.
* 1 mg vitamin K may be given orally to rapidly reduce the INR to the therapeutic range within 24 h in all patients with an INR above the therapeutic range and no bleeding.

Table 21.8 Fibrinolytic agents—plasminogen activators

Streptokinase (SK)
Tissue plasminogen activator (tPA)
Single-chain urokinase-type plasminogen activator (SCU-PA)
Acylated plasminogen–streptokinase activator complex (APSAC)

Table 21.9 Contraindications to thrombolytic therapy

Absolute contraindications	Relative contraindications
Active gastrointestinal bleeding	Traumatic cardiopulmonary resuscitation
Aortic dissection	
Head injury or cerebrovascular accident in the past 2 months	Major surgery in the past 10 days
	Past history of gastrointestinal bleeding
Neurosurgery in the past 2 months	Recent obstetric delivery
Intracranial aneurysm or neoplasm	Prior arterial puncture
	Prior organ biopsy
Proliferative diabetic retinopathy	Serious trauma
	Severe arterial hypertension (systolic pressure >200 mmHg, diastolic pressure >110 mmHg)
	Bleeding diathesis

ANTIPLATELET DRUGS

Antiplatelet agents are gaining an increasing role in clinical medicine. It is now clear that aspirin is valuable in the secondary prevention of vascular disease. Several other agents are being investigated and the sites of action of the antiplatelet drugs are illustrated in Fig. 21.8.

Aspirin Aspirin inhibits platelet cyclo-oxygenase irreversibly, thus reducing the production of platelet thromboxane A_2. It has been suggested that vascular endothelial cyclo-oxygenase is less sensitive to aspirin than platelet cyclo-oxygenase. Low-dose therapy (e.g. 75 mg daily) is more effective than standard doses at enhancing the prostacyclin : thromboxane A_2 ratio and may have a greater antithrombotic effect. It is used in patients who have a history of coronary artery or cerebrovascular disease. It may also be useful in preventing thrombosis in patients with thrombocytosis.

Dipyridamole (Persantin) This drug is a phosphodiesterase inhibitor thought to elevate cyclic adenosine monophosphate (cAMP) levels in circulating platelets which decreases their sensitivity to activating stimuli. Dipyridamole has been shown to reduce thromboembolic complications in patients with prosthetic heart valves and to improve the results in coronary bypass operations.

Sulphinpyrazone This drug is a competitive inhibitor of cyclo-oxygenase. It has been effective in reducing the frequency of blockage in arteriovenous shunts in chronic dialysis patients.

Ticlopidine This is an antiplatelet drug that was used following coronary angioplasty. Side-effects

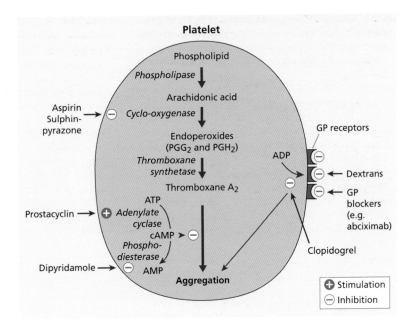

Fig. 21.8 Sites of action of antiplatelet drugs. Aspirin acetylates the enzyme cyclo-oxygenase irreversibly. Sulphinpyrazone inhibits cyclo-oxygenase reversibly. Dipyridamole inhibits phosphodiesterase, increases cyclic adenosine monophosphate (cAMP) levels and inhibits aggregation. Inhibition of adenosine uptake by red cells allows adenosine accumulation in plasma which stimulates platelet adenylate cyclase. Prostacyclin (epoprostenol) stimulates adenylate cyclase. The lipid-soluble β blockers inhibit phospholipase. Calcium channel antagonists block the influx of free calcium ions across the platelet membrane. Dextrans coat the surface interfering with adhesion and aggregation. GP, glycoprotein.

include neutropenia or thrombocytopenia. It has been replaced by clopidogrel.

Clopidogrel This is an antiplatelet agent in use for reduction of ischaemic events in patients with ischaemic stroke, myocardial infarction or peripheral vascular disease. It is used after coronary artery stenting or angioplasty.

Abciximab This drug is a monoclonal antibody which inhibits the platelet GPIIb/IIIa receptor. It is used in conjunction with heparin and aspirin for the prevention of ischaemic complications in high-risk patients undergoing percutaneous transluminal coronary angioplasty. It can be used once only.

Specific antithrombotic agents Recently introduced agents have been developed to alter the balance of physiological prostaglandin metabolism. Intravenous prostacyclin has been used in clinical trials in patients with peripheral vascular disease and thrombotic thrombocytopenic purpura. It has also reduced arteriovenous shunt blockage in haemodialysis patients.

BIBLIOGRAPHY

Baglin T. *et al.* (1998) Guidelines on oral anticoagulation: third edition. *Br. J. Haematol.* **101**, 374–87.

Bertina R.M. *et al.* (1994) Mutation in blood coagulation factor V associated with resistance to activated protein C. *Nature* **369**, 64–7.

British Society for Haematology (1992) Guidelines on the use and monitoring of heparin: second revision. *J. Clin. Pathol.* **46**, 97–103.

Dahlback B. *et al.* (1993) Familial thrombophilia due to poor anticoagulant response to activated protein C. *Proc. Natl. Acad. Sci. USA* **90**, 1004–8.

Epstein F.H. (1998) Homocysteine and atherothrombosis. *N. Engl. J. Med.* **338**, 1042–50.

Guidelines on the investigation and management of the antiphospholipid syndrome (2000) *Br. J. Haematol.* **109**, 704–15.

Hirsh J. and Weitz J. (1999) New antithrombotic agents. *Lancet.* **353**, 1431–5.

Kearon C. and Hirsh J. (1997) Management of anticoagulation before and after elective surgery. *N. Engl. J. Med.* **336**, 1506–11.

Lane D.A. and Grant P.J. (2000) Role of hemostatic gene polymorphisms in venous and arterial thrombotic disease. *Blood* **95**, 1517–32.

Lensing A.W.A. *et al.* (1999) Deep-vein thrombosis. *Lancet* **353**, 479–85.

Levine M. *et al.* (1996) A comparison of low molecular weight heparin administered primarily at home with unfractionated heparin administered in the hospital for proximal deep vein thombosis. *N. Engl. J. Med.* **334**, 677–81.

MacCallum P.K. and Meade T.W. (eds) (1999) Thrombophilia. *Clin. Haematol.* **12**, 329–603.

Meijers J.C.M., Tekelenburg W.L.H., Bouma B.N. *et al.* (2000) High levels of coagulation factor XI as a risk factor for venous thrombosis. *N. Engl. J. Med.* **342**, 696–701.

Perry D.J. (1999) Hyperhomocysteinaemia. *Clin. Haematol.* **12**, 451–78.

Prandoni P. and Mannucci P.M. (1999) Deep-vein thrombosis of the lower limbs: diagnosis and management. *Clin. Haematol.* **12**, 533–44.

Rosendaal F.R. (1999) Venous thrombosis: a multicausal disease. *Lancet* **353**, 1167–73.

Shapiro S.S. (1996) The lupus anticoagulant/antiphopholipid syndrome. *Ann. Rev. Med.* **47**, 533–53.

Simonneau G. *et al.* (1997) A comparison of low molecular weight heparin with unfractionated heparin for acute pulmonary embolism. *N. Engl. J. Med.* **337**, 663–9.

Thorogood M. (1998) Oral contraceptives and thrombosis. *Curr. Opin. Haematol.* **5**, 350–54.

Weitz J. (1997) Low molecular-weight heparins. *N. Engl. J. Med.* **337**, 688–98.

Wood K. (ed) For the British Committee for Standards in Haematology (2000) *Standard Haematology Practice 2: Guidelines in Oral Anticoagulation.* Blackwell Science, Oxford; pp. 104–29.

CHAPTER 22

Haematological changes in systemic disease

ANAEMIA OF CHRONIC DISORDERS

Many of the anaemias seen in clinical practice occur in patients with systemic disorders and are the result of a number of contributing factors. The anaemia of chronic disorders is of central importance and occurs in patients with a variety of chronic inflammatory and malignant diseases (Table 22.1). Usually both the erythrocyte sedimentation rate (ESR) and C-reactive protein (CRP) are raised. It may be complicated by additional features which may be because of disease affecting particularly one or other system.

The characteristic features are as follows:
1 Normochromic, normocytic or mildly microcytic indices (mean corpuscular volume (MCV) 77–82 fl) and red cell morphology (see also p. 38).
2 Mild and non-progressive anaemia (haemoglobin rarely less than 9.0 g/dl) — the severity being related to the severity of the underlying disease.
3 Both the serum iron and total iron-binding capacity (TIBC) are reduced.
4 The serum ferritin is normal or raised.
5 Bone marrow (reticuloendothelial) storage iron is normal but incorporation of iron into erythroblasts is reduced.

The pathogenesis of this anaemia appears to be related to the decreased release of iron from macrophages to plasma and so to erythroblasts, reduced red cell lifespan and an inadequate erythropoietin response to anaemia. The plasma levels of various cytokines, especially interleukin-1 (IL-1), IL-6 and tumour necrosis factor (TNF) are raised and probably reduce erythropoietin secretion. The anaemia is corrected by the successful treatment of the underlying disease. It does not respond to iron therapy despite the low serum iron. Responses to recombinant erythropoietin therapy may be obtained, e.g. in rheumatoid arthritis or cancer, but this alone does not correct the anaemia completely. In many conditions the anaemia is complicated by anaemia from other causes, e.g. iron or folate deficiency, renal failure, bone marrow infiltration, hypersplenism or endocrine abnormality.

MALIGNANT DISEASES (OTHER THAN PRIMARY BONE MARROW DISEASES)

Anaemia

Contributing factors include anaemia of chronic disorders, blood loss and iron deficiency, marrow infiltration (Fig. 22.1) often associated with a leucoerythroblastic blood film (nucleated red cells and granuloctye precursors in the blood film), folate deficiency, haemolysis and marrow suppression from radiotherapy or chemotherapy (Table 22.2). Other causes of a leucoerythroblastic anaemia include myelofibrosis, acute and chronic leukaemias, and severe haemolytic or megalo-blastic anaemia.

Microangiopathic haemolytic anaemia (p. 68) occurs with mucin-secreting adenocarcinoma (Fig. 22.2), particularly of the stomach, lung and

Fig. 22.1 Metastatic carcinoma in bone marrow aspirates: (a) breast; (b) stomach; (c) colon and bone marrow trephine biopsies; (d) prostate; (e) stomach; (f) kidney.

Table 22.1 Causes of anaemia of chronic disorders

Chronic inflammatory diseases
Infectious, e.g. pulmonary abscess, tuberculosis, osteomyelitis, pneumonia, bacterial endocarditis
Non-infectious, e.g. rheumatoid arthritis, systemic lupus erythematosus and other connective tissue diseases, sarcoid, Crohn's disease, cirrhosis

Malignant disease
e.g. carcinoma, lymphoma, sarcoma, myeloma

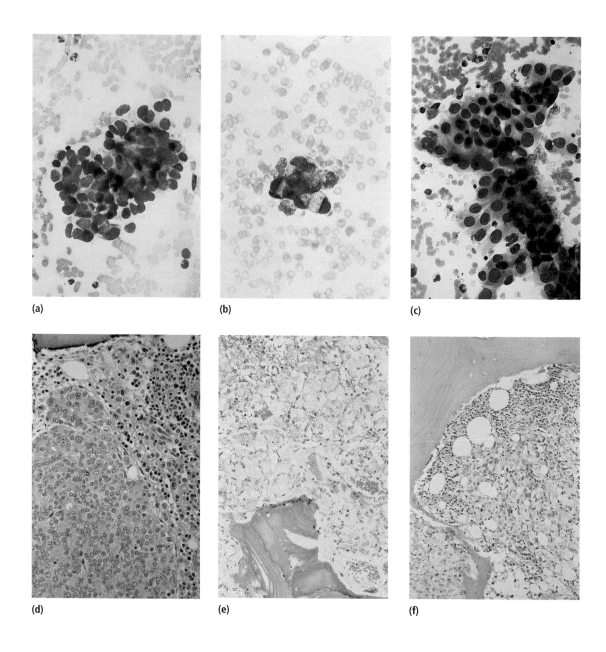

(a)

(b)

(c)

(d)

(e)

(f)

Table 22.2 Haematological abnormalities in malignant disease

Haematological abnormality	Tumour or treatment associated
Pancytopenia	
Marrow hypoplasia	Chemotherapy, radiotherapy
Myelodysplasia	Chemotherapy, radiotherapy
Leucoerythroblastic	Metastases in marrow
Megaloblastic	Folate deficiency
	B_{12} deficiency (carcinoma of stomach)
Red cells	
Anaemia of chronic disorders	Most forms
Iron deficiency anaemia	Especially gastrointestinal, uterine
Pure red cell aplasia	Thymoma
Immune haemolytic anaemia	Lymphoma, ovary, other tumours
Microangiopathic haemolytic anaemia	Mucin-secreting carcinoma
Polycythaemia	Kidney, liver, cerebellum, uterus
White cells	
Neutrophil leucocytosis	Most forms
Leukaemoid reaction	Disseminated tumours, those with necrosis
Eosinophilia	Hodgkin's disease, others
Monocytosis	Various tumours
Platelets and coagulation	
Thrombocytosis	Gastrointestinal tumours with bleeding, others
Disseminated intravascular coagulation	Mucin-secreting carcinoma, prostate
Activation of fibrinolysis	Prostate
Acquired inhibitors of coagulation	Most forms
Paraprotein interfering with platelet function	Lymphomas, myeloma

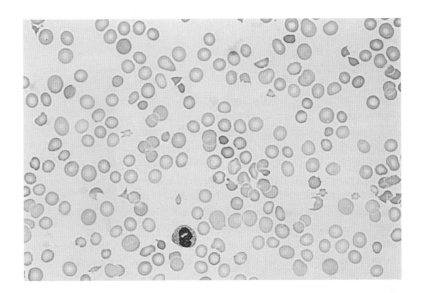

Fig. 22.2 Peripheral blood film in metastatic mucin-secreting adenocarcinoma of the stomach showing red cell polychromasia and fragmentation and thrombocytopenia. The patient had disseminated intravascular coagulation.

breast. Less common forms of anaemia with malignant disease include autoimmune haemolytic anaemia with malignant lymphoma and, rarely, with other tumours; primary red cell aplasia with thymoma or lymphoma; and myelodysplastic syndromes secondary to chemotherapy. There is also an association of pernicious anaemia with carcinoma of the stomach.

The anaemia of malignant disease may respond partly to erythropoietin. Folic acid should only be given if there is definite megaloblastic anaemia caused by the deficiency; it might 'feed' the tumour.

Polycythaemia

Secondary polycythaemia is occasionally associated with renal, hepatic, cerebellar and uterine tumours (p. 231).

White cell changes

Leukaemoid reactions (p. 121) may occur with tumours showing widespread necrosis and inflammation. Hodgkin's disease is associated with a variety of white cell abnormalities including eosinophilia, monocytosis and leucopenia. In non-Hodgkin's lymphoma, malignant cells may circulate in the blood (p. 198).

Platelet and blood coagulation abnormalities

Patients with malignant disease may show either thrombocytosis or thrombocytopenia. Disseminated tumours, particularly mucin-secreting adenocarcinomas, are associated with disseminated intravascular coagulation (DIC) (p. 268) and generalized haemostatic failure. Activation of fibrinolysis occurs in some patients with carcinoma of the prostate. Occasional patients with malignant disease have spontaneous bruising or bleeding caused by an acquired inhibitor of one or other coagulation factor, most frequently factor VIII

or to a paraprotein interfering with platelet function.

RHEUMATOID ARTHRITIS (AND OTHER CONNECTIVE TISSUE DISORDERS)

In patients with rheumatoid arthritis the anaemia of chronic disorders is proportional to the severity of the disease. It is complicated in some patients by iron deficiency caused by gastrointestinal bleeding related to therapy with salicylates, nonsteroidal anti-inflammatory agents or corticosteroids. Bleeding into inflamed joints may also be a factor. Marrow hypoplasia may follow therapy with gold. In Felty's syndrome splenomegaly is associated with neutropenia (Fig. 22.3). Anaemia and thrombocytopenia may also be present. In systemic lupus erythematosus (SLE) there may be

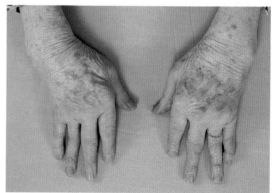

(a)

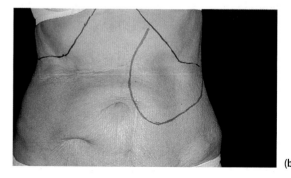

(b)

Fig. 22.3 Felty's disease: (a) the typical deformities of rheumatoid arthritis of the hand and (b) splenomegaly.

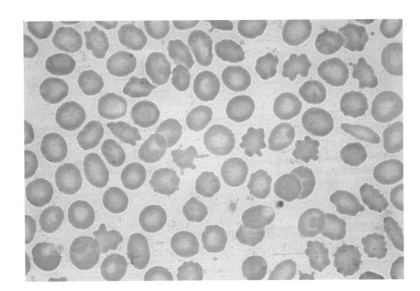

Fig. 22.4 Peripheral blood film in chronic renal failure showing red cell acanthocytosis and numerous 'burr' cells.

anaemia of chronic disorders and 50% of patients are leucopenic with reduced neutrophil and lymphocyte counts often associated with circulating immune complexes. Renal impairment and drug-induced gastrointestinal blood loss also contribute to the anaemia. Autoimmune haemolytic anaemia (typically with immunoglobulin G (IgG) and the C3 component of complement on the surface of the red cells) occurs in 5% of patients and may be the presenting feature of the syndrome. There may be autoimmune thrombocytopenia in 5% of patients. The lupus anticoagulant is described on p. 279. This circulating anticardiolipin interferes with blood coagulation by altering the binding of coagulation factors to platelet phospholipid and predisposes to both arterial and venous thrombosis and recurrent abortions. The antibody may be responsible for a false positive Wassermann reaction. Tests for antinuclear factor (ANF) and anti-DNA antibodies are usually positive.

Patients with temporal arteritis and polymyalgia rheumatica have a markedly elevated ESR, pronounced red cell rouleaux in the blood film and a polyclonal immunoglobulin response. These and other collagen vascular disorders are associated with anaemia of chronic disorders.

RENAL FAILURE

Anaemia

A normochromic anaemia is present in most patients with chronic renal failure. Generally there is a 2 g/dl fall in haemoglobin level for every 10 mmol/l rise in blood urea. There is impaired red cell production as a result of defective erythropoietin secretion (see Fig. 2.5). Uraemic serum has also been shown to contain factors which inhibit proliferation of erythroid progenitors but, in view of the excellent response to erythropoietin in most patients, the clinical relevance of these is doubtful. Variable shortening of red cell lifespan occurs and in severe uraemia the red cells show abnormalities including spicules (spurs) and 'burr' cells (Fig. 22.4). Increased red cell 2,3-diphosphoglycerate (2,3-DPG) levels in response to the anaemia and hyperphosphataemia result in decreased oxygen affinity and a shift of the haemoglobin oxygen dissociation curve to the right (p. 18), which is augmented by uraemic acidosis. The patient's symptoms are therefore relatively mild for the degree of anaemia.

Other factors may complicate the anaemia of

Table 22.3 Haematological abnormalities in renal failure

Anaemia
Reduced erythropoietin production
Aluminium excess in dialysis patients
Anaemia of chronic disorders
Iron deficiency
    blood loss, e.g. dialysis, venesection, defective platelet function
Folate deficiency
    chronic haemodialysis without replacement therapy

Abnormal platelet function

Thrombocytopenia
Immune complex-mediated, e.g. systemic lupus erythematosus,
    polyarteritis nodosa
Some cases of acute nephritis and following allograft
Haemolytic uraemic syndrome and thrombotic thrombocytopenic
    purpura

Thrombosis
Some cases of the nephrotic syndrome

Polycythaemia
In renal allograft recipients
Rarely in renal cell carcinoma, cysts, arterial disease

---

chronic renal failure (Table 22.3). These include the anaemia of chronic disorders, iron deficiency from blood loss during dialysis or caused by bleeding because of defective platelet function, and folate deficiency in some chronic dialysis patients. Aluminium excess in patients on chronic dialysis also inhibits erythropoiesis. Patients with polycystic kidneys usually have retained erythropoietin production and may have less severe anaemia for the degree of renal failure.

Treatment

Erythropoietin therapy has been found to correct the anaemia in patients on dialysis or in chronic renal failure, providing that iron and folate deficiency, aluminium excess and infections have been corrected. The dosage of erythropoietin usually required is 50–150 units/kg three times a week intravenously or by subcutaneous infusion. The response is faster after intravenous administration, but greater with the subcutaneous route. Maintenance by 75 units/kg/week subcutaneously is typical. Complications of therapy have been initial transient flu-like symptoms, hyper-

tension, clotting of the dialysis lines and, rarely, fits. A poor response to erythropoietin suggests iron or folate deficiency, infection, aluminium toxicity or hyperparathyroidism.

Platelet and coagulation abnormalities

A bleeding tendency with purpura, gastrointestinal or uterine bleeding occurs in 30–50% of patients with chronic renal failure and is marked in patients with acute renal failure. The bleeding is out of proportion to the degree of thrombocytopenia and has been associated with abnormal platelet or vascular function which can be reversed by dialysis. Correction of the anaemia with erythropoietin also improves the bleeding tendency. Immune complex-mediated thrombocytopenia occurs in some patients with acute nephritis, SLE and polyarteritis nodosa and also following renal allografts. Renal allografts may also lead to polycythaemia in 10–15% of patients.

The haemolytic uraemic syndrome and thrombotic thrombocytopenic purpura are discussed on p. 255. Patients with the nephrotic syndrome have an increased risk of venous thrombosis.

LIVER DISEASE

The haematological abnormalities in liver disease are listed in Table 22.4. Chronic liver disease is associated with anaemia which is mildly macrocytic and often accompanied by target cells mainly as a result of increased cholesterol in the membrane (Fig. 22.5a). Contributing factors to the anaemia may include blood loss (e.g. bleeding varices) with iron deficiency, dietary folate deficiency and direct suppression of haemopoiesis by alcohol. Alcohol may have an inhibiting effect on folate metabolism and is occasionally associated with (ring) sideroblastic changes which disappear when alcohol is withdrawn.

Haemolytic anaemia may occur in patients with alcohol intoxication (Zieve's syndrome) (Fig. 22.5b) and in Wilson's disease (caused by copper oxidation of red cell membranes) and autoimmune haemolytic anaemia is found in some patients with chronic immune hepatitis. Viral hepatitis (usually non-A, non-B, non-C) is associated with aplastic anaemia.

The acquired coagulation abnormalities associated with liver disease are described on p. 269. There are deficiencies of vitamin K-dependent factors (II, VII, IX and X) and, in severe disease, of factor V and fibrinogen. Thrombocytopenia may occur from hypersplenism or from immune complex-mediated platelet destruction. Abnormalities of platelet function may also be present. Dysfibrinogenaemia with abnormal fibrin polymerization may occur as a result of excess sialic acid in the fibrinogen molecules. A consumptive coagulopathy may be superimposed. These haemostatic defects may contribute to major blood loss from bleeding varices caused by portal hypertension.

Table 22.4 Haematological abnormalities in liver disease

Liver failure ± obstructive jaundice ± portal hypertension
Refractory anaemia—usually mildly macrocytic, often with target cells; may be associated with:
    Blood loss and iron deficiency
    Alcohol (± ring sideroblastic change)
    Folate deficiency
    Haemolysis, e.g. Zieve's syndrome, Wilson's disease, immune
        hypersplenism from portal hypertension
Bleeding tendency
    Deficiency of vitamin K-dependent factors; also of factor V and
        fibrinogen
    Thrombocytopenia hypersplenism, immune platelet function
        defects
    Functional abnormalities of fibrinogen
    Increased fibrinolysis
    Portal hypertension—haemorrhage from varices

Viral hepatitis
Aplastic anaemia

Tumours
Polycythaemia
Neutrophil leucocytosis and leukaemoid reactions

HYPOTHYROIDISM

A moderate anaemia is usual and may be caused by lack of thyroxine. T_3 and T_4 potentiate the action of erythropoietin. There is also a reduced oxygen need and thus reduced erythropoietin secretion. The anaemia is often macrocytic and the MCV falls with thyroxine therapy. Autoimmune thyroid disease, especially myxoedema or Hashimoto's disease, is associated with pernicious anaemia. Iron deficiency may also be present, particularly in women with menorrhagia.

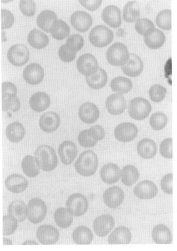
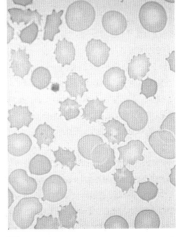

Fig. 22.5 Liver disease: peripheral blood film showing (a) macrocytosis and target cells; and (b) marked acanthocytosis in Zieve's syndrome.

(a)   (b)

Table 22.5 Blood abnormalities associated with infections

Haematological abnormality	Infection associated
Anaemia	
Anaemia of chronic disorders	Chronic infections especially tuberculosis
Aplastic anaemia	Viral hepatitis
Transient red cell aplasia	Human parvovirus
Marrow fibrosis	Tuberculosis
Immune haemolytic anaemia	Infectious mononucleosis, *Mycoplasma pneumoniae*
Direct red cell damage or microangiopathic	Bacterial septicaemia (associated DIC), *Clostridium perfringens*, malaria, bartonellosis
	Viruses—haemolytic-uraemic syndrome and TTP
Hypersplenism	Chronic malaria, tropical splenomegaly syndrome, leishmaniasis, schistosomiasis
White cell changes	
Neutrophil leucocytosis	Acute bacterial infections
Leukaemoid reactions	Severe bacterial infections particularly in infants
	Tuberculosis
Eosinophilia	Parasitic diseases, e.g. hookworm, filariasis, schistosomiasis, trichinosis, etc.
	Recovery from acute infections
Monocytosis	Chronic bacterial infections: tuberculosis, brucellosis, bacterial endocarditis, typhoid
Neutropenia	Viral infections—HIV, hepatitis, influenza
	Fulminant bacterial infections, e.g. typhoid, miliary tuberculosis
Lymphocytosis	Infectious mononucleosis, toxoplasmosis, cytomegalovirus, rubella, viral hepatitis, pertussis, tuberculosis, brucellosis
Lymphopenia	HIV infection
	Legionella pneumonophilia
Thrombocytopenia	
Megakaryocytic depression, immune complex-mediated and direct interaction with platelets	Acute viral infections particularly in children, e.g. measles, varicella, rubella, malaria, severe bacterial infection

DIC, disseminated intravascular coagulation; HIV, human immunodeficiency virus; TTP, thrombotic thrombocytopenic purpura.

INFECTIONS

Haematological abnormality is usually present in patients with infections of all types (Table 22.5).

Bacterial infections

Acute bacterial infections are the most common cause of neutrophil leucocytosis. Toxic granulation, Doehle bodies and metamyelocytes may be present in the blood. Leukaemoid reactions with a white cell count $> 50 \times 10^9/l$ and granulocyte precursors in the blood may occur in severe infec-

tions, particularly in infants and young children. The neutrophil alkaline phosphatase (NAP) score is raised in contrast to the low NAP score in chronic myeloid leukaemia. Mild anaemia is common if the infection is prolonged. Severe haemolytic anaemia occurs in bacterial septicaemias particularly due to Gram-negative organisms, where there is usually associated DIC (p. 268).

Clostridium perfringens organisms produce an α toxin, a lecithinase acting directly on the circulating red cells (Fig. 22.6). Haemolysis in bartonellosis (Oroya fever) is caused by direct red cell infection. With severe acute bacterial infections there may be thrombocytopenia. *Mycoplasma*

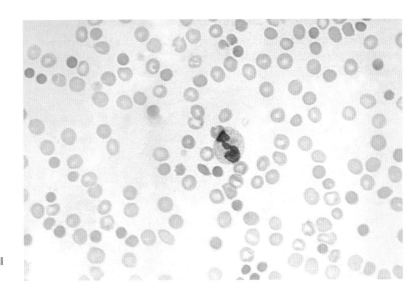

Fig. 22.6 Peripheral blood film in a patient with haemolytic anaemia in clostridial septicaemia showing red cell contraction and spherocytosis.

pneumoniae infections are associated with autoimmune haemolytic anaemia of the 'cold' type (p. 66).

Chronic bacterial infections are associated with the anaemia of chronic disorders. In tuberculosis, additional factors in the pathogenesis of anaemia include marrow replacement and fibrosis associated with miliary disease and reactions to antituberculous therapy (e.g. isoniazid is a pyridoxine antagonist and may cause sideroblastic anaemia). Disseminated tuberculosis is associated with leukaemoid reactions and patients with involvement of bone marrow may show leucoerythroblastic changes in the peripheral blood film.

Viral infections

Acute viral diseases are often associated with a mild anaemia. An immune haemolytic anaemia with an anti-i autoantibody is associated with infectious mononucleosis (p. 138). Viral infections, as well as syphilis, have been associated with paroxysmal cold haemoglobinuria (p. 67). Viruses have also been linked to the pathogenesis of the haemolytic uraemic syndrome, thrombotic thrombocytopenic purpura (pp. 255 and 257) and the haemophagocytic syndrome (pp. 125). Aplas-

tic anaemia may occur with viral A or more usually non-A, non-B, non-C hepatitis. Transient red cell aplasia is associated with human parvovirus infection and this may result in severe anaemia in patients with a haemolytic anaemia because of the shortened red cell survival, e.g. in hereditary spherocytosis or sickle cell disease (see p. 96).

Acute thrombocytopenia is not uncommon in rubella, morbilli and varicella infections. Rubella and cytomegalovirus (CMV) infections may cause a reactive lymphocytosis similar to that found in infectious mononucleosis. CMV may be responsible for a post-transfusion mononucleosis-like syndrome, CMV being transmitted by leucocytes. CMV infections in infants are associated with massive hepatosplenomegaly. In bone marrow transplant recipients or other immunosuppressed patients CMV infections may cause pancytopenia as well as other severe disorders, e.g. pneumonitis or hepatitis (p. 108). Haematological abnormalities associated with human immunodeficiency virus (HIV) infection and acquired immune deficiency syndrome (AIDS) are dealt with in Chapter 10.

Malaria

Some degree of haemolysis is seen in all types of malarial infection. The most severe abnormalities are found in *Plasmodium falciparum* infections

(Fig. 22.7). In the worst cases DIC occurs and intra-vascular haemolysis is marked with haemo-globinuria. This may be associated with quinine therapy ('blackwater fever'). Thrombocytopenia is commonly found in acute malaria. Patients with chronic malaria have an anaemia of chronic disorders; hypersplenism may contribute to the anaemia and result in moderate thrombocyto-penia and neutropenia. Tropical splenomegaly (p. 303) is probably a chronic immune reaction to malaria. Dyserythropoiesis in the marrow, folate deficiency and protein-calorie malnutrition may contribute to the anaemia.

Toxoplasmosis

Toxoplasmosis in children and adults is asso-ciated with lymphadenopathy and large numbers of atypical lymphocytes in the blood. Congenital disease may be confused with hydrops fetalis in a severely anaemic hydropic infant with gross hepatosplenomegaly, thrombocytopenia or a leucoerythroblastic blood film.

Kala-azar (visceral leishmaniasis)

The visceral form of leishmaniasis is associated with pancytopenia, hepatosplenomegaly and lymphadenopathy. Bone marrow or splenic

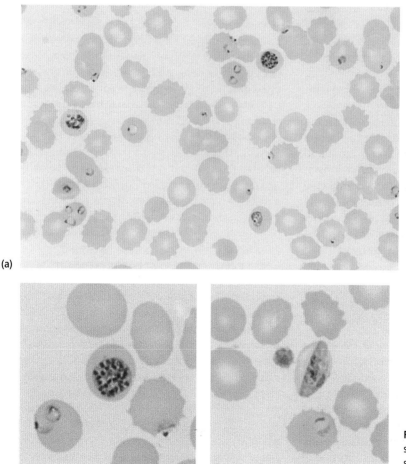

(a)

(b)

(c)

Fig. 22.7 Malaria: peripheral blood in severe *Plasmodium falciparum* infection showing: (a) many ring forms and a meront; and at higher magnification: (b) a meront, and (c) a gametocyte.

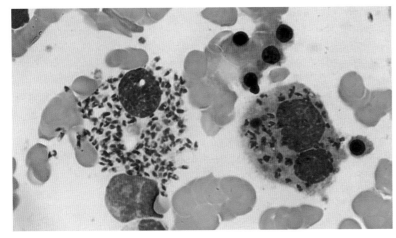 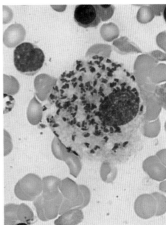

Fig. 22.8 Kala-azar: bone marrow aspirates showing macrophages containing Leishman–Donovan bodies.

aspirates may show large numbers of parasitized macrophages (Fig. 22.8).

Other parasitic diseases

In the acute phase of both African and South American trypanosomiasis, organisms are found in the peripheral blood (Fig. 22.9). Microfilaria of bancroftian filariasis and loiasis are also detected during blood film examination (Fig. 22.10). In chronic schistosomiasis, hypersplenism follows the splenic enlargement associated with portal hypertension. In many parasitic diseases there is eosinophilia (Table 22.5).

SPLENOMEGALY

With few exceptions disease involvement of the spleen results in its enlargement. Splenomegaly is consequently a frequent and important clinical sign and a palpable spleen is at least twice its normal size. Table 22.6 presents a simple classification of splenomegaly. In some of the diseases listed splenic enlargement is only found occasionally and when it occurs it is seldom marked, e.g. in acute septicaemias, the megaloblastic anaemias, most collagen disorders and amyloidosis.

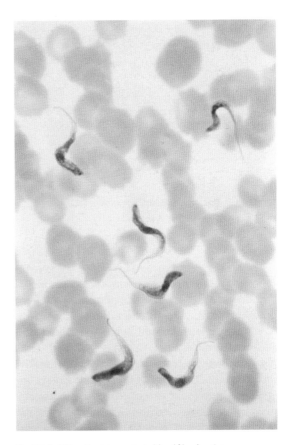

Fig. 22.9 African trypanosomiasis: blood film showing *Trypanosoma brucei*.

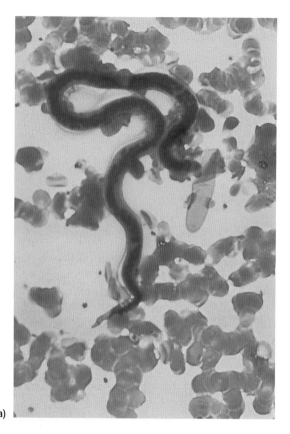

(a)

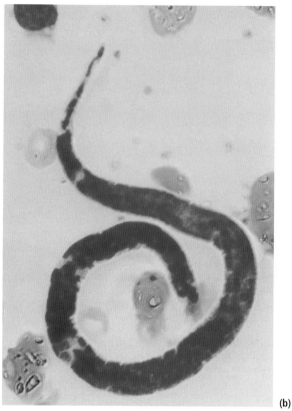

(b)

Fig. 22.10 Peripheral blood films showing microfilariae of (a) *Wuchereria bancrofti* and (b) *Loa loa*.

The relative incidence of the causes of splenomegaly are subject to enormous geographical variation. In the UK the leukaemias, malignant lymphomas, myeloproliferative disorders, haemolytic anaemias and portal hypertension account for most cases. Infective endocarditis is also relatively frequent. In tropical countries, the incidence of these haematological causes of splenomegaly is far exceeded by the frequency of splenic enlargement caused by the parasitic tropical infections: malaria, leishmaniasis and schistosomiasis. Portal hypertension remains an important cause of splenomegaly in most tropical countries but is especially prevalent in north-eastern India and southern China. The 'tropical splenomegaly syndrome' is seen in large numbers of patients in New Guinea and Central Africa. Among the causes of splenomegaly as a result of blood disorders the haemoglobinopathies become relatively more important in some countries. Haemoglobin C disease in West Africa and haemoglobin E disease in the Far East are associated with splenomegaly and the thalassaemia syndromes have a wide distribution throughout the tropics. Because of the multiplicity of factors responsible for splenomegaly in such countries, more than one pathology may contribute to splenomegaly in a particular patient.

Hypersplenism: haematological effects of splenomegaly

Splenic enlargement is asociated with anaemia, leucopenia and thrombocytopenia (pancytopenia) caused by an enhanced capacity of the

Table 22.6 Causes of splenomegaly

Haematological
Chronic myeloid leukaemia*
Chronic lymphocytic leukaemia
Acute leukaemia
Malignant lymphoma*
Chronic myelofibrosis*
Polycythaemia vera
Hairy cell leukaemia
Thalassaemia major or intermedia*
Sickle cell anaemia (before splenic infarction)
Haemolytic anaemias
Megaloblastic anaemia

Portal hypertension
Cirrhosis
Hepatic, portal, splenic vein thrombosis

Storage diseases
Gaucher's disease*
Niemann–Pick disease
Histiocytosis X

Systemic diseases
Sarcoidosis
Amyloidosis
Collagen diseases — systemic lupus erythematosus, rheumatoid
  arthritis
Systemic mastocytosis

Infections
Acute
  septicaemia, bacterial endocarditis, typhoid, infectious
    mononucleosis
Chronic
  tuberculosis, brucellosis, syphilis, tropical:* malaria,*
    leishmaniasis,* schistosomiasis

* Possible causes of massive (> 20 cm) splenomegaly.

enlarged spleen for pooling, sequestering and destroying blood cells and also leading to an increased plasma volume. The term 'hypersplenism' is used to describe this reduction in blood cell counts. In many conditions causing splenomegaly, factors other than the enlarged spleen may also contribute to the pancytopenia. Many haemolytic anaemias and myeloproliferative or lymphoproliferative disorders are associated with splenic enlargement. Although intrinsic red cell defects, immunological abnormalities or bone marrow failure are the primary causes of the reduction of blood elements in these disorders the associated splenomegaly may also contribute to the observed cytopenias.

INBORN ERRORS OF METABOLISM

Gaucher's, Tay–Sachs and Niemann–Pick diseases all result from hereditary deficiency of the enzymes required for glycolipid breakdown.

Gaucher's disease

Gaucher's disease is an uncommon autosomal recessive disorder characterized by an accumulation of glucocerebroside in reticuloendothelial cells as a result of deficiency of lysosomal glucocerebrosidase. Three types occur: a chronic adult type (type I); an acute infantile neuronopathic type (type II); and a subacute neuronopathic type with onset in childhood or adolescence (type III). Type I is caused by a variety of mutations in the glucocerebrosidase gene, one type of which is particularly common in Ashkenazi Jews and explains the high incidence of the disease in this group. In type I the outstanding physical sign is splenomegaly. Moderate liver enlargement and pingueculae (conjunctival deposits) are other characteristic findings. In many cases bone deposits cause bone pain and pathological fractures. Expansion of the lower end of the femur may produce the 'Erlenmeyer flask deformity' (Fig. 22.11c).

The clinical manifestations are caused by the accumulation of glucocerebroside-laden macrophages in the spleen, liver and bone marrow (Fig. 22.11a,b,c). Gaucher's disease at all ages is commonly associated with marked anaemia, leucopenia and thrombocytopenia occurring singly or in combination. Splenectomy can result in haematological improvement but following this operation there is often increased deposition of cerebroside in extrasplenic tissue, particularly bones. Diagnosis is made by assay of white cell glucocerebrosidase and DNA analysis. Lysosomal enyzmes, chitotriosidase and acid phosphatase are raised and useful in monitoring therapy. Enzyme replacement therapy with glucocerebrosidase either purified from placenta or

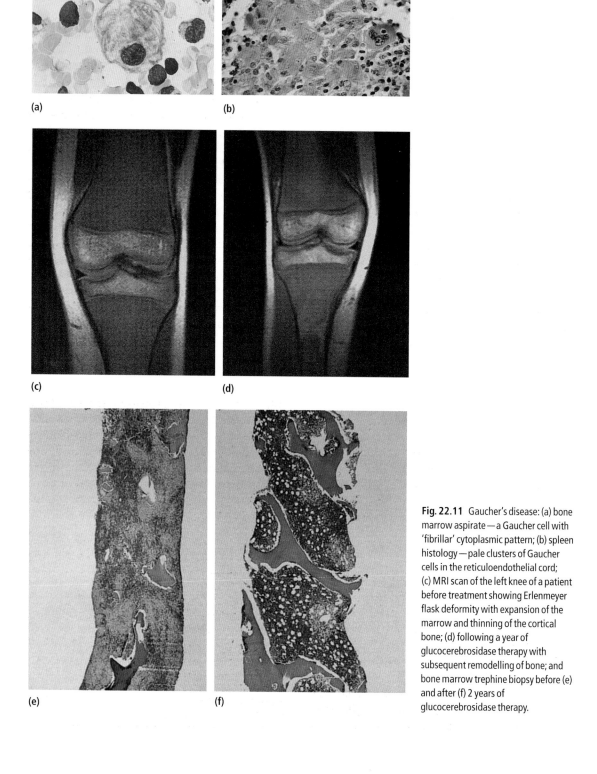

Fig. 22.11 Gaucher's disease: (a) bone marrow aspirate—a Gaucher cell with 'fibrillar' cytoplasmic pattern; (b) spleen histology—pale clusters of Gaucher cells in the reticuloendothelial cord; (c) MRI scan of the left knee of a patient before treatment showing Erlenmeyer flask deformity with expansion of the marrow and thinning of the cortical bone; (d) following a year of glucocerebrosidase therapy with subsequent remodelling of bone; and bone marrow trephine biopsy before (e) and after (f) 2 years of glucocerebrosidase therapy.

made by recombinant technology is very effective in treating the disease with shrinkage of spleen, rise in blood count and improved bone structure (Fig. 22.11d, f). Stem cell transplantation has been carried out successfully in severely affected patients, usually with type II or III disease.

Niemann–Pick disease

Niemann–Pick disease shows certain clinical and pathological similarities to Gaucher's disease. It is caused by a sphingomyelinase deficiency. The majority of patients are infants who die in the first few years of life although occasional patients survive to adult life. Massive hepatosplenomegaly occurs and there is usually lung and nervous system involvement with retarded physical and mental development. A 'cherry-red' spot is commonly seen in the retina of affected infants. Pancytopenia is a regular feature and in marrow aspirates 'foam cells' of similar size to Gaucher cells are seen. Chemical analysis of the tissues reveals that the disorder is caused by an accumulation of sphingomyelin and cholesterol.

TROPICAL SPLENOMEGALY SYNDROME

A syndrome of massive splenomegaly of uncertain aetiology has been frequently found in many malarious zones of the tropics including Uganda, Nigeria, New Guinea and the Congo. Smaller numbers of patients with this disorder are seen in southern Arabia, the Sudan and Zambia. Previously such terms as 'big spleen disease', 'cryptogenic splenomegaly' and 'African macroglobulinaemia' have been used to describe this syndrome.

While it seems probable that malaria is the fundamental cause of tropical splenomegaly syndrome, this disease is not the result of active malarial infection as parasitaemia is usually scanty and malarial pigment is not found in biopsy material from the liver and spleen. The available evidence suggests that an abnormal host response to the continual presence of malarial antigen results in a reactive and relatively benign lymphoproliferative disorder which predominantly affects the liver and spleen.

Splenomegaly is usually gross and the liver is also enlarged. Portal hypertension may be a feature. The anaemia is often severe and the lowest haemoglobin levels are found in subjects with the largest spleens. While leucopenia is usual, some patients develop a marked lymphocytosis. The moderate degree of thrombocytopenia present does not often cause spontaneous bleeding. Serum IgM levels are high and fluorescent techniques reveal high titres of malarial antibody.

Although splenectomy corrects the pancytopenia there is an increased risk of fulminant malarial infection. Trials of antimalarial prophylaxis, e.g. proguanil and other antimalarial drugs, have proved successful in the management of many affected patients supporting the view that a continuing presence of malarial antigen is needed for the perpetuation of the lymphoproliferation associated with this syndrome. Resistant cases have also been treated successfully with chemotherapy.

SPLENECTOMY AND HYPOSPLENISM

Splenectomy is undertaken in a number of disorders (Table 22.7) and the effects often depend on the underlying disease. Functional hyposplenism may also occur in a variety of diseases including sickle cell disease and gluten-induced enteropathy (Table 22.8). Characteristic changes occur in the blood irrespective of the underlying pathology (Fig. 22.12).

Table 22.7 Indications for elective splenectomy (some cases only)

Chronic immune thrombocytopenia (failed steroids)
Haemolytic anaemia
Hereditary spherocytosis
Autoimmune haemolytic anaemia (failed steroids)
Thalassaemia major or intermedia
Chronic lymphocytic leukaemia
Lymphoma
Myelofibrosis
Tropical splenomegaly
Systemic mast cell syndrome

Table 22.8 Causes of hyposplenism and blood film features

Causes	Blood film features
Splenectomy	**Red cells**
Sickle cell disease	Target cells
Essential thrombocythaemia	Acanthocytes
Adult gluten-induced	Irregularly contracted or crenated
enteropathy	cells
Dermatitis herpetiformis	Howell–Jolly bodies (DNA remnants)
Rarely	Siderotic (iron) granules
ulcerative colitis	(Pappenheimer bodies)
Crohn's disease	**White cells**
	± Mild lymphocytosis, monocytosis
	Platelets
	± Thrombocytosis

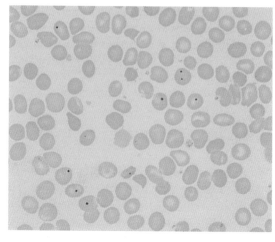

Fig. 22.12 Splenic atrophy: peripheral blood film showing Howell–Jolly bodies, Pappenheimer bodies and misshapen cells.

Haematological effects

Red cell changes

The changes in red cell morphology include the presence of Howell–Jolly bodies and Pappenheimer (siderotic) granules (p. 24) in some of the cells and the appearance of target cells (Fig. 22.12 and Table 22.8). In a proportion of subjects irregularly contracted or crenated acanthocytic forms are also a feature. Occasional erythroblasts may be seen. These red cell changes are often referred to as hyposplenism (Table 22.8). The presence of red cell inclusions reflects the absence of the splenic 'pitting' function.

Leucocyte changes

After splenectomy there is a rise in the total leucocyte count. A neutrophil leucocytosis in the immediate postoperative period is, in the majority of subjects, later replaced by a small but significant and permanent increase in both lymphocytes and monocytes.

In response to infection, splenectomized subjects produce a greater leucocytosis than persons with intact spleens and often there is a marked left shift in the differential leucocyte count with myelocytes and occasionally more primitive cells.

Platelet changes

The spleen normally pools a third of the circulating platelets. In the immediate postoperative period in uncomplicated splenectomized patient, the platelet count rises steeply to a maximum of usually less than 1000×10^9/l with a peak at 7–12 days. The thrombocytosis is usually transitory and a fall to a level one-third higher than in normal subjects over the following 1–2 months is the rule. Occasional large and bizarre platelets can be seen in the blood films of many splenectomized subjects; their presence suggests that these particular platelets are normally removed by the spleen. In a number of patients thrombocytosis persists indefinitely after splenectomy and this appears to be usually a consequence of continuing anaemia with a hypercellular marrow.

Immunological effects and infection prophylaxis

The spleen plays an important part in immunoglobulin synthesis, and a fall in the IgM fraction of the serum immunoglobulins is commonly found postsplenectomy.

Fulminant, potentially life-threatening infection is a major long-term risk after splenectomy and in those with hyposplenism. Infection with encapsulated bacteria such as *Streptococcus pneu-*

moniae, Haemophilus influenzae type b and *Neisseria meningitidis* are a particular risk. Individuals are also at significantly increased risk of severe malarial infection.

Pneumococcal vaccination should be given to all hyposplenic patients who have not received it and preferably 1 month before splenectomy. Reimmunization is recommended every 5–10 years. In addition, patients not previously immunized should receive *Haemophilus influenzae* type b (HIB) vaccine. Life-long prophylactic antibiotics should be offered in all cases. It is particularly vital in children aged up to 16. Typical regimes for adults would include phenoxymethylpenicillin 250 mg 12-hourly or erythromycin 250 mg daily. It is also useful for patients to have a store of antibiotics to keep at home to take if they develop an acute febrile illness.

NON-SPECIFIC MONITORING OF SYSTEMIC DISEASE

The inflammatory response to tissue injury includes changes in plasma concentrations of proteins known as acute phase proteins. These proteins include fibrinogen and other clotting factors, complement components and CRP (p. 306), haptoglobin, serum amyloid A (SAA) protein, ferritin and others. The rise in these liver-derived proteins is part of a wider response which includes fever, leucocytosis and increased immune reactivity. The acute phase response is mediated by cytokines, e.g. IL-1 (see Fig. 1.5) and TNF, released from macrophages and possibly other cells. Patients with chronic disease may show periodic or continuous evidence of the acute phase response depending upon the extent of inflammation. Quantitative measurements of acute phase proteins are valuable indicators of the presence and extent of inflammation and of its response to treatment. When short-term (less than 24 h) changes in the inflammatory response are expected CRP is the test of choice. Long-term changes in the acute phase proteins are monitored by either the ESR or plasma viscosity. These tests are influenced by plasma proteins that are either slowly responding acute phase reactants, e.g. fibrinogen, or are not acute phase proteins, e.g. immunoglobulins.

Erythrocyte sedimentation rate

This commonly used but non-specific test measures the speed of sedimentation of red cells in plasma over a period of 1 h. The speed is mainly dependent on the plasma concentration of large proteins, e.g. fibrinogen and immunoglobulins. The normal range in men is 1–5 mm/h and in women 5–15 mm/h but there is a progressive increase in old age. The ESR is raised in a wide variety of systemic inflammatory and neoplastic diseases and in pregnancy. It is useful for diagnosing and monitoring temporal arteritis and polymyalgia rheumatica and for monitoring patients with Hodgkin's disease. High values (>100 mm/h) have a 90% predictive value for serious disease including infections, collagen vascular disease or malignancy (particularly myeloma). A raised ESR is associated with marked rouleaux formation of red cells in the peripheral blood film (see Fig. 16.5). Changes in the ESR can be used to monitor the response to therapy.

Lower than expected readings occur in polycythaemia vera because of the high red cell concentration. Higher than expected values may occur in severe anaemia because of the low red cell concentration.

Plasma viscosity

In many laboratories measurement of ESR has been replaced by plasma viscosity measurement. Plasma viscosity is affected by the concentration of plasma proteins of large molecular size, especially those with pronounced axial asymmetry—fibrinogen and some immunoglobulins. Normal values at room temperature are usually in the range of 1.50–1.70 mPa/s. Lower levels are found in neonates because of lower levels of proteins particularly fibrinogen. Viscosity increases only slightly in the elderly as fibrinogen increases. There is no difference in values between men and women. Other advantages over the ESR test in-

Table 22.9 Advantages and disadvantages of the tests used to monitor the acute phase response

Advantages	Disadvantages
CRP*	
Specific test of acute phase protein	More than one protein required to measure acute (CRP) and chronic inflammation
Fast response (6 h) to change in disease activity	Costly when assayed in small numbers
High sensitivity — owing to large incremental change	Sophisticated equipment and antisera required
Can be measured on stored serum	
Small sample volumes	
Automated analysis	
ESR and plasma viscosity	
Useful in chronic disease	Not sensitive to acute changes (<24 h)
ESR inexpensive, easy, no electrical power required	Not specific for acute phase response
Plasma viscosity — result obtained quickly (15 min)	Slow to change with alteration in disease activity and insensitive to small changes in activity
Plasma viscosity not affected by anaemia	Fresh samples (<2 h) required for ESR

* C-reactive protein (CRP) is normally present in low concentrations (<5 mg/l). Levels are not influenced by anaemia, pregnancy or heart failure. During severe acute infection the plasma concentration may rise 100-fold.
ESR, erythrocyte sedimentation rate.

clude independence from the effects of anaemia and results that are available within 15 min.

C-reactive protein

Phylogenetically CRP is a crude 'early' immunoglobulin which initiates the inflammatory reaction. CRP–antigen complexes can substitute for antibody in the fixation of Clq and trigger the complement cascade initiating the inflammatory response to antigens or tissue damage, Subsequent binding of C3b on the surface of microorganisms opsonizes them for phagocytosis.

After tissue injury, an increase in CRP, SAA protein and other acute phase reactants may be detected within 6–10 h. Increase in fibrinogen may not occur until 24–48 h following injury. Immunoassays of CRP are now widely used for early detection of acute inflammation or tissue injury and for the monitoring of remission, e.g. response of infection to an antibiotic.

Table 22.9 lists the advantages and disadvantages of the tests used to assess the acute phase response.

BIBLIOGRAPHY

Bain B.J., Clark D.M. and Lampert I.A. (1992) *Diagnostic Bone Marrow Pathology*. Blackwell Scientific Publications, Oxford.

Balicki D. *et al.* (1995) Gaucher disease. *Medicine* **74**, 305–23.

Beutler E. (1997) Gaucher disease. *Curr. Opin. Haematol.* **4**, 19–23.

Bowdler A.J. (ed.) (1990) *The Spleen: Structure, Function and Clinical Significance*. Chapman & Hall, London.

Frenkel E.P. *et al.* (1996) Anemia of malignancy. *Hematol. Oncol. Clin. North Am.* **10**, 861–73.

Lowe G.D. (1994) Should plasma viscosity replace the ESR? *Br. J. Haematol.* **86**, 6–11.

Mehta A.B. and McIntyre N. (1998) Hematological disorders in liver disease. *Forum* **8.1**, 8–25.

Phillips R.E. and Pavsol G. (1992) Anaemia of *Plasmodium falciparum* malaria. *Clin. Haematol.* **5**, 315–30.

Spivak J.L. (2000) The blood in systemic diseases. *Lancet* **355**, 1707–12.

Wickramasinghe S.N. (ed.) (2000) Haematological aspects of infection. *Clin. Haematol.* **13**, 151–326.

Working Party of the BCSH. (1996) Guidelines for the prevention and treatment of infection in patients with an absent or dysfunctional spleen. *Br. Med. J.* **312**, 430–4.

RED CELL ANTIGENS AND BLOOD GROUP ANTIBODIES

Approximately 400 red blood cell group antigens have been described. The clinical significance of blood groups in blood transfusion is that individuals who lack a particular blood group antigen may produce antibodies reacting with that antigen which may lead to a transfusion reaction. The different blood group antigens vary greatly in their clinical significance with the ABO and rhesus (Rh) groups being the most important. Some other systems are listed in Table 23.1.

Blood group antibodies

Naturally occurring antibodies occur in the plasma of subjects who lack the corresponding antigen and who have not been transfused or been pregnant. The most important are anti-A and anti-B. They are usually immunoglobulin M (IgM), and react optimally at cold temperatures (4°C) so, although reactive at 37°C, are called cold antibodies.

Immune antibodies develop in response to the introduction—by transfusion or by transplacental passage during pregnancy—of red cells possessing antigens which the subject lacks. These antibodies are commonly IgG, although some IgM antibodies may also develop—usually in the early phase of an immune response. Immune antibodies react optimally at 37°C (warm antibodies). Only IgG antibodies are capable of transplacental passage from mother to fetus. The most important immune antibody is the Rh antibody, anti-D.

ABO system

This consists of three allelic genes: A, B and O. The A and B genes control the synthesis of specific enzymes responsible for the addition of single carbohydrate residues (N-acetyl galactosamine for group A and D-galactose for group B) to a basic antigenic glycoprotein or glycolipid with a terminal sugar L-fucose on the red cell, known as the H substance (Fig. 23.1). The O gene is an amorph and does not transform the H substance. Although there are six possible genotypes, the absence of a specific anti-O prevents the serological recognition of more than four phenotypes (Table 23.2). The two major subgroups of A (A_1 and A_2) complicate the issue but are of minor clinical significance. A_2 cells react more weakly than A_1 cells with anti-A and patients who are A_2B can be wrongly grouped as B.

The A, B and H antigens are present on most body cells including white cells and platelets. In the 80% of the population who possess secretor genes, these antigens are also found in soluble form in secretions and body fluids, e.g. plasma, saliva, semen and sweat.

Naturally occurring antibodies to A and/or B antigens are found in the plasma of subjects whose red cells lack the corresponding antigen (Table 23.2 and Fig. 23.2).

Rh system

The Rh blood group locus is composed of two related structural genes, *RhD* and *RhCE*, which encode the membrane proteins that carry the D, Cc and Ee antigens. The *RhD* gene may be either present or absent, giving the Rh D+ or Rh D– phenotype respectively. Alternative RNA splicing from the *RhCE* gene generates two proteins, which encode the C, c, E or e antigens (Fig. 23.3). A shortened nomenclature for Rh phenotype is commonly used (Table 23.3).

Rh antibodies rarely occur naturally; most are immune, i.e. they result from previous transfusion or pregnancy. Anti-D is responsible for most of the clinical problems associated with the system and a simple subdivision of subjects into Rh D positive and Rh D negative using anti-D is sufficient for routine clinical purposes. Anti-C, anti-c, anti-E and anti-e are occasionally seen and may cause both transfusion reactions and haemolytic disease of the newborn. Anti-d does not exist. Rh haemolytic disease of the newborn is described in Chapter 24.

Other blood group systems

Other blood group systems are less frequently of

Table 23.1 Clinically important blood group systems

Systems	Frequency of antibodies	Cause of haemolytic transfusion reaction	Cause of haemolytic disease of newborn
ABO	Very common	Yes (common)	Yes (usually mild)
Rh	Common	Yes (common)	Yes
Kell	Occasional	Yes (occasional)	Yes
Duffy	Occasional	Yes (occasional)	Yes (occasional)
Kidd	Occasional	Yes (occasional)	Yes (occasional)
Lutheran	Rare	Yes (rare)	No
Lewis	Occasional	Yes (rare)	No
P	Occasional	Yes (rare)	Yes (rare)
MN	Rare	Yes (rare)	Yes (rare)
Li	Rare	Unlikely	No

Table 23.2 The ABO blood group system

Phenotype	Genotype	Antigens	Naturally occurring antibodies	Frequency (UK) (%)
O	OO	O	Anti-A, anti-B	46
A	AA or AO	A	Anti-B	42
B	BB or BO	B	Anti-A	9
AB	AB	AB	None	3

Fig. 23.1 Structure of ABO blood group antigens. Each consists of a chain of sugars attached to lipids or proteins which are an integral part of the cell membrane. The H antigen of the O blood group has a terminal fucose (fuc). The A antigen has an additional *N*-acetyl galactosamine (galnac), and the B antigen has an additional galactose (gal). glu, glucose.

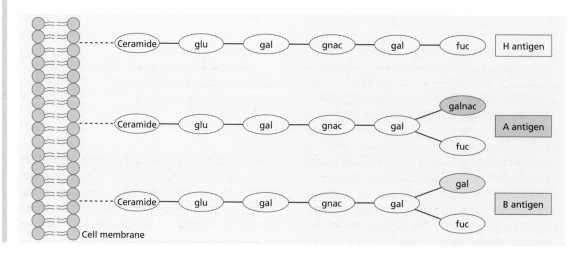

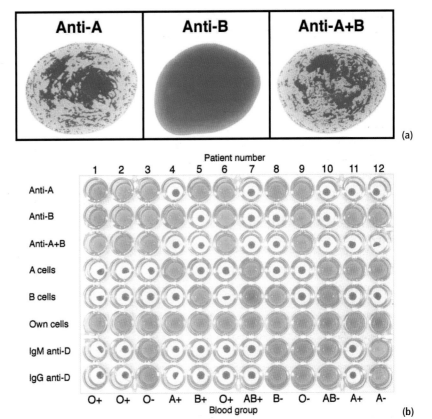

(a)

(b)

Fig. 23.2 (a) The ABO grouping in a group A patient. The red cells suspended in saline agglutinate in the presence of anti-A or anti-A + B (serum from a group O patient). (b) Routine grouping in a 96-well microplate. Positive reactions show as sharp agglutinates; in negative reactions the cells are dispersed. Rows 1–3, patient cells against antisera; rows 4–6, patient sera against known cells; rows 7–8, anti-D against patient cells.

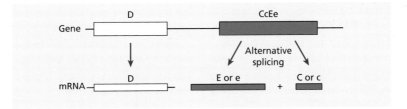

Fig. 23.3 Molecular genetics of the rhesus blood group. The locus consists of two closely linked genes, *RhD* and *RhCcEe*. The *RhD* gene codes for a single protein which contains the RhD antigen whereas *RhCcEe* mRNA undergoes alternative splicing to three transcripts. One of these encodes the E or e antigen whereas the other two (only one is shown) contain the C or c epitope. A polymorphism at position 226 of the *RhCcEe* gene determines the Ee antigen status whereas the C or c antigens are determined by a four amino acid allelic difference. Some individuals do not have an *RhD* gene and are therefore RhD negative.

clinical importance. Although naturally occurring antibodies of the P, Lewis and MN system are not uncommon they usually only react at low temperatures and hence are of no clinical consequence. Immune antibodies against antigens of these systems are detected infrequently. Many of the antigens are of low antigenicity and others (e.g. Kell), although comparatively immunogenic, are of relatively low frequency and therefore provide few opportunities for isoimmunization except in multiply transfused patients.

Table 23.3 The Rh system of genotypes

CDE nomenclature	Short symbol	Caucasian frequency (%)	Rh D status
cde/cde	rr	15	Negative
CDe/cde	R_1r	32	Positive
CDe/CDe	R_1R_1	17	Positive
cDE/cde	R_2r	13	Positive
CDe/cDE	R_1R_2	14	Positive
cDE/cDE	R_2R_2	4	Positive
Other genotypes		5	Positive (almost all)

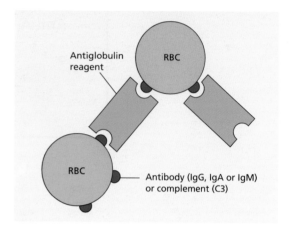

Fig. 23.4 The antiglobulin test for antibody or complement on the surface of red blood cells (RBC). The antihuman globulin (Coombs) reagent may be broad spectrum or specific for immunoglobulin G (IgG), IgM, IgA or complement (C3).

TECHNIQUES IN BLOOD GROUP SEROLOGY

The most important technique is based on the agglutination of red blood cells. Saline agglutination is important in detecting IgM antibodies, usually at room temperature and 4°C, e.g. anti-A, anti-B (Fig. 23.2). Addition of colloid to the incubation or proteolytic enzyme treatment of red cells increases the sensitivity of the indirect antiglobulin test, as does low ionic strength saline (LISS). These latter methods can detect a range of IgG antibodies.

The antiglobulin (Coombs) test is a fundamental and widely used test in both blood group serology and general immunology. Antihuman globulin (AHG) is produced in animals following the injection of human globulin, purified complement or specific immunoglobulin (e.g. IgG, IgA or IgM). Monoclonal preparations are also now available. When AHG is added to human red cells coated with immunoglobulin or complement components, agglutination of the red cells indicates a positive test (Fig. 23.4).

The antiglobulin test may be either direct or indirect. The direct antiglobulin test is used for detecting antibody or complement on the red cell surface where sensitization has occurred *in vivo*. The AHG reagent is added to washed red cells and agglutination indicates a positive test. A positive test occurs in haemolytic disease of the newborn, autoimmune or drug-induced immune haemolytic anaemia and haemolytic transfusion reactions.

The indirect antiglobulin test is used to detect antibodies that have coated the red cells *in vitro*. It is a two-stage procedure: the first step involves the incubation of test red cells with serum; in the second step, the red cells are washed and the AHG reagent is added. Agglutination implies that the original serum contained antibody which has coated the red cells *in vitro*. This test is used as part of the routine antibody screening of the recipient's serum prior to transfusion and for detecting blood group antibodies in a pregnant woman.

Most of the above methods were originally developed for tube techniques but 96-well microplates and gel-based spin columns are now widely used (Fig. 23.5).

CROSS-MATCHING AND PRETRANSFUSION TESTS

A number of steps are taken to ensure that patients receive compatible blood at the time of transfusion.

From the patient

1 The ABO and Rh blood group is determined.
2 Serum is screened for important antibodies by an indirect antiglobulin test on a large panel of antigenically-typed red cells.

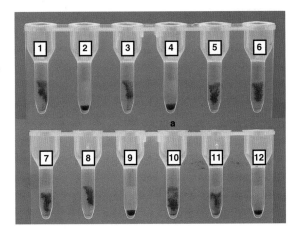

Fig. 23.5 Patient antibody screening using the microcolumn (gel) system: 10 tests with two controls (tube 11 is the positive control and tube 12 the negative control) are shown. The patient's serum is tested against screening cells with known red cell phenotype. Tubes 1, 3, 5, 6, 7, 8 and 10 show positive results. The patient's serum contained anti-Fyª. (Courtesy of Mr G. Hazlehurst.)

From the donor

An appropriate ABO and Rh unit is selected. Donor (blood) testing is described on p. 313.

At the cross-match (Table 23.4)

The patient's serum is added to donor red cells and spun down to exclude agglutination (the 'immediate spin'). Some units also perform an indirect antiglobulin test of patient serum on donor red cells.

COMPLICATIONS OF BLOOD TRANSFUSION (Table 23.5)

Haemolytic transfusion reactions

Haemolytic transfusion reactions may be immediate or delayed. Immediate life-threatening reactions associated with massive intravascular haemolysis are the result of complement-activating antibodies of IgM or IgG classes, usually with ABO specificity. Reactions associated with extravascular haemolysis (e.g. immune antibodies

Table 23.4 Techniques used in compatibility testing. Donor cells tested against recipient serum and agglutination detected visually or microscopically after mixing and incubation at the appropriate temperature

---

For detecting clinically significant IgM antibodies
Saline 37°C

For detecting immune antibodies (mainly IgG)
Indirect antiglobulin test at 37°C
Low ionic strength saline at 37°C
Enzyme-treated red cells at 37°C

Ig, immunoglobulin.

Table 23.5 Complications of blood transfusion

Early	Late
Haemolytic reactions	*Transmission of disease*
immediate	Virus
delayed	hepatitis A, B, C and others
Reactions caused by infected blood	HIV
Allergic reactions to white cells,	CMV
platelets or proteins	Bacteria
Pyrogenic reactions (to plasma	*Treponema pallidum*
proteins or caused by HLA	*Brucella*
antibodies)	*Salmonella*
Circulatory overload	Parasites
Air embolism	malaria
Thrombophlebitis	*Toxoplasma*
Citrate toxicity	microfilaria
Hyperkalaemia	
Clotting abnormalities (after	*Transfusional iron overload*
massive transfusion)	
Transfusion-related acute lung	*Immune sensitization*
injury	e.g. to red cells, platelets or
	Rh D antigen
	Transfusion-associated graft-versus-host disease

CMV, cytomegalovirus; HIV, human immunodeficiency virus; HLA, human leucocyte antigen.

of the Rh system which are unable to activate complement) are generally less severe but may still be life-threatening. The cells become coated with IgG and are removed in the reticuloendothelial system. In mild cases, the only signs of a transfusion reaction may be a progressive unexplained anaemia with or without jaundice. In some cases where the pretransfusion level of an antibody was too low to be detected in a cross-match, a patient may be reimmunized by transfusion of incompatible red cells and this will lead to a delayed transfusion reaction with accelerated clearance of the red cells. There may be rapid appearance of anaemia with mild jaundice.

Clinical features of a major haemolytic transfusion reaction

Haemolytic shock phase This may occur after only a few millilitres of blood have been transfused or up to 1–2 h after the end of the transfusion. Clinical features include urticaria, pain in the lumbar region, flushing, headache, precordial pain, shortness of breath, vomiting, rigours, pyrexia and a fall in blood pressure. If the patient is anaesthetized this shock phase is masked. There is increasing evidence of blood destruction and haemoglobinuria, jaundice and disseminated intravascular coagulation (DIC) may occur. Moderate leucocytosis, e.g. $15–20 \times 10^9$/l is usual.

The oliguric phase In some patients with a haemolytic reaction there is renal tubular necrosis with acute renal failure.

Diuretic phase Fluid and electrolyte imbalance may occur during the recovery from acute renal failure.

Investigation of an immediate transfusion reaction

If a patient develops features suggesting a severe transfusion reaction the transfusion should be stopped and investigations for blood group incompatibility and bacterial contamination of the blood must be initiated.

1 Most severe reactions occur because of clerical errors in the handling of donor or recipient blood specimens. Therefore it must be established that the identity of the recipient is the same as that stated on the compatibility label and that this corresponds with the actual unit being transfused.

2 The unit of donor blood and post-transfusion samples of the patient's blood should be sent to the laboratory who will:

(a) repeat the group on pre- and post-transfusion samples and on the donor blood, and repeat the cross-match;

(b) perform a direct antiglobulin test on the post-transfusion sample;

(c) check the plasma for haemoglobinaemia;

(d) perform tests for DIC; and

(e) examine the donor sample directly for evidence of gross bacterial contamination and set up blood cultures from it at 20 and 37°C.

3 A post-transfusion sample of urine must be examined for haemoglobinuria.

4 Further samples of blood are taken 6 h and/or 24 h after transfusion for a blood count and bilirubin, free haemoglobin and methaemalbumin estimations.

5 In the absence of positive findings, the patient's serum is examined 5–10 days later for red cell or white cell antibodies.

Management of patients with major haemolysis

The principal object of initial therapy is to maintain the blood pressure and renal perfusion. Intravenous dextran, plasma or saline and frusemide are sometimes needed. Hydrocortisone 100 mg intravenously and an antihistamine may help to alleviate shock. In the event of severe shock, support with intravenous adrenaline 1 : 10 000 in small incremental doses may be required. Further compatible transfusions may be required in severely affected patients. If acute renal failure occurs this is managed in the usual way, if necessary with dialysis until recovery occurs.

Other transfusion reactions

Febrile reactions because of white cell antibodies Human leucocyte antigen (HLA) antibodies (see below and Chapter 8) are usually the result of sensitization by pregnancy or a previous transfusion. They produce rigors, pyrexia and, in severe cases, pulmonary infiltrates. They are minimized by giving leucocyte-depleted (i.e. filtered) packed cells (see below).

Febrile or non-febrile non-haemolytic allergic reactions
These are usually caused by hypersensitivity to donor plasma proteins and if severe can result in anaphylactic shock. The clinical features are urticaria, pyrexia and, in severe cases, dyspnoea, facial oedema and rigors. Immediate treatment is with antihistamines and hydrocortisone. Adrenaline is also useful. Washed red cells or frozen red cells may be needed for further transfusions if the majority of plasma-removed blood (e.g. saline, adenine, glucose, mannitol (SAG-M) blood causes reactions.

Post-transfusion circulatory overload The management is that of cardiac failure. These reactions are prevented by a slow transfusion of packed red cells or of the blood component required, accompanied by diuretic therapy.

Transfusion of bacterially contaminated blood This is very rare but may be serious. It can present with circulatory collapse.

Viral transmission Post-transfusion hepatitis may be caused by one of the hepatitis viruses, although cytomegalovirus (CMV) and Epstein–Barr virus (EBV) have also been implicated. Post-transfusion hepatitis and human immunodeficiency virus (HIV) infection is seen less frequently now because of routine screening of all blood donations.

Other infections Toxoplasmosis, malaria and syphilis may all be transmitted by blood transfusion. As yet, no case of transfusion-transmitted new variant Creutzfeld–Jakob disease (nvCJD) has been identified.

Post-transfusional iron overload Repeated red cell transfusions over many years, in the absence of blood loss, cause deposition of iron initially in reticuloendothelial tissue at the rate of 200–250 mg/unit (450 ml) of whole blood. After 50 units in adults, and lesser amounts in children, the liver, myocardium and endocrine glands are damaged with clinical consequences. This is a major problem in thalassaemia major and other severe chronic refractory anaemias (see Chapter 6).

BLOOD PRODUCTS

A blood donation is taken by an aseptic technique into plastic bags containing an appropriate amount of anticoagulant—usually citrate, phosphate, dextrose (CPD). The citrate anticoagulates the blood by combining with the blood calcium. Before issue the following tests are carried out: ABO and RhD blood grouping, red cell antibody screen and serological tests to exclude syphilis, hepatitis B surface antigen (Hb_SAg), hepatitis C virus (HCV) and HIV 1 and 2. Currently HCV and HIV are excluded by detection of appropriate antiviral antibodies, and the introduction of polymerase chain reaction (PCR)-based detection of viral nucleic acid has increased the sensitivity of screening by identifying infected individuals in the 'window period' prior to antibody formation.

Blood is stored at 4–6°C for up to to 35 days, depending on the preservative. After the first 48 h there is a slow progressive K^+ loss from the red cells into the plasma. In cases where infusion of K^+ could be dangerous, fresh blood should be used, e.g. for exchange transfusion in haemolytic disease of the newborn. During red cell storage there is a fall in 2,3-diphosphoglycerate (2,3-DPG) but after transfusion 2,3-DPG levels return to normal within 24 h. Optimum additive solutions have been developed to increase the shelf life of plasma-depleted red cells by maintaining both adenosine triphosphate (ATP) and 2,3-DPG levels. SAG-M medium allows red cells to be used up to 35 days after donation.

Blood is usually processed and separated into its components before use (Fig. 23.6). Whole blood is very rarely used.

Leucodepletion

In many countries, including Britain, blood products are now routinely filtered to remove the majority of white cells, a process known as leucodepletion. This is usually performed soon after collection and prior to processing (Fig. 23.7) and is more effective than filtration of blood at the bedside. A blood product is defined as leucocyte

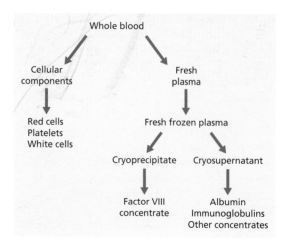

Fig. 23.6 The preparation of blood components from whole blood.

depleted if there are less than 5×10^6 white cells present (Table 23.6).

Leucodepletion reduces the incidence of febrile transfusion reactions and alloimmunization. It is effective at preventing transmission of CMV infection and in addition should reduce the theoretical possibility of transmission of nvCJD in countries where this has been reported.

Red cells

Packed (plasma-depleted) red cells are the treatment of choice for most transfusions (Fig. 23.8a). In older subjects, a diuretic is often given simultaneously and the infusion should be

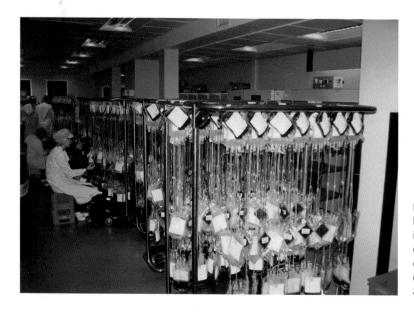

Fig. 23.7 Leucofiltration of blood: leucofiltration of individual donor units is carried out by gravity through a depleting filter in a closed system. It is commenced 8 h after obtaining the donor blood to allow phagocytosis of any possible contaminating bacteria.

Table 23.6 Number of white cells present in different blood components

Red cell components	Packed cells $>2 \times 10^9$	Buffy coat removed $5{-}10 \times 10^8$	Leucocyte depleted $5{-}10 \times 10^5$
Platelets	Prepared from buffy coat 10^8	Prepared by apheresis 10^8	Leucocyte depleted $<10^6$

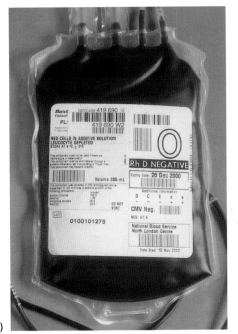

(a)

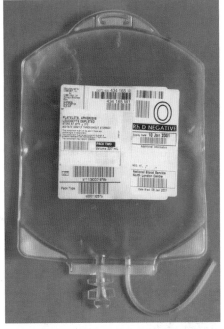

(b)

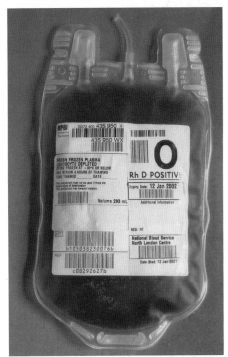

(c)

Fig. 23.8 Blood components: (a) plasma-depleted red cells; (b) platelets; and (c) fresh frozen plasma.

sufficiently slow to avoid circulatory overload. Iron chelation therapy should be considered with patients on a regular transfusion programme to avoid iron overload.

Whole blood is occasionally used for treating acute blood loss or for exchange transfusions.

Red cell substitutes are under development but have not yet proven clinically valuable. These synthetic oxygen-carrying substitutes are often fluorinated hydrocarbons and stromal-free pyridoxylated and polymerized haemoglobin solutions.

Autologous donation and transfusion

Anxiety over acquired immune deficiency syndrome (AIDS) and other infections has increased the demand for autotransfusion. There are three ways of administering an autologous transfusion.
1 Predeposit—blood is taken from the potential recipient in the weeks immediately prior to elective surgery.
2 Haemodilution—blood is removed immediately prior to surgery once the patient has been anaesthetized and then reinfused at the end of the operation.
3 Salvage—blood lost during the operation is collected during heavy blood loss and then reinfused.

The increasing demand is for predeposit autotransfusion. Autotransfusion is the safest form of transfusion with regard to transmission of disease. The individual involved must be fit enough to donate blood and the predicted operative replacement transfusion should be between 2 and 4 units. Larger replacement transfusions would require blood to be collected over a longer period and red cells stored in the frozen state, which is both labour intensive and expensive. Although autotransfusion is the safest form of transfusion, the high cost and initial restriction of its use to patients undergoing elective surgery means that it will benefit only a minor proportion of the total number of blood recipients.

Granulocyte concentrates

These are prepared as buffy coats or on blood cell separators from normal healthy donors or from patients with chronic myeloid leukaemia. They have been used in patients with severe neutropenia ($<0.5\times10^9/l$) who are not responding to antibiotic therapy but it is not usually possible to give sufficient amounts. They may transmit CMV infection.

Platelet concentrates

These are harvested by cell separators or from individual donor units of blood (Fig. 23.8b). Platelet transfusion is used in patients who are thrombocytopenic or have disordered platelet function and who are actively bleeding (therapeutic use) or are at serious risk of bleeding (prophylactic use).

For prophylaxis the platelet count should be kept above $5-10\times10^9/l$ unless there are additional risk factors such as sepsis, drug use or coagulation disorders for which the threshold should be higher. For minor invasive procedures, e.g. liver biopsy or lumbar puncture, the platelet count should be raised to above $50\times10^9/l$.

Therapeutic use is indicated in bleeding associated with platelet disorders. In massive haemorrhage the count should be kept above $50\times10^9/l$.

Platelet transfusions should be avoided in autoimmune thrombocytopenic purpura unless there is serious haemorrhage. They are contraindicated in heparin-induced thrombocytopenia, thrombotic thrombocytopenic purpura and haemolytic uraemic syndrome (p. 255).

Refractoriness to platelet transfusions is defined by a poor platelet increment posttransfusion ($<7.5\times10^9/l$ at 1 h or $<4.5\times10^9/l$ at 24 h). The causes are either immunological (mostly HLA alloimmunization) or nonimmunological (sepsis, hypersplenism, DIC, drugs). Platelets express HLA class I (but not class II) antigens and HLA-matched or crossmatch-compatible platelets are needed for patients with HLA antibodies.

Human plasma preparations

Plasma is a useful volume expander. The risk of hepatitis has been reduced by the introduction of more sensitive tests for hepatitis B and C. Frozen plasma is usually prepared from single donor units.

Fresh frozen plasma (FFP) Rapidly frozen plasma separated from fresh blood is stored at less than $-30°C$. Its main use is for the replacement of coagulation factors (e.g. when specific concentrates are unavailable) or after massive transfusions, in liver disease and DIC, after cardiopulmonary bypass surgery, to reverse a warfarin effect, and in thrombotic thrombocytopenic purpura (see Table 20.6). Virally inactivated forms of FFP are now available.

Human albumin solution (4.5%)

This contains human albumin and its main use is in the treatment of hypovolaemic shock. It is a useful plasma volume expander when a sustained osmotic effect is required prior to the administration of blood, but it should not be given in excess. It is also used for plasma replacement in patients undergoing plasmapheresis and sometimes for protein replacement in selected patients with hypoalbuminaemia.

Human albumin solution (20%) (salt-poor albumin)

This expensive purified preparation is not recommended as a general plasma volume expander although its usefulness for this purpose is undoubted. It may be used in severe hypoalbuminaemia when it is necessary to use a product with minimal electrolyte content. Principal indications for its use are patients with nephrotic syndrome or liver failure.

Cryoprecipitate

This is obtained by thawing fresh frozen plasma at $4°C$ and contains concentrated factor VIII and fibrinogen. It is stored at less than $-30°C$ or, if lyophylized, at $4–6°C$, and was used widely as replacement therapy in haemophilia A and von Willebrand's disease before more purified preparations of factor VIII became available.

Freeze-dried factor VIII concentrates

These are also used for treating haemophilia A or von Willebrand's disease. The small volume makes them ideal for children, surgical cases, patients at risk from circulatory overload and for those on home treatment. Their use is declining as recombinant forms of factor VIII become available.

Freeze-dried factor IX–prothrombin complex concentrates

A number of preparations are available which contain variable amounts of factors II, VII, IX and X. They are mainly used for treating factor IX deficiency (Christmas disease) but are also used occasionally in patients with liver disease or in life-threatening haemorrhage following overdose with oral anticoagulants or in patients with factor VIII inhibitors. There is a risk of thrombosis.

Protein C concentrate

This is used in severe sepsis with disseminated intravascular coagulation, e.g. meningococcal septicaemia to reduce thrombosis resulting from depletion of protein C.

Immunoglobulin

Pooled immunoglobulin is a valuable source of antibodies against common viruses. It is used in hypogammaglobulinaemia for protection against viral and bacterial disease. It may also be used in immune thrombocytopenia and other acquired immune disorders, e.g. post-transfusion purpura or alloimmune neonatal thrombocytopenia.

Specific immunoglobulin

This may be obtained from donors with high titres of antibody, e.g. anti-RhD, antihepatitis B, antiherpes zoster or antirubella.

ACUTE BLOOD LOSS

As mentioned on p. 20, until 3–4 h after a single episode of blood loss the haemoglobin and packed cell volume remain normal because there is initial vasoconstriction with a reduction in total blood volume. After 3–4 h, however, the plasma volume begins to expand and the haemoglobin and packed cell volume fall and there is a rise in neutrophils and platelets. The reticulocyte response begins on the second or third day and lasts 8–10 days. The haemoglobin begins to rise by about the seventh day but, if iron stores have become depleted, the haemoglobin may not rise subsequently to normal. Clinical assessment is needed to gauge whether blood transfusion is needed, but this is usually unnecessary in adults with losses of 500 ml or less unless haemorrhage is continuing. Blood transfusion is not without risks and should not be undertaken lightly. The problems of massive blood loss and massive transfusion are considered on p. 257.

BIBLIOGRAPHY

Anderson K.C. and Ness P.M. (1999) *Scientific Basis of Transfusion Medicine.* W.B. Saunders, Philadelphia.

British Committee for Standards in Haematology Guidelines (1999) The administration of blood and blood components and the management of transfused patients. *Transfus. Med.* **9**, 227–38.

Chang T.M.S. (2000) Red blood cell substitutes. *Clin. Haematol.* **13**, 651–68.

Consensus Conference on Autologous Transfusion (1996) *Transfusion* **36**, 667.

Contreras M. (ed.) (2000) New aspects of blood transfusion. *Clin. Haematol.* **13**, 485–688.

Corash L. (2000) New technologies for the inactivation of infectious pathogens in cellular blood components and the development of platelet substitutes. *Clin. Haematol.* **13**, 549–63.

Goodnough L.T., Brecher M.E. and Kanter M.H. (1999) Transfusion medicine. *N. Engl. J. Med.* **340**, 438–46; 525–33.

Issitt P. (1993) *Applied Blood Group Serology,* 3rd edn. Montgomery Scientific, Miami, Florida.

Mollison P.L., Engelfriet C.P. and Contreras M. (1993) *Blood Transfusion in Clinical Medicine,* 9th edn. Blackwell Scientific Publications, Oxford.

Mouro I. *et al.* (1993) Molecular basis of the human Rhesus blood group. *Nature Genet.* **5**, 62.

Navarette C.V. (2000) The HLA system in blood transfusion. *Clin. Haematol.* **13**, 511–32.

Norfolk D.R. *et al.* (1998) Consensus conference on platelet transfusion. *Br. J. Haematol.* **101**, 609–17.

Prusiner S.B. (1998) The prion diseases. *Brain Pathol.* **8**, 499–513.

Reid M.E. (2000) Blood group antigens: molecular biology, functions and clinical applications. *Semin. Hematol.* **37**, 111–216.

Reid M.E. and Yahalom V. (2000) Blood groups and their function. *Clin. Haematol.* **13**, 485–510.

Vamvakus E.C. and Pineda A.A. (2000) Autologous transfusion and other approaches to reduce allogeneic blood exposure. *Clin. Haematol.* **13**, 533–47.

Pregnancy and paediatric haematology

HAEMATOLOGY OF PREGNANCY

Pregnancy places extreme stresses on the haematological system and an understanding of the physiological changes that result is obligatory in order to interpret any need for therapeutic intervention.

Physiological anaemia

Physiological anaemia is the term often used to describe the fall in haemoglobin (Hb) concentration that occurs during normal pregnancy (Fig. 24.1). Blood plasma volume increases by around 1250 ml, or 45%, above normal by the end of gestation and although the red cell mass itself increases by some 25% this still leads to a fall in Hb concentration. Values below 10 g/dl are probably abnormal and require investigation.

Iron deficiency anaemia

Up to 600 mg of iron is required for the increase in red cell mass and a further 300 mg for the fetus. Despite an increase in iron absorption, few women avoid severe depletion of iron reserves by the end of pregnancy.

In uncomplicated pregnancy the mean corpuscular volume (MCV) typically rises by around 4 fl. A fall in red cell MCV is the earliest sign of iron deficiency. Later the mean corpuscular haemoglobin (MCH) falls and finally anaemia results. Early iron deficiency is likely if the serum ferritin is below 15 μg/l together with serum iron < 10 μmol/l and

should be treated with oral iron supplements. The use of routine iron supplementation in pregnancy is often debated but iron is probably better avoided until Hb falls below 10 g/dl or MCV below 82 fl in the third trimester.

Folate deficiency

Folate requirements are increased approximately twofold in pregnancy and serum folate levels fall to about half the normal range with a less dramatic fall in red cell folate. In some parts of the world megaloblastic anaemia during pregnancy is common because of a combination of poor diet and exaggerated folate requirements. Given the protective effect of folate against neural tube defects folic acid 400 μg daily should be taken periconceptually and throughout pregnancy. Food fortification with folate is now being practised in several countries. Vitamin B_{12} deficiency is rare during pregnancy although serum vitamin B_{12} levels fall to below normal in 20–30% of pregnancies and low values are sometimes the cause of diagnostic confusion.

Thrombocytopenia in pregnancy

The platelet count typically falls by around 10% in an uncomplicated pregnancy. In about 7% of women this fall is more severe and can result in thrombocytopenia (platelet count $<150\times10^9/l$). In over 75% of cases this is mild and of unknown cause, a condition referred to as incidental thrombocytopenia of pregnancy. Around 21% of cases

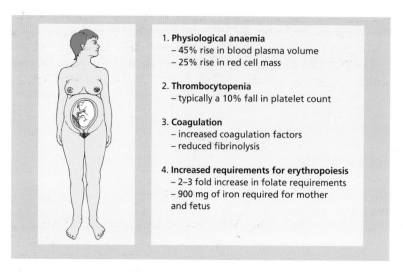

1. **Physiological anaemia**
   – 45% rise in blood plasma volume
   – 25% rise in red cell mass

2. **Thrombocytopenia**
   – typically a 10% fall in platelet count

3. **Coagulation**
   – increased coagulation factors
   – reduced fibrinolysis

4. **Increased requirements for erythropoiesis**
   – 2–3 fold increase in folate requirements
   – 900 mg of iron required for mother and fetus

Fig. 24.1 Haematological changes during pregnancy.

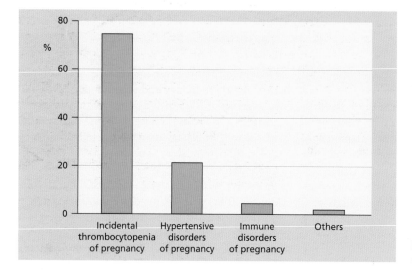

Fig. 24.2 Causes of thrombocytopenia during pregnancy.

are secondary to a hypertensive disorder and 4% are associated with immune thrombocytopenic purpura (ITP) (Fig. 24.2).

Incidental thrombocytopenia of pregnancy This is a diagnosis of exclusion and is usually detected at the time of delivery. The platelet count is always above $70 \times 10^9/l$ and recovers within 6 weeks. No treatment is required and the infant is not affected.

Thrombocytopenia of hypertensive disorders This is variable in severity but the platelet count rarely falls below $40 \times 10^9/l$. It is more severe when asso-

ciated with pre-eclampsia and if severe the primary treatment is as rapid a delivery as possible. The platelet count falls for a day or two after delivery and then recovers rapidly. The HELLP syndrome (*h*aemolysis, *e*levated *l*iver enzymes and *l*ow *p*latelets) is a subtype of this cagtegory.

Idiopathic thrombocytopenic purpura (see p. 253) In pregnancy ITP represents a particular problem, both to the mother and to the fetus as the antibody crosses the placenta and the fetus may become severely thrombocytopenic.

Like all adults, pregnant women with ITP and

platelet counts $>50\times10^9/l$ do not usually need treatment. Treatment is required for women with platelet counts $<10\times10^9/l$ and for those with platelet counts of $10\times10^9/l$ to $30\times10^9/l$ who are in their second or third trimester or who are bleeding. Treatment is with steroids, intravenous immunoglobulin G (IgG) and splenectomy as appropriate.

At delivery umbilical vein blood sampling or fetal scalp vein sampling to measure the fetal platelet count may be offered although their exact role is unclear. In general, caesarean section is not indicated when the maternal platelet count is $>50\times10^9/l$ unless the fetal platelet count is known to be$<20\times10^9/l$. Platelet transfusion may be given to mothers in labour with very low platelet counts or who are actively bleeding.

Newborns of mothers with ITP should have a blood count measured for the first 4 days of life as the platelet count may progressively drop. A count greater than $50\times10^9/l$ is reassuring. Cerebral ultrasounds may be performed to look for intracranial haemorrhage (ICH). In newborns without evidence of ICH, treatment with intravenous IgG is appropriate if the infant's platelet count is $<20\times10^9/l$. Neonates with thrombocytopenia and ICH should be treated with steroids and intravenous IgG therapy.

Haemostasis and thrombosis during pregnancy

Pregnancy leads to a hypercoaguable state with consequent increased risks of thromboembolism and disseminated intravascular coagulation (DIC, p. 268). There is an increase in plasma factors VII, VIII, X and fibrinogen and fibrinolysis is suppressed. These changes last for up to 2 months into the puerperal period and the incidence of thrombosis during this period is increased.

Treatment of thrombosis in pregnancy

Warfarin has little role in management. It crosses the placenta and in addition is associated with embryopathy, especially between 6 and 12 weeks of gestation. Heparin does not cross the placenta but a significant side-effect of prolonged use is maternal osteoporosis. Low molecular weight heparin is now the treatment of choice because it can be given once daily and is less likely to cause osteoporosis.

NEONATAL HAEMATOLOGY

Normal blood count

The cord blood Hb varies between around 16.5 and 17.1 g/dl and is influenced by the timing of cord clamping (Fig. 24.3). MCV averages 119 fl but falls to adult levels by around 9 weeks. The reticulocyte count is initially high (2–6%) but falls to below 0.5% at 1 week. This is associated with a progressive fall in Hb to around 10–11 g/dl at 8 weeks from which point it recovers to 12.5 g/dl at around 6 months. In the blood film nucleated red cells will be seen for the first 4 days and for up to 1 week in preterm infants. Numbers are increased in cases of hypoxia, haemorrhage or haemolytic disease of the newborn (HDN). Neutrophils are initially high at birth and fall to plateau at 4 days—from this point on the lymphocyte count is higher than neutrophils throughout childhood.

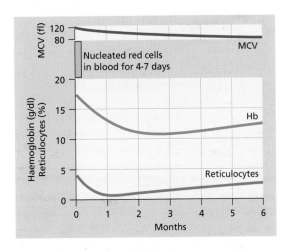

Fig. 24.3 Typical profile of the blood count in the neonatal period.

Anaemia in the neonate

Causes to be considered include the following.
1 Haemorrhage—fetomaternal, twin–twin, cord, placenta.
2 Increased destruction—haemolysis (immune or non-immune) or infection.
3 Decreased production—congenital red cell aplasia, infection.

Generally anaemia at birth is usually secondary to immune haemolysis or haemorrhage with non-immune causes of haemolysis appearing within 24 h. Impaired red cell production is usually not apparent for at least 3 weeks. Haemolysis is often associated with severe jaundice and the causes include HDN, autoimmune haemolytic anaemia (AIHA) in the mother and congenital disorders of red cell membrane or metabolism.

Red cell transfusion may be needed for symptomatic anaemia with Hb <10.5 g/dl or a higher threshold if there is severe cardiac or respiratory disease.

Fetomaternal alloimmune thrombocytopenia

Fetomaternal alloimmune thrombocytopenia (FMAIT) results from an immunological process similar to that which causes HDN. Fetal platelets which possess a paternally inherited antigen (HPA-1a in 80%; HPA-5b in 15%) which is not present on maternal platelets can sensitize the mother to make antibodies that cross the placenta, coat the platelets which are then destroyed by the reticuloendothelial system and lead to serious bleeding, including intracranial haemorrhage (ICH). Alloimmune thrombocytopenia differs from HDN in that 50% of cases occur in the first pregnancy. Its incidence is around one in 1000–5000 births.

Thrombocytopenia can lead to serious, sometimes fatal, bleeding *in utero* or after birth. Treatment is unsatisfactory. Severe postnatal cases may be treated with a platelet transfusion that is negative for the relevant antigen. Antenatal treatment may be either maternal (intravenous immunoglobulin, corticosteroids or a combination of the two) or fetal (platelet transfusions or steroids) and these are being assessed in trials.

Coagulation

Standard tests need to be interpreted with caution in the neonate. The activated partial thromboplastin time (APTT) is prolonged because of reduced levels of activation factors and returns to normal at around 3 months. The prothrombin time (PT) and thrombin time (TT) are comparable with adult values. Antithrombin (AT) levels are around 60% of normal for the first 3 months. Although homozygous AT deficiency is probably incompatible with life, homozygous protein C deficiency is associated with fulminant purpura fulminans in early life. Therapeutic protein C concentrates are now available.

HAEMOLYTIC DISEASE OF THE NEWBORN

HDN is the result of the passage of IgG antibodies from the maternal circulation across the placenta into the circulation of the fetus where they react with fetal red cells and lead to their destruction by the fetal reticuloendothelial system.

Before 1967, when the prophylactic use of anti-D IgG was introduced, anti-D Rh HDN was responsible for about 800 stillbirths and neonatal deaths each year in the UK. Anti-D was responsible for 94% of Rh HDN; other cases were usually caused by anti-c and anti-E, with a wide range of antibodies found in occasional cases (for examples see Table 23.1). The incidence of Rh HDN is now dramatically lower and the proportion of cases caused by anti-c and anti-E has increased substantially.

The most frequent causes of HDN are now immune antibodies of the ABO blood group system—most commonly anti-A produced by a group O mother against a group A fetus. However, this form of HDN is usually mild. Occasional cases of HDN are caused by antibodies of other blood group systems, e.g. anti-Kell.

Rhesus HDN

Pathogenesis

When an Rh D-negative (Rh d/d or rr) woman has a pregnancy with an Rh D-positive fetus, Rh D-positive fetal red cells cross into the maternal circulation (usually at parturition) and sensitize the mother to form anti-D. Sensitization is more likely if the mother and fetus are ABO compatible. The mother could also be sensitized by a previous miscarriage, amniocentesis or other trauma to the placenta or by blood transfusion.

Anti-D crosses the placenta to the fetus during the next pregnancy with an Rh D-positive fetus, coats the fetal red cells with antibody and results in reticuloendothelial system destruction of these cells, causing anaemia and jaundice. If the father is heterozygous for D antigen (D/d) there is a 50% probability that the fetus will be D positive.

Clinical features

1 Severe disease: intrauterine death from hydrops fetalis.
2 Moderate disease: the baby is born with severe anaemia and jaundice and may show pallor, tachycardia, oedema and hepatosplenomegaly. When the unconjugated bilirubin level exceeds 250 μmol/l, bile pigment deposition in the basal ganglia may lead to kernicterus—central nervous system damage with generalized spasticity and possible subsequent mental deficiency, deafness and epilepsy. This problem becomes acute after birth as maternal clearance of fetal bilirubin ceases and conjugation of bilirubin by the neonatal liver has not yet reached full activity.
3 Mild disease: mild anaemia with or without jaundice.

Laboratory findings at birth

1 Cord blood. Variable anaemia (haemoglobin < 16/dl) with a high reticulocyte count; the baby is Rh D positive, the direct antiglobulin test is positive and the serum bilirubin raised. In moderate and severe cases many erythroblasts are seen in the blood film (Fig. 24.4)—erythroblastosis fetalis.
2 The mother is Rh D negative with a high plasma level of anti-D.

Treatment

Exchange transfusion may be necessary; the indications for this include the following.
1 Clinical features: obvious pallor, jaundice and signs of heart failure.
2 Laboratory findings: haemoglobin <14.0 g/dl with a positive direct antiglobulin test; a cord serum bilirubin >60 μmol/l or infant serum bilirubin >300 μmol/l or bilirubin level rising rapidly

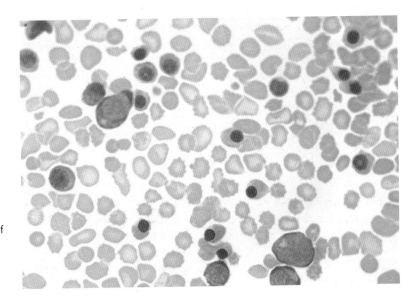

Fig. 24.4 Rhesus haemolytic disease of the newborn (erythroblastosis fetalis): peripheral blood film showing large numbers of erythroblasts, polychromasia and crenated cells.

and positive antiglobulin test. Premature babies are more liable to kernicterus and should be exchange transfused at lower bilirubin levels (e.g. > 200 μmol/l).

In infants with moderate disease, more than one exchange transfusion may be required. Exchange transfusions performed soon after birth are used to replace the infant's red cells and reduce the rate of bilirubin rise. Subsequent exchange transfusions may be required to remove unconjugated bilirubin. The procedure of removing and replacing one equivalent blood volume will remove 60% of the pre-existing constituents in the blood. The blood for the exchange transfusion should be < 7 days old, Rh D negative and ABO compatible with the baby and with the mother's serum by cross-match. Normally, 500 ml is sufficient for each exchange. Phototherapy (exposure of the infant to bright light of appropriate wavelength) has been used to photodegrade the bilirubin to permit urinary excretion, thus reducing the likelihood of kernicterus.

Management of pregnant women

Prevention of Rh immunization

At the time of booking all pregnant women should have their ABO and Rh group determined and serum screened for antibodies at least twice during the pregnancy. Passively administered IgG anti-D suppresses primary immunization in the majority of Rh D-negative women and all non-sensitized Rh D-negative women should be routinely given 500 i.u. of anti-D at 28 and 34 weeks of pregnancy to reduce the risk of sensitization because of fetomaternal haemorrhage. In addition, at birth the babies of Rh D-negative women who do not have antibodies must have their cord blood grouped for ABO and Rh. If the baby's blood is Rh D negative the mother will require no further treatment. If the baby is Rh D positive, prophylactic anti-D should be administered at a dose of 500 i.u. intramuscularly within 72 h of delivery. A Kleihauer test should also be performed in this situation to estimate the severity of the fetomaternal haemorrhage (FMH). This uses differential staining to estimate the number of fetal cells in the maternal circulation (Fig. 24.5). The chance of developing antibodies is related to the number of fetal cells found. The dose of anti-D is increased if the Kleihauer test shows greater than 4 ml transplacental haemorrhage. Anti-D IgG (125 i.u.) is given for each 1 ml of FMH greater than 4 ml.

Sensitizing episodes during pregnancy Anti-D IgG should be given to Rh D-negative women who have potentially sensitizing episodes during

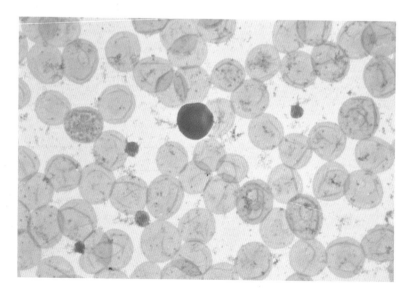

Fig. 24.5 Kleihauer test for fetal red cells; a deeply eosin-staining cell containing fetal haemoglobin is seen at the centre. Haemoglobin has been eluted from the other red cells by an incubation at acid pH and these appear as colourless ghosts.

pregnancy: 250 i.u. is given if the event occurs up to week 20 of gestation and 500 i.u. thereafter, followed by a Kleihauer test. Potentially sensitizing events include therapeutic termination of pregnancy, spontaneous miscarriage after 12 weeks' gestation, ectopic pregnancy and invasive antenatal diagnostic procedures.

Treatment of established anti-D sensitization

If any anti-D antibodies are detected during pregnancy they should be identified and quantified at regular intervals (e.g. 2–3 weekly, and more often in late pregnancy or if antibody levels are rising or high). The strength of anti-D present in maternal serum is related to the clinical severity of HDN but this is also affected by such factors as the IgG subclass, rate of rise of antibody and past history. As a rough guide, levels below 1.0 i.u./ml (0.2 μg/ml) require no action. A level of 10 i.u./ml (2.0 μg/ml) usually reflects a seriously affected infant as does a level of 5 i.u./ml (1.0 μg/ml) which is rising rapidly. These latter two situations and any history of a previously affected infant are indications for amniocentesis. Other antibodies are monitored by serological titration using the antiglobulin method. As a rough guide, titres in excess of 1/20 involving anti-c or anti-Kell are causes for concern.

The severity of the haemolytic disease can be assessed by spectroscopic estimation of bile pigment derivatives in the amniotic fluid obtained by amniocentesis. If this shows severe haemolysis the fetus can be kept alive by intrauterine transfusion of fresh (<7-day-old) Rh D-negative blood after 24 weeks and by premature delivery after 35 weeks. Suitable fresh blood should be available at the time of induction in preparation for exchange transfusion.

ABO haemolytic disease of the newborn

In 20% of births, a mother is ABO incompatible with the fetus. Group A and group B mothers usually have only IgM ABO antibodies. The majority of cases of ABO HDN are caused by 'immune' IgG antibodies in group O mothers. Although 15% of pregnancies in white people involve a group O mother with a group A or group B fetus, most mothers do not produce IgG anti-A or anti-B and very few babies have severe enough haemolytic disease to require treatment. Exchange transfusions are needed in only one in 3000 infants. The mildness of ABO HDN is partly explained by the A and B antigens not being fully developed at birth and by partial neutralization of maternal IgG antibodies by A and B antigens on other cells, in the plasma and tissue fluids.

In contrast to Rh HDN, ABO disease may be found in the first pregnancy and may or may not affect subsequent pregnancies. The direct antiglobulin test on the infant's cells may be negative or only weakly positive. Examination of the blood film shows autoagglutination and spherocytosis, polychromasia and erythroblastosis.

BIBLIOGRAPHY

Christiensen R.D. (2000) *Hematological Problems in the Neonate*. W.B. Saunders, Philadelphia.

Hann I.M., Lake D.B., Lilleyman J. and Pritchard J. (1996) *Colour Altas of Paediatric Haematology*, 3rd edn. Oxford University Press, Oxford.

Joint Working Group of the BBTS/RCOG (1999) Recommendations for the use of anti-D immunoglobulin for Rh prophylaxis. *Transf. Med.* **9**, 93–7.

Lanzkowsky P. (1999) *Manual of Pediatric Hematology and Oncology*, 3rd edn. Academic Press, San Diego.

Lilleyman J.S. (ed.) (2000) Paediatric haematology. *Clin. Haematol.* **13**, 327–483.

Luban N.L.C. (1998) Hemolytic disease of the newborn: progenitor cells and late effects. *N. Engl. J. Med.* **338**, 830.

Nathan D.G. and Orkin S.H. (eds) (1997) *Nathan and Orkin's Hematology of Infancy and Childhood*, 5th edn. W.B. Saunders, Philadelphia.

Appendix 1

Principal features of known cluster differentiation (CD) molecules

Cluster	Main cellular distribution	Name/comments/function/diagnostic value
CD1a	Thymocytes, dendritic cells	Ligand for some $\gamma\delta$ T cells
CD1b	Thymocytes, dendritic cells	Ligand for some $\gamma\delta$ T cells
CD1c	Thymocytes, dendritic cells	Ligand for some $\gamma\delta$ T cells
CD2	Pan T cell, NK cells	SRCR, adhesion (LFA-2) binds LFA-3
CD3	Pan T cell	Signal transduction from the T-cell receptor
CD4	T-helper subset	Adhesion (binds class II MHC)
CD5	Pan T cell, B-cell subset	Expressed on B-CLL
CD6	Subset of T cells	
CD7	Subset of T cells	
CD8	Cytotoxic T cell	Adhesion (binds class I MHC)
CD9	Pre-B cells, monocytes, platelets	
CD10	Precursor B and some mature B cells	Expressed in c-ALL (CALLA), kidney, intestine, neural tissue
CD11a	Leucocytes	Adhesion (combines with CD18 to form LFA-1 integrin)
CD11b	Granulocytes, monocytes, NK cells	Adhesion (combines with CD18 to form Mac-I integrin)
CD11c	Granulocytes, monocytes, NK cells	Adhesion (combines with CD18 to form p150,95 [$\alpha_x\beta_2$] integrin)
CD11d	Peripheral blood leucocytes	Adhesion (combines with CD18 to form $\alpha_D\beta_2$ integrin)
CD12	Monocytes, granulocytes	
CD13	Monocytes, granulocytes	An aminopeptidase
CD14	Monocytes, macrophages	Binds LPS
CD15	Granulocytes	Lewis X antigen (carbohydrate epitope)
CD16	NK cells, granulocytes, macrophages	FcγRIII
CD17	Granulocytes, monocytes, platelets	
CD18	Leucocytes	Adhesion (β chain of LFA-1 integrin family)
CD19	B cells	Modulates the threshold for signalling through B-cell receptor
CD20	B cells	
CD21	Mature B cells	CR2, C3dR, receptor for EBV. Complexes with CD19
CD22	B cells	Down-regulates B-cell activation
CD23	Activated B cells, macrophages, FDC	FcϵRII
CD24	B cells, granulocytes	
CD25	Activated T cells, B cells, macrophages	α chain of IL-2 receptor
CD26	Activated T cells, B cells, macrophages	

continued

Cluster	Main cellular distribution	Name/comments/function/diagnostic value
CD27	T cells, plasma cells	
CD28	T cells	Co-stimulation
CD29	Broad	Integrin β_1 subunit. Forms heterodimers with many integrin α subunits, e.g. CD49
CD30	Activated T and B cells	Reed–Sternberg cells express; Ki detects
CD31	Monocytes, platelets, endothelium	Platelet endothelial cell adhesion molecule 1 (PECAM-1)
CDw32	Monocytes, platelets	FcγRII (receptor for aggregated IgG)
CD33	Monocytes, myeloid progenitors	
CD34	Precursors of haemopoietic cells	Marrow progenitors
CD35	Granulocytes, monocytes, B cells	C3b receptor, CR1
CD36	Monocytes, platelets	Platelet GPIIIb
CD37	Pan-13, some T cells, FDC	
CD38	Thymocytes, activated T cells, plasma cells	Plasma cell tumours
CD39	B cells	
CD40	B cells	Important costimulatory molecule for B cells
CD41	Platelets	Platelet GPIIb (forms complex with GPIIIa [CD61]), mutated in Glanzmann thrombasthenia
CD42a & b	Platelets	Form GPIb (platelet adhesion to von Willebrand factor)
CD43	Leucocytes	
CD44	Leucocytes, erythrocytes	
CD45	Leucocytes	Leucocyte common antigen
CD46	Leucocytes, epithelial cells, fibroblasts	Regulates complement activation
CD47	Broad	
CD48	Leucocytes	Binds CD2
CD49a–f	T cells, monocytes, platelets	α-integrin subunits. They can all form heterodimers with CD29 (to generate VLA1–6)
CD50	Leucocytes	ICAM-3
CD51	Platelets, megakaryocytes, activated T cells	Integrin α_V subunit. Can form heterodimers with β_1, β_3, β_5, β_6 or β_8
CD52	Lymphocytes and monocytes	Target for CAMPATH antibody (see p. 195)
CD53	Leucocytes	
CD54	Leucocytes	Adhesion (ICAM-1 ligand for LFA-1)
CD55	Leucocytes and endothelium	Complement decay-accelerating factor (DAF)
CD56	Some T and B cells, neural and muscle tissue	NCAM
CD57	NK cells, subset of T cells	
CD58	Leucocytes, epithelial cells	Adhesion (LFA-3) ligand for CD2
CD59	Broad	Membrane inhibitor of reactive lysis (MIRL)
CDw60	T subset, platelets	
CD61	Platelets, megakaryocytes	Integrin β_3 subunit (associates with CD41 to form GPIIb/IIIa)
CD62 E, L and P	Endothelium (E), leucocytes (L), megakaryocytes and platelets (P)	Selectins. Recruit leucocytes to inflammation
CD63	Activated platelets, monocytes	
CD64	Monocytes, macrophages	FcγRI (high-affinity Fcγ receptor)
CD65	Granulocytes	
CD66a–e	Granulocytes (a–d)	Carcinoembryonic antigen (CEA) family. CEA is CD66e

continued p. 328

Cluster	Main cellular distribution	Name/comments/function/diagnostic value
CD68	Monocytes, macrophages	
CD69	Activated B, T cells, macrophages, NK cells	
CDw70	Activated B, T cells	CD27Lm
CD71	Proliferating cells	Transferrin receptor
CD72	B cells	
CD73	B subset, T subset	Ecto 5′-nucleotidase
CD74	B cells, monocytes	MHC class II-associated invariant chain (Ii)
CDw75	Mature B cells	
CD76	Mature B cells	
CD77	Germinal centre B cells	
CD79a	B cells	Associated with B-cell antigen receptor complex (Igα)
CD79b	B cells	Associated with B-cell antigen receptor complex (Igβ)
CD80	Monocytes/dendritic cells/B cells	B7-1. Involved in T-cell activation via CD28 and CD152
CD81	General expression	
CD82	General expression	
CD83	Dendritic cells/germinal centre B cells	
CD84	Macrophages and platelets	
CD85	Plasma cells/monocytes	Many lymphoid leukaemias
CD86	Dendritic cells and B cells	B7-2. Binds CD28 and CD152
CD87	Monocytes/granulocytes	Urokinase plasminogen activator receptor
CD88	Myeloid cells	Binds C5a
CD89	Phagocytic cells	IgA receptor, FcαR
CD90	Prothymocytes	Thy-1
CD91	Phagocytes	α_2-macroglobulin receptor
CD92	Myeloid	
CD93	Granulocytes, monocytes, endothelial cells	
CD94	NK cells, subset of T cells	Inhibitory receptor. Complexes with NKG2 and then binds HLA-E
CD95	Activated lymphocytes, monocytes, neutrophils	Fas. Triggers apoptosis
CD96	NK and T cells	
CD97	Granulocytes, macrophages	
CD98	Monocytes	
CD99	Leucocytes	
CD100	B, T and NK cells. Myeloid cells	
CD101	Monocytes, granulocytes and T cells	
CD102	Leucocytes and endothelium	ICAM-2. Ligand for CD11a/CD18 (LFA-1)
CD103	Intraepithelial lymphocytes	Integrin α_E subunit—with β_7 it binds to E-cadherin
CD104		Integrin β_4 subunit
CD105	Endothelial cells	Endoglin. Binds to TGF-β. Mutated in hereditary haemorrhagic telangiectasia
CD106	Endothelium	VCAM-1. Binds the integrins $\alpha_4\beta_1$ and $\alpha_4\beta_7$
CD107	Wide distribution	Lysosomal proteins
CD108	Lymphoid, myeloid, stroma	
CD109	Platelets	Can be target for alloantibodies
CD114	Myeloid cells, endothelium, platelets	G-CSFR

continued

Cluster	Main cellular distribution	Name/comments/function/diagnostic value
CD115	Monocytes, macrophages	Macrophage colony-stimulating factor receptor (M-CSFR)
CD116	Monocytes, neutrophils, eosinophils, endothelial cells	α chain of GM-CSFR
CD117		c-kit, steel factor receptor
CD118	Broad	Interferon α/β receptor
CD119	Broad	α chain of IFN-γR
CD120	Broad	TNFRI, TNFRII
CD121	Broad	Components of the IL-1 receptor
CD122	B, T and NK cells	β chain of IL-2 receptor, IL-15R
CD123	Early and committed bone marrow progenitors	α chain of IL-3 receptor
CD124	Broad	α chain of IL-4R and component of IL-13R
CD125	Eosinophils and basophils	α chain of IL-5 receptor
CD126	Activated B cells, plasma cells and myeloma	α chain of IL-6 receptor
CD127	Lymphoid precursors and T cells	α chain of IL-7 receptor
CD128	Neutrophils	Component of IL-8 receptor
CD129	Erythroid and myeloid precursors, lymphocytes	α chain of IL-9 receptor
CD130	Broad	β chain of IL-6R, IL-11R
CD131		β chain of GM-CSFR, IL-3R and IL-5R
CD132		β chain of IL-7R, IL-9R, IL-15R
CD134	Activated T cells	OX40
CD135	Haemopoietic stem cells	FLT-3
CD136		Macrophage-stimulating protein receptor
CD137	Activated lymphocytes, monocytes	4-1BB
CD138	Pre-B cells and plasma cells	Syndecan-1. Detected by Mab BB4 and useful in the diagnosis of myeloma
CD139	Germinal centre B cells	
CD140	Broad	PDGF receptor
CD141	Endothelium	Thrombomodulin
CD142	Activated monocytes and endothelium	Tissue factor
CD143	Endothelium	Angiotensin-converting enzyme
CD144		VE-cadherin
CD145	Endothelium/stroma	
CD146	Endothelium/activated T cells	MUC-18
CD147	Broad	Extracellular matrix metalloproteinase inducer
CD148	Myeloid cells	
CD149	Broad	
CD150	Activated B and T cells	SLAM
CD151	Platelets, moncytes and endothelium	PETA-3
CD152	Activated T cells	CTLA-4. Binds CD80 and CD86
CD153	Activated T cells	CD30L
CD154	Activated T cells	CD40L. Mutations lead to hyper-IgM syndrome
CD155	Monocytes, macrophages, thymocytes	Poliovirus receptor
CD156	Monocytes, macrophages, granulocytes	ADAM-8
CD157	Monocytes, neutrophils, endothelium	BST-1

continued

Cluster	Main cellular distribution	Name/comments/function/diagnostic value
CD158	NK cells and T-cell subsets	Killer inhibitory receptors (KIR)
CD161	NK cells and some T cells	NKR-P1 family
CD162	Lymphocytes, neutrophils and monocytes	P-selectin glycoprotein ligand
CD163	Monocyte macrophage lineage	
CD164	Haemapoietic cells	MGC-24
CD165	Thymocytes, thymic epithelial cells	AD2/gp37
CD166	Thymic epithelial cells, activated T cells	CD6L

ADAM, A disintegrin and metalloprotease; B-CLL, B-chronic lymphocytic leukaemia; c-ALL, common (CD10+) acute lymphoblastic leukaemia; CD, cluster differentiation; C3dR, complement 3d receptor; EBV, Epstein–Barr virus; FcR, immunoglobulin Fc fragment receptor; FDC, follicular dendritic cell; G-CSFR, granulocyte colony-stimulating factor receptor; GM-CSFR, granulocyte–macrophage colony-stimulating factor; GP, glycoprotein; ICAM, intercellular adhesion molecule; IFN, interferon; Ig, immunoglobulin; IL, interleukin; Ki, antibody to CD30; LFA, leucocyte function-associated antigen; LPS, lipopolysaccharide; Mac-I, integrin molecule; MHC, major histocompatibility complex; NK, natural killer; PDGF, platelet-derived growth factor; SRCR, sheep red cell receptor; TGF, transforming growth factor; TNFR, tumour necrosis factor receptor; VLA, very late antigens; w, workshop.

For an updated CD list up to CD166 see Barclay *et al.* (1997) *The Leucocyte Antigen Facts Book*, 2nd edn. Academic Press, London.

Appendix 2

Normal values

	Males	Females	Males and females
Haemoglobin	13.5–17.5 g/dl	11.5–15.5 g/dl	
Red cells (erythrocytes)	$4.5–6.5 \times 10^{12}/l$	$3.9–5.6 \times 10^{12}/l$	
PCV (haematocrit)	40–52%	36–48%	
MCV			80–95 fl
MCH			27–34 pg
MCHC			20–35 g/dl
White cells (leucocytes)			
total			$4.0–11.0 \times 10^{9}/l$
neutrophils			$2.5–7.5 \times 10^{9}/l$
lymphocytes			$1.5–3.5 \times 10^{9}/l$
monocytes			$0.2–0.8 \times 10^{9}/l$
eosinophils			$0.04–0.44 \times 10^{9}/l$
basophils			$0.01–0.1 \times 10^{9}/l$
Platelets			$150–400 \times 10^{9}/l$
Red cell mass	30 ± 5 ml/kg	27 ± 5 ml/kg	
Plasma volume	45 ± 5 ml/kg	45 ± 5 ml/kg	
Serum iron			10–30 μmol/l
Total iron-binding capacity			40–75 μmol/l (2.0–4.0 g/l as transferrin)
Serum ferritin*	40–340 μg/l	14–150 μg/l	
Serum vitamin B_{12}*			160–925 ng/l
Serum folate*			3.0–15.0 μg/l
Red cell folate*			160–640 μg/l

* Normal ranges differ with different commercial kits.

MCH, mean corpuscular haemoglobin; MCHC, mean corpuscular haemoglobin concentration; MCV, mean corpuscular volume; PCV, packed cell volume.

Appendix 3

Table 1 Proposed World Health Organization (WHO) classification of myeloid neoplasms*

Myeloproliferative disease (MPD)
Chronic myelogenous leukemia, Philadelphia chromosome (Ph1)
  [t(9;22)(qq34;q11), BCR/ABL] +
Chronic neutrophilic leukaemia
Chronic eosinophilic leukaemia/hypereosinophilic syndrome
Chronic idiopathic myelofibrosis
Polycythaemia vera
Essential thrombocythaemia
Myeloproliferative disease, unclassifiable

Myelodysplastic/myeloproliferative diseases
Chronic myelomonocytic leukaemia (CMML)
Atypical chronic myelogenous leukaemia (aCML)
Juvenile myelomonocytic leukaemia (JMML)

Myelodysplastic syndromes (MDS)
Refractory anaemia (RA)
  with ringed sideroblasts (RARS)
  without ringed sideroblasts
Refractory cytopenia (myelodysplastic syndrome) with multilineage
  dysplasia (RCMD)
Refractory anemia (myeldysplastic syndrome) with excess blasts
  (RAEB)
5q-syndrome
Myelodysplastic syndrome, unclassifiable

Acute myeloid leukaemias (AML)*
Acute myeloid leukemias with recurrent cytogenetic translocations
  AML with t(8;21)(q22;q22), AML1(CBFα)/ETO
  Acute promyelocytic leukaemia (AML with t(15;17)(q22;q11–12)
    and variants, PML/RAXα)
  AML with abnormal bone marrow eosinophils (inv(16)(p13q22) or
    t(16;16)(p13;q11), CBFβ/MYH11X)
  AML with 11q23 (MLL) abnormalities

Acute myeloid leukemia with multilineage dysplasia
  with prior myelodysplastic syndrome
  without prior myelodysplastic syndrome

*Acute myeloid leukemia and myelodysplastic syndrome, therapy
  related*
  Alkylating agent related
  Epipodophyllotoxin related (some may be lymphoid)
  Other types

Acute myeloid leukemia not otherwise categorized
  AML minimally differentiated
  AML without maturation
  AML with maturation
  Acute myelomonocytic leukaemia
  Acute monocytic leukaemia
  Acute erythroid leukaemia
  Acute megakaryocytic leukaemia
  Acute basophilic leukaemia
  Acute panmyelosis with myelofiborisis

Acute biphenotypic leukaemias

* Only major disease categories are listed.

Table 2 Proposed World Health Organization (WHO) classification of lymphoid neoplasms*

B-CELL NEOPLASMS
Precursor B-cell neoplasm
Precursor B-lymphoblastic leukaemia / lymphoma (precursor B-cell acute lymphoblastic leukaemia)
Mature (peripheral) B-cell neoplasms**
B-cell chronic lymphocytic leukaemia / small lymphocytic lymphoma
B-cell prolymphocytic leukaemia
Lymphoplasmacytic lymphoma
Splenic marginal zone B-cell lymphoma (+/− villous lymphocytes)
Hairy cell leukemia
Plasma cell myeloma/plasmacytoma
Extranodal marginal zone B-cell lymphoma of MALT type
Nodal marginal zone B-cell lymphoma (+/− monocytoid B cells)
Follicular lymphoma
Mantle cell lymphoma
Diffuse large B-cell lymphoma
Mediastinal large B-cell lymphoma
Primary effusion lymphoma
Burkitt lymphoma/Burkitt cell leukaemia

T AND NK-CELL NEOPLASMS
Precursor T-cell neoplasm
Precursor T-lymphoblastic lymphoma / leukaemia (precursor T-cell acute lymphoblastic leukaemia)

T AND NK-CELL NEOPLASMS (*Cont.*)
Mature (peripheral) T-cell neoplasms**
T-cell prolymphocytic leukaemia
T-cell granular lymphocytic leukaemia
Aggressive NK-cell leukaemia
Adult T-cell lymphoma / leukaemia (HTLV1+)
Extranodal NK/T-cell lymphoma, nasal type
Enteropathy-type T-cell lymphoma
Hepatosplenic $\gamma\delta$ T-cell lymphoma
Subcutaneous panniculitis-like T-cell lymphoma
Mycosis fungoides / Sézary syndrome
Anaplastic large cell lymphoma, T / null cell, primary cutaneous type
Peripheral T-cell lymphoma, not otherwise characterized
Angioimmunoblastic T-cell lymphoma
Anaplastic large cell lymphoma, T / null cell, primary systemic type

HODGKIN LYMPHOMA (HODGKIN DISEASE)
Nodular lymphocyte predominance Hodgkin lymphoma
Classical Hodgkin lymphoma
Nodular sclerosis Hodgkin lymphoma (Grades 1 and 2)
Lyphocyte-rich classical Hodgkin lymphoma
Mixed cellularity Hodgkin lymphoma
Lymphocyte depletion Hodgkin lymphoma

* More common entities are in italics; ** B- and T / NK-cell neoplasms are grouped according to major clinical presentations (predominantly disseminated/leukaemic, primary extranodal, predominantly nodal).

Table 3 Mast cell diseases

Cutaneous mastocytosis
Systematic mast cell disease (+/− skin involvement)
Systematic mast cell disease with associated hematological disorder (+/− skin involvement)
Mast cell leukaemia/sarcoma

Table 4 Histiocytic and dendritic-cell neoplasms

Macrophage/histiocytic neoplasm
Histiocytic sarcoma

Dendritic-cell neoplasms
Langerhans cell histiocytosis
Langerhans cell sarcoma
Interdigitating dendritic cell sarcoma/tumor
Follicular dendritic cell sarcoma/tumor
Dendritic cell sarcoma, not otherwise specified (NOS)

Table 5 Plasma cell disorders: subtypes and variants

Monoclonal gammopathy of undetermined significance (MGUS)

Plasma cell myeloma variants:
- Indolent myeloma
- Smoldering myeloma
- Osteosclerotic myeloma (POEMS syndrome)
- Plasma cell leukaemia
- Non-secretory myeloma

Plasmacytoma variants:
- Solitary plasmacytoma of bone
- Extramedullary plasmacytoma

Table 6 Immunosecretory disorders (clinical manifestations of diverse lymphoid neoplasms)

Clinical syndrome	Underlying neoplasm
Waldenström's macro-globulinemia	Lymphoplasmacytic lymphoma
Heavy chain diseases (HCD)	
gamma HCD	Lymphoplasmacytic lymphoma
alpha HCD	Extranodal marginal zone lymphoma (immunoproliferative small intestinal disorder)
Mu HCD	B-cell chronic lymphocytic leukaemia
Immunoglobulin deposition diseases:	
Systemic light chain disease	Plasma cell myeloma, monoclonal gammopathy
Primary amyloidosis	Plasma cell myeloma, monoclonal gammopathy

Glossary of molecular genetics

alleles Alternative forms of the gene found at a particular locus (e.g. β^A, β^S, β^E, β^{thal}, etc.). There may be many different alleles in a population, but two at the most in one individual.

amplification Production of additional copies of a particular DNA sequence, which may be extrachromosomal or become integrated in a chromosome.

aneuploidy A cell that has additions or deletions of a small number of whole chromosomes from the expected balanced diploid number.

anticipation Refers to the younger age or increased severity of a disease in successive generations and has been observed in some families with leukaemia.

anticodon A triplet of nucleotides in a special position in the structure of tRNA that is complementary to the codon(s) in mRNA to which that tRNA binds.

antisense oligonucleotides Short sequences of nucleotides that are designed to bind to specific nucleotide sequences within the cell and therefore block gene function.

autosome Any chromosome that is not a sex chromosome.

base pair (bp) A partnership of A with T or of C with G in a DNA double helix; in RNA, A pairs with U.

cell-specific genes Genes coding for proteins involved in specialized functions and synthesized sometimes in large amounts in particular cells types. Also sometimes referred to as luxury genes.

cDNA A single-stranded DNA molecule complementary to an RNA molecule; usually synthesized from it *in vitro* by the use of the enzyme reverse transcriptase.

cDNA clone A molecular clone in which a cDNA has been copied from a molecule of mature mRNA. It may differ from a *genomic clone (q.v.)* corresponding to the same region, because of the processing that takes place in the pathway from the primary transcript to mature mRNA.

centromere The constricted region of a chromosome to which the spindle fibres attach during division.

chromatid One of the two replicas produced by chromosome replication in mitosis or meiosis.

chromosome walking The sequential isolation of clones carrying overlapping sequences of DNA to span large regions of the chromosome (often in order to reach a particular locus).

***cis*-acting** A DNA sequence that affects the expression of a gene on the same chromosome but not on the homologous chromosome.

clone, cellular The progeny of a single cell. Cells belonging to the same clone are often referred to as a *monoclonal population*. Because a neoplastic growth is mostly monoclonal, the two terms are often regarded as synonymous. This is not the case; for instance, all the cells proceeding from a single haemopoietic stem cell are normal clones; all the cells proceeding from the proliferation of a single antibody-producing lymphocyte are also normal clones. An individual is a clone of her/his mother's egg fertilized by her/his father's sperm cell.

clone, molecular A large number of identical DNA molecules. The term is most commonly used to describe a sequence (for instance a gene or a portion of a gene) obtained by recombinant DNA methods. In this case the large number of identical DNA molecules is obtained by growing up a culture from a single bacterial cell or from a single bacteriophage containing that molecule. Hence a molecular clone is derived from a cellular clone.

codon A triplet of nucleotides that specifies an amino acid or a termination signal.

comparative genomic hybridization (CGH) DNA is extracted from tumour cells and normal cells and labelled with different fluorescent dyes. These are then mixed and hybridized to chromosome spreads and chromosomal regions that are under- or over-represented in the tumour samples can be detected.

consensus sequence This is an idealized DNA sequence serving a particular function in which each position represents the base most often found when many actual sequences are compared.

degeneracy In the genetic code, this refers to the fact that several codons specify the same amino acid. Therefore, certain mutations in a gene may not affect the respective amino acid in the protein encoded.

deletion This constitutes removal of a sequence of DNA, the regions on either side being joined together.

diploid The state of having each chromosome in two copies per nucleus or cell.

domain A discrete continuous part of the amino acid sequence of a protein to which a particular function can be attributed.

dominant An allele which determines the phenotype displayed in a heterozygote, the other allele being recessive.

enhancer A DNA sequence that increases the expression of a gene in *cis*-configuration. It can function in many locations, upstream or downstream, relative to the promoter.

eukaryocytes More complex organisms, e.g. fungi, plants, animals. Eukaryocyte cells have a nucleus.

exon A segment of an interrupted gene present in its respective mRNA.

fluorescence *in situ* hybridization (FISH) Specific cDNA probes are labelled by fluorescent dyes and hybridized to metaphase cells. The fluorescent spots correlate with gene copy number and chromosomal location and the technique is useful for detecting chromosomal rearrangements.

footprinting A technique for identifying the site on DNA to which some protein binds, based on the protection exerted by the protein against attack by nucleases in this region.

gene The unit of inheritance. In biochemical terms, a gene specifies the structure of a polypeptide chain, or protein, which can be regarded as its product. In molecular terms, the gene is a stretch of DNA that is transcribed in one block, and therefore it can be regarded usually as a *transcription unit*.

genetic code The dictionary whereby a certain triplet of bases, called a codon, calls for a particular amino acid during the process of translation. Because in many cases several triplets call for the same amino acid, the genetic code is said to be *degenerate*.

genome The entire complement of genetic material in a chromosome set.

genomic clone A molecular clone consisting of a portion of cellular DNA (as opposed to cDNA).

genotype The genetic constitution of an individual. With respect to a particular locus, the two genes present at that locus in that individual (for instance, β^A/β^S is the genotype, at the β-globin locus on chromosome 11 of a person with sickle cell trait).

haploid The state of having one copy of each chromosome per nucleus or cell.

haplotype A set of closely linked allelic genes or sites within a short region of one chromosome. Because they are closely linked they are almost invariably inherited as a single block. Examples are antigenic determinants of the Rh (rhesus) system, such as cDe; HLA genes, such as *A10-B12*; or numerous restriction sites in and around a globin gene or any other gene.

heterozygote An individual with two different alleles on homologous chromosomes at a particular locus.

housekeeping genes Genes expressed in all cells because they provide basic functions needed for sustenance of essential functions, such as cell structure, cell division and intermediary metabolism.

hybridization The pairing of complementary

RNA or DNA strands to give an RNA–DNA hybrid or a DNA duplex.

interphase The cell cycle stage between nuclear divisions when chromosomes are extended and functionally active.

intron A segment of DNA that is transcribed, but is removed from within the primary transcript by splicing together the sequences (exons) on either side of it.

kb Abbreviation for 1000 base pairs of DNA or 1000 bases of RNA.

leader The non-translated sequence at the 5′ end of mRNA that precedes the initiation codon.

library A set of cloned DNA fragments representing together the entire genome, or a portion thereof, or a population of RNA molecules. It is important to distinguish genomic libraries from cDNA libraries (see cDNA clone; genomic clone). Gene libraries are also referred to as gene banks.

linkage The property of genes to be inherited together as a result of their neighbouring location on the same chromosome; it is measured by percentage recombination between loci.

linkage disequilibrium A situation whereby two linked alleles are found in a population to be in *cis*, or in tandem to each other, more frequently than would be expected by chance. At least two explanations are possible: (a) the mutation giving rise to one of the alleles is rather recent (therefore recombination has not yet had the time to cause equilibration with other linked genes); (b) the arrangement in tandem of the two alleles is favoured by selection.

locus The position on a chromosome where a particular gene is located. In diploid organisms, like humans, there are at each locus two genes (one on each of the two homologous chromosomes); with the only exception being most of the X chromosome in males, who are haploid for this region.

locus control region (LCR) A DNA segment located upstream of the β-globin gene cluster and required for its high-level expression in erythroid cells. LCRs may exist for other cell-specific genes.

metaphase The stage of nuclear division when chromosomes align along the equatorial plane of the cell spindle.

mutations These are changes in the sequence of genomic DNA. *Missense* mutations result in the substitution of an incorrect amino acid. *Nonsense* mutations cause termination of the peptide chain and *frameshift* mutations shift the reading frame of the triplet sequence.

nonsense codon See termination codon.

Northern blotting A technique for transferring RNA from an agarose gel to a nitrocellulose filter on which it can be recognized by a suitable probe. Widely used to identify expression of an individual gene.

open reading frame A series of triplets coding for amino acids and thus potentially translatable into protein.

penetrance This is defined as the proportion of individuals with a specific genetic alteration who will express the associated trait.

phage (bacteriophage) A bacterial virus.

phenotype The appearance of an individual person. In relation to a particular genetic character, the phenotype reflects the genotype conferring that character, plus the possible effects of the environment. In addition, the phenotype (what appears) depends on what we analyse (the way we look at it). Thus, while genotype is an absolute concept, phenotype is a relative concept.

plasmid An autonomously replicating extra-chromosomal circular supercoiled DNA.

polymerase chain reaction (PCR) A technique for amplifying *in vitro* by a very large factor (10^5 or more) an individual DNA sequence. The reaction must be primed by using specific oligonucleotides, and therefore prior sequence information is necessary for the procedure to be carried out.

polymorphism The difference in DNA sequence among individuals.

probe (gene probe) A nucleic acid sequence that can be used, by hybridization, to recognize a specific cellular DNA sequence or a specific RNA molecule (usually a gene, or its vicinity, or its cognate mRNA).

prokaryocyte Simple organism such as a bacteria.

promoter A DNA sequence located upstream of

the transcribed portion of a gene, and essential for its transcription because it is the binding site for RNA polymerase.

real time PCR A form of PCR (see above) in which a fluorescent signal is released during each round of the amplification process. Continuous measurement of the fluorescence released during the reaction permits an evaluation of the degree of amplification in 'real-time'. Real time PCR allows *quantitative* measurement of the amount of template in the reaction and is therefore widely used.

recessive An allele which is obscured in the phenotype of a heterozygote by the dominant allele, often because of inactivity or absence of the product of the recessive allele.

recombinant DNA Any DNA molecule constructed artificially by bringing together DNA segments of different origin.

recombination An event whereby two non-allelic genes, located in tandem on a chromosome, are not transmitted together to the offspring because a cross-over with the homologous chromosome has taken place at meiosis. It is possible that a similar event may take place sometimes in somatic cells (mitotic recombination).

restriction enzymes These recognize specific short sequences (mostly four or six bases) of DNA and cleave the duplex wherever those sequences are found. These sequences are therefore called restriction sites.

reverse transcription Synthesis of DNA on a template of RNA; accomplished by the enzyme, reverse transcriptase.

restriction fragment length polymorphism (RFLP) Genetic variation in the size of a DNA fragment detectable, after digestion with a particular restriction enzyme, by a particular probe. RFLP results from a point mutation in a restriction site, or from a shift in its position because of a deletion or a duplication.

ribozyme An RNA molecule that can itself degrade RNA by recognising a specific nucleotide sequence.

Southern blotting The procedure for transferring denatured DNA from an agarose gel to a nitrocellulose filter, where it can be recognized by an appropriate probe.

splicing Describes the removal of introns from an RNA primary transcript and joining of the exons; thus introns are spliced out, while exons are spliced together.

telomerase A DNA polymerase that maintains the length of telomeres.

telomere The end of a chromosome.

terminal deoxynucleotide transferase (Tdt) An enzyme that adds random nucleotides to the junctions of gene segments as they join during the rearrangement of immunoglobulin or T cell receptor genes.

termination codon This is one of three triplet sequences, UAG, UAA or UGA, that cause termination of protein synthesis; these are also called stop codons or nonsense codons.

trans Configuration of two sites is called *trans* when their location is on two different chromosomes.

transcription This is synthesis of RNA on a DNA template.

transcription factors These are proteins that regulate other genes.

transcription unit See gene.

transfection This is the acquisition by eukaryotic cells of new genetic properties or markers by incorporation of added DNA.

transformation This refers to the conversion of eukaryotic cells to a state of unrestrained growth in culture, resembling or identical with neoplastic growth.

transgenic Animals produced by introducing new DNA sequences into the germline by microinjection into the egg or into the blastocyst.

translation Synthesis of protein on an mRNA template.

translocation The state whereby part of a chromosome becomes attached to a different chromosome.

vector A DNA molecule capable of replication and specially engineered to facilitate cloning of another DNA molecule of interest. The vector is mostly a plasmid, a phage or a YAC (see below), but may also be an animal virus, such as a retrovirus.

yeast artificial chromosomes (YAC) Eukaryocyte vectors suitable for cloning large pieces of DNA (up to 2000 kb).

Index

Note: page numbers in *italic* refer to figures, page numbers in **bold** refer to tables.